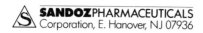

SANDOZPHARMACEUTICALS
Corporation, E. Hanover, NJ 07936

Dear Colleague:

When I completed the editing of the enclosed book, *Drug Therapy for Headache*, I knew it would be an invaluable reference for physicians who treat headache.

Now, thanks to the support of Sandoz Pharmaceuticals, the book is available to a broad audience of practicing physicians.

The evaluation and treatment of the patient with frequently recurring, disabling headaches can often be difficult because we are unsure of what we are going to encounter. Another factor is that no two headache patients are exactly alike.

This book was developed not as a theoretical thesis, but rather as a hands-on guide for the practicing physician. Within the limited arsenal of available therapeutic agents, it provides a broad range of options that may be useful for the headache types you are currently diagnosing.

The esteemed group of physicians who contributed to this book has spent several lifetimes' worth of experience treating patients with serious headaches and offers a plethora of options for successful outcomes.

I am grateful for all their contributions and to Sandoz Pharmaceuticals for making the book more broadly available to the medical profession.

Sincerely,

R. Michael Gallagher
University Headache Center
Moorestown, New Jersey

INFLAMMATORY DISEASE AND THERAPY

Series Editor

Daniel E. Furst
*University of Medicine and Dentistry
of New Jersey
Robert Wood Johnson Medical School
New Brunswick, New Jersey
and Pharmaceuticals Division
CIBA-GEIGY Corporation
Summit, New Jersey*

Drug Therapy for Headache

edited by

R. Michael Gallagher

University Headache Center
Moorestown, New Jersey

University of Medicine & Dentistry of New Jersey
School of Osteopathic Medicine
Stratford, New Jersey

MARCEL DEKKER, INC.   New York • Basel • Hong Kong

Library of Congress Cataloging--in--Publication Data

Drug therapy for headache/edited by R. Michael Gallagher.
    p.   cm. -- -- (Inflammatory diseases and therapy; 6)
    Includes bibliographical references.
    Includes index.
    ISBN 0-8247-8179-1 (alk. paper)
    1. Headache-- --Chemotherapy. 2. Migraine-- --Chemotherapy.
3. Headache. I. Gallagher, R. Michael.   II. Series
    [DNLM: 1. Headache-- --drug therapy. W1 IN41LA v. 6 / WL 342 D7945]
RB128.D785   1990
616.8'491061-- --dc20
DNLM/DLC
for Library of Congress   90-14029
                                                                            CIP

This book is printed on acid-free paper.

MARCEL DEKKER, INC.
270 Madison Avenue, New York, New York 10016

Current printing (last digit):
10 9 8 7 6 5 4 3 2

PRINTED IN THE UNITED STATES OF AMERICA

To Joanne

Foreword

The practice of medicine is an art,
not a trade; a calling, not a business;
a calling in which your heart will be
exercised equally with your head.
Sir William Osler

The care of a person suffering from frequently recurring headache of disabling severity requires all the skill, patience, empathy, understanding, and good will that a physician can command. In this volume Dr. Gallagher and his colleagues have well delineated the medications available to the physician that, when mixed with his or her skills, will help to control the problem. Like any other tool or implement, the result of the effort will depend largely on the skill with which these medications are employed.

Before one can be an artist—an essential in treating the patient with headache—one must first become thoroughly familiar with the available materials. Only when this has been achieved can their application be guided carefully—by a combination of science and instinct.

The popular explanation for the superb tone of the instruments produced by Stradivarius is based on his use of some secret ingredient in the varnish with which they were coated. I suspect it was not a secret ingredient in the varnish but rather the skill, determination, and dedication by which it was applied.

Study well the lessons contained herein so that familiarity with the pharmacology of these medications may become second nature. Only then will the powers of the Intellect and Spirit be free to employ them appropriately. Affectionate support remains an essential ingredient to every prescription.

Perry S. MacNeal, M.D.
Associate Professor of Medicine
University of Philadelphia
Philadelphia, Pennsylvania
Distinguished Clinician and Former President
American Association for the Study of Headache

Preface

The evaluation and treatment of the headache patient can be a challenging and sometimes frustrating experience for both the patient and the physician. Unfortunately, there are no sure diagnostic markers nor are there sure therapeutic regimens. Each headache sufferer is a unique individual who may not respond to treatment in the same fashion as others who experience similar symptoms. For this reason, it is necessary for physicians who desire to help headache sufferers not only to be familiar with headache syndromes but to possess an expanded armamentarium of pharmacological agents with appropriate alternatives.

There are only a handful of medications specifically indicated for the headache diagnosis. Practitioners have had to be resourceful, selecting medications for headache treatment from among those commonly utilized for other medical conditions. This book of drug treatment for headache patients was created to be an easily understood reference text for all physicians interested in helping these sufferers. The majority of this text discusses various pharmacological agents used by specialists in treating the more commonly encountered chronic headache conditions. Outstanding clinicians and researchers of international reputation have contributed their expertise by presenting appropriate therapies with alternatives in a simple and logical manner.

R. Michael Gallagher

Contents

Contributors

J. Keith Campbell, M.D.   Associate Professor, Department of Neurology, Mayo Medical School, Rochester, Minnesota

James R. Couch, M.D., Ph.D.   Professor and Chief of Neurology, Department of Medicine, Southern Illinois University School of Medicine, Springfield, Illinois

P. T. G. Davies, M.A., M.R.C.P.   Registrar in Neurology, Department of Neurology, Charing Cross Hospital, London, England

Seymour Diamond, M.D.   Director, Diamond Headache Clinic, Chicago, and Adjunct Professor, Pharmacology and Molecular Biology Department, Chicago Medical School, North Chicago, Illinois

Frank J. DiSerio, Ph.D.   Executive Director, Clinical Research Department, Sandoz Research Institute, East Hanover, New Jersey

John Edmeads, M.D.   Professor, Department of Medicine (Neurology), Sunybrook Medical Center, University of Toronto, Toronto, Ontario, Canada

Arthur H. Elkind, M.D. Director, Elkind Headache Center, Mount Vernon, New York, and Clinical Assistant Professor, Department of Medicine, New York Medical College, Valhalla, New York

Frederick G. Freitag, D.O. Associate Director, Diamond Headache Clinic, and Clinical Associate, Department of Internal Medicine, University of Chicago School of Medicine, Chicago, Illinois

R. Michael Gallagher, D.O. Director, University Headache Center, Moorestown, New Jersey, and Assistant Dean for Clinical Affairs and Professor of Clinical Medicine, University of Medicine and Dentistry of New Jersey—School of Osteopathic Medicine, Stratford, New Jersey

Gerald S. Golden, M.D. Director, Boling Center for Develomental Disabilities, University of Tennessee, Memphis, Tennessee

Makoto Ichijo, M.D. Research Associate, Cerebral Blood Flow Laboratory, Veterans Administration Medical Center, and Baylor College of Medicine, Houston, Texas

Masahiro Kobari, M.D. Research Associate, Cerebral Blood Flow Laboratory, Veterans Administration Medical Center, and Baylor College of Medicine, Houston, Texas

Jamshid Lofti, M.D. Research Associate, Neurology Department and Cerebrovascular Research Laboratories, Baylor College of Medicine, and Physician, Neurology Department, St. Luke's Episcopal Hosptial, Houston, Texas

Ninan T. Mathew, M.D. Houston Headache Clinic, Veteran Administration Medical Center, Houston, Texas

John Sterling Meyer, M.D. Director, Cerebral Blood Flow Laboratory, Veterans Administration Medical Center, and Professor, Neurology Department, Baylor College of Medicine, Houston, Texas

Eugene Mochan, Ph.D., D.O. Professor and Chairman, Department of Family Practice, University of Medicine and Dentistry of New Jersey—School of Osteopathic Medicine, Stratford, New Jersey

Brian E. Mondell, M.D. Medical Director, Baltimore Headache Institute, and Assistant Professor, Neurology Department, The Johns Hopkins University School of Medicine, Baltimore, Maryland

F. Clifford Rose, F.R.C.P. Director, Princess Margaret Migraine Clinic, Charing Cross Hospital, London, England

Glen D. Solomon, M.D. Headache Section, Cleveland Clinic Foundation, Cleveland, Ohio, and Clinical Associate Professor of Medicine, Pennsylvania State University College of Medicine, Hershey, Pennsylvania

William G. Speed, III, M.D. Speed Headache Associates, P.A., and Associate Professor, Depatment of Medicine, The Johns Hopkins University School of Medicine, Baltimore, Maryland

Drug Therapy for Headache

1

The Treatment of Headache:
A Historical Perspective

John Edmeads
Sunnybrook Medical Center
University of Toronto
Toronto, Ontario, Canada

INTRODUCTION

The study of headache is a complex and occasionally confusing endeavor. Often, treatments are introduced because they make sense according to the pathophysiology of the day; that doctrine in time falls from favor, but the therapy it spawned sometimes endures for that most incontestable of reasons—because it works. This is not an isolated situation. It is a theme that has recurred since antiquity.

ANCIENT APPROACHES

In antiquity, diseases were explained through the agency of supernatural forces, and treated by magical methods, which included prayers to countervailing deities, and the application, often to the suffering head, of objects designed to propitiate the malevolent spirit.

The Sumerian prescription of 4000 B.C. for headaches was:

> Take the hair of a virgin kid. Let a wise woman spin it on the right side and double it on the left, and tie twice seven knots. Perform the incantation of Eridu. Bind therewith the head of the sick man ... cast therewith the water of incantation over him, that the headache may ascend to heaven.

Clearly, this treatment was efficacious, for a closely similar prescription, dating from about 2500 B.C., was found in a temple in Thebes, Egypt:

> The physician shall bind a crocodile made of clay, with an eye of faience, and straw in its mouth, to the head using a strip of fine linen upon which has been inscribed the names of the gods, and he shall pray (Fig. 1).

In modern scientific terms we recognize two elements in the success of this therapy: the placebo effect and the compression of the scalp, possibly collapsing painfully distended vessels.

In the GrecoRoman era, although the gods were still important in the genesis of disease, increasing emphasis was placed upon humors and vapors that permeated the body, causing adverse effects. Hippocrates (400 B.C.) advocated bleeding as a treatment for headaches to remove the offending humors, to be followed by the application of the herb, hellebore, to the head. Galen (150 A.D.) recommended purging, presumably to rid the body of noxious influences by another route. The idea of placing magical substances in proximity to the aching head persisted in the work of Pliny the Elder (70 A.D.), who treated headache by tying a hangman's noose around the head, or by suspending from the neck, on a red string, some moss scraped from the head of a statue.

THE MEDIEVAL ERA

Some of the magical concoctions used by physicians became increasingly bizarre during the Middle Ages. Around 800 A.D., when the vulture was much prized as an agent of healing, there appeared in the text *Incipit Epistula Vulturis* the following medical observation:

> The bones from its head wrapped in deer skin will cure any pain and headache; its brain, mixed with the best of oil and put in the nose, will expel all ailments of the head.

Less dramatic methods of treatment gradually evolved, so that in 13th century Italy, headache sufferers had a poultice of opium and vinegar placed upon their throbbing heads. (There is some evidence that the vinegar aided the percutaneous absorption of the opium.)

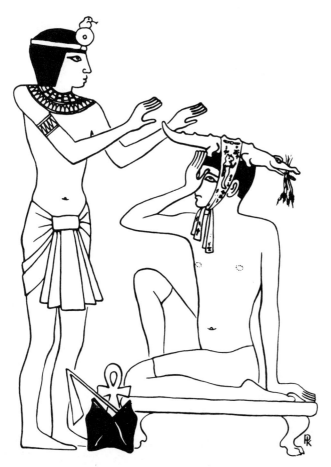

Figure 1 An early Egyptian cure recommended for headache.

The Arabian physician, Abulcasis (936–1013 A.D.) directed a more surgical approach to the problem of headache, applying a hot iron to the affected forehead, or incising the painful temple and appying garlic to the wound. The parallel to the cryosurgery of superficial temporal arteries practiced in North America in the 20th century is evident.

The magic of the New World was somewhat different from that of the Old, but remarkably similar systems of treatment apparently evolved independently and were traditional by the time the European explorers of the 16th and 17th century recorded them. The Incas of South America, when treating headache, would incise the scalp, and drip coca juice into the incision; the active ingredient of coca juice, cocaine, probably functioned as a potent local anesthetic. There is some evidence that the ancient civilizations of South America were proficient in the technique of trephination of the skull. Instruments have been found, in both Incan and Mayan sites, that were clearly used for placing holes in the skull, for the instructions were engraved upon the instruments. Also, skulls have been found in South America (and in Neolithic Europe) with surgical holes in them and with some evidence of survival beyond surgery, in the form of new bone proliferation around the margins of the craniotomies. Why these craniotomies were done is not known; there has been speculation that they were a primitive surgical treatment for headache, but there is no proof of this. We do know however (see later) that in 17th century Europe trephination was, on rare occasions, practiced for the relief of intractable headache.

The Indians of North America practiced a slighly less invasive brand of headache medicine. Samuel de Champlain, the founder of New France (17th century) wrote that the Indians of the Atlantic Coast gave him the head of a gar pike so that if he had a headache, he could scratch that part with it. For particularly severe headache, these Indians used the teeth of the pike to apply to the head, by scarification, a decoction of the root of the water hemlock. Use of this plant for local application (taken orally it was poisonous) was widespread among neighboring tribes. The Chippewa had an apparatus that incorporated several needles fastened at the end of a wooden handle. This was used to apply, by scarification in mild cases, the juice of the painted trillium; in severe cases of headache, sticks of cedarwood were burnt to a charcoal and mixed with an equal quantity of the dried gall of a bear; this was moistened with water and worked into the temple with needles. The dark spots in the temples of some Indians, left by the charcoal, identified them as headache sufferers (much as the indoor wearing of sunglasses identifies the migraineurs of today).

Although bizarre in modern terms, all of these primitive American therapies must have been at least partly efficacious. They stood the test of time; it is impossible to believe that pragmatic civilizations that flourished in such harsh environments would carry with them through generations the excess baggage of treatments that did not work. We see in these primitive treatments the rudiments of local surgical attack on the scalp, possibly interrupting nerve pathways, and some elements of pharmacotherapy—and, undoubtedly, the ubiquitous placebo response.

RENAISSANCE HEADACHE TREATMENT

Back across the Atlantic, European medicine was evolving slowly toward a scientific basis, but still used those appurtenances of traditional medicine that seemed to be helpful. Bleeding was still much in vogue. The painful temple would be incised and a heated glass globe would be applied over it; as the globe cooled, setting up a vacuum within it, blood (and possibly maleficent humors) were sucked from the head into the globe. Sometimes, the globes were applied without incisions, drawing blood to the surface (cupping). Surgical division and ligation of the superficial temporal artery was popular in the 17th and 18th centuries. Thomas Willis (1660) treated his eminent patient, Lady Conway, with mercurials, venesections, and one arteriotomy. He was, however, not in favor of more aggressive treatments. The same Lady Conway was also under treatment for her intractable migraine by her cousin, William Harvey, who made certain recommendations with which Willis did not agree. Willis wrote

> The opening of the skull cry'd up by many, but rarely attempted ... this our most ingenious Harvey endeavoured to persuade a Noble Lady labouring with a most grievous inveterate headache, promising a cure from thence ... but neither she nor any other would admit that administration ... I think opening of the skull will profit little or nothing.

There were even some critics of the more conservative temporal arteriotomy. Fordyce, in his book *De Hemicrania* (1758) argued against arteriotomy, making the point that not infrequently a patient would obtain temporary relief from an arteriotomy on one side of the head, only to have the pain begin anew in other areas of the head—an observation evidently unheeded by many 20th century surgeons.

Pharmacotherapy during the Renaissance was herbal, with drugs such as valerian and opium widely prescribed; in addition, mercurials and other mineral substances were used; they were prescribed empirically, with little apparent rationale and with little apparent efficacy.

THE 19TH CENTURY

At the opening of the 1800s, headache treatment was simply a shadow cast by preceding centuries. For example, William Heberden (1802), the foremost physician of his day, treated headaches with methods that were 200 years old, including blistering the head, bleeding, cupping, and emetics. Slowly, with the advent of the new science of chemistry, and with increasing communication between physicians with greater opportunity for exchange of ideas, new treatments for headache evolved. These were largely pharmacologic. Sometimes they worked—although seldom did those prescribing them know why. Another feature of 19th century medicine was a welcome conservatism, exemplified by the statements of one of the neurological giants of the day, Romberg (1853), about the treatment of headache: "We must avoid everything that is unnecessary," and "The local abstraction of blood is to be avoided." Also, there was new emphasis on life-style in the treatment of headache, as exemplified in the first statement by William Gowers (1888) in his passage on the treatment of migraine: "If any error in mode of life or defect in general health can be traced, the removal of this is the first and most essential step in treatment."

Gowers was one of the first physicians to divide the treatment of headache into prophylactic and episodic.

> The special treatment consists first in the continuous administration of drugs, with the object of rendering the attacks less frequent and less severe, and, secondly, the treatment of the attacks themselves.

He was obliged, however, to confess that the drugs available were not dramatic in their effectiveness. Gowers found bromide useful as a migraine prophylactic medication in some patients, often given as part of the famous "Gowers' mixture." For the treatment of acute attacks, he advocated a larger dose of bromide, often in combination with Indian hemp (*Cannabis indica*, or marijuana). Other treatments mentioned by Gowers for the acute attack of headache include a sedative dose of chloral, and a hypodermic injection of morphia. Gowers felt that "... drugs that cause contraction of the arteries are almost powerless; all that a full dose of ergotin does is to lessen the throbbing intensification of the pain complained of by some patients"; Gowers, of course, was using a crude extract of ergot, probably of low potency.

William Osler (1892) made very similar recommendations, which attests to the more rapid transfer of information among physicians. He particularly favored *Cannabis indica*, calling it "probably the most satisfactory remedy." He noted that antipyrin and phenacetin (the forerunners of acetylsalicyclic acid and acetaminophen) were sometimes effective when given at the very outset of the attack.

The headache treatment of the 19th century was a momentous advance on everything that had gone before. It recognized the influence of life-style on the production of headaches, it disparaged aggressive surgical adventures on the head, and it introduced a pharmacotherapy that was based on empiricism rather than dogma. It was the foundation of today's treatment.

THE PRESENT TREATMENT OF HEADACHE

With the 20th century came the application of the experimental method to the study of headache, the waxing (and waning) of various pathophysiologic theories, and increasing expertise and resourcefulness of a pharmaceutical industry that could design drugs to treat what were viewed as the pathophysiologic aberrations in migraine and other headaches. The results of this benificent troika were not always predictable, as exemplified by the saga of ergotamine.

An aqueous extract of the crude rye fungus, ergot, was used for painful afflictions of the head, including migraine, as early as 1868. In 1875 a partially purified extract, (ergotin) was available for the treatment of headache but, as noted previously, it was not considered particularly efficacious. However, in 1925 Rothlin purified a potent alkaloid of ergot, ergotamine, and this was applied to the therapy of migraine by Maier in 1925 and Tzank in 1929. This potent purified product proved a major advance in the treatment of migraine. As a commentary on how a good drug can overcome any obstacle, one notes the rationale expressed by Maier for using ergotamine for the treatment of migraine, which was that, since migraine was caused by vasoconstricction, and ergotamine was a vasodilator, ergotamine was likely to be useful in the treatment of migraine.

Equally illuminating is the example of methysergide, a potent serotonin (5-HT) antagonist, which was introduced into the headache pharmacopeia 30 years ago because of the then prevalent belief that migraine was characterized biochemically by excessive serotoninergic activity. Its efficacy appears not to be impaired by the current belief that migraine is characterized by deficiency of serotonin.

Currently undergoing wide clinical trials is a specific agonist of the 5-HT$_1$ receptor, with preliminary results indicating a high degree of efficacy in relieving acute attacks of migraine.

Clinicians, by and large, are philosophical about these apparent contradictions, and they are happy to use all of these medications as long as they are safe and efficacious. One physician, Che Guevara, wrote in his monograph on guerilla warfare: "The most important thing about a strategy is not that it is conventional, ingenious or legitimate, but simply that it works."

Also strengthening the hand of the 20th century clinician in treating migraine has been the force of serendipity, as exemplified by the introduction of β-blocking agents, and tricyclic antidepressants as powerful migraine prophylactic medications. Nobody knows how or why these medications work in migraine. Some of the more ingenious theoreticians have seized upon one or a few of the many pharmacologic actions of these drugs and, from them, woven a tissue of pathophysiologic speculation. One is irresistibly reminded of the Victorian physician, Locock, who adduced the efficacy of bromide, which is an anaphrodisiac, in the treatment of epilepsy, as evidence that the cause of epilepsy was excessive sexual activity.

These occasional intellectual pratfalls have in no way diminished the remarkable advances made in this century in our ability to treat patients with headaches. Indeed, they have had a beneficial effect in stimulating caution when examining and interpreting theories, and in pointing out that the important thing about a treatment is not why it should work, but whether and how well it does work.

CONCLUSION

Arnold Friedman, one of the great headache physicians of the 20th century, looked back through history and traced our ideas of headache from the times of magic to the present age of the molecule. He concluded

It is astonishing how successful we have been in treating headache without really knowing what pain is or being able to define accurately how drugs can relieve it. This perhaps is our present-day magic.

2

Classification of Headache

R. Michael Gallagher
University Headache Center
Moorestown, New Jersey, and
University of Medicine & Dentistry of New Jersey—
School of Osteopathic Medicine
Stratford, New Jersey

INTRODUCTION

To classify headaches or patients who suffer from headache is a most difficult
and often confusing task. Many patients suffer not just from one type of headache,
but from two or more. Some patients experience headaches that may conceivably
fall into more than one category (e.g., migraine with some symptoms that resemble cluster) or evolve or change over a lifetime (e.g., classic migraine that changes
to common migraine).

In 1962, the Ad Hoc Committee on Classification of Headache [1] developed
a workable and useful classification of this disorder. It divided headache into
vascular, muscle contraction, and traction and inflammatory categories. This system
was workable and established a basis for communication, research, and treatment.
However, as more interest developed in headache research and treatment, this
system became somewhat inadequate.

Various other systems have been developed since 1962. None of these have
been completely adequate, which is understandable, given the enormity and complexity of the problem. In 1988, the Headache Classification Committee of the

9

International Headache Society put forth a new detailed system. This classification entitled *Classification and Diagnostic Criteria for Headache Disorders, Cranial Neuralgias and Facial Pain* [2] is based on a four-digit hierarchial system. It allows headache disorders to be classified at different levels of sophistication, depending on the specificity of the clinician. However, this system is quite lengthy and cumbersome for purposes of this text. For simplicity and ease of understanding, I have elected to follow a simple classification modified from the Ad Hoc Committee [1] and the *Practicing Physician's Approach to Headache* [3].

CLASSIFICATION

Vascular Headaches

Cerebral vascular dilatation is a feature characteristic of this group of headaches. The dilatation can be intracranial or extracranial, and vasoconstriction can be a part of the headache complex.

Migraine

Migraine is the so-called Rolls Royce of headaches and is more than simply a severe headache. These headaches are more prevalent in women by 3:1 in the adult-aged groups [4] and about equal in male/female distribution in children [5]. The pain is most often unilateral and is associated with other symptoms. Other symptoms can include nausea, pallor, vomiting, yawning, throbbing, photophobia, irritability, constipation, cold extremities, personality changes, or fluid balance changes. Attacks occur from as infrequently as one or two a year to several a month. The headaches are often incapacitating and last from hours to several days.

Most migraine sufferers experience one of two types: classic or common. Differentiating these headaches is a characteristic aura of classic migraine. The classic migraine aura precedes the pain by 10–30 min and is characterized by some type of sensory disturbance, such as fortification spectra, teichopsia, photopsia, tunnel vision, visual field defects, paresthesias, dysphasia, or olfactory symptoms. The common migraine is most often associated with no aura, but some patients can experience personality changes, fluid retention, food cravings, or exceptional feelings of well-being 1–2 days before an attack. This vague prodrome of common migraine sometimes is noticed by family or friends before the patient is aware that an attack is imminent.

Hemiplegic, ophthalmoplegic, and basilar artery migraine are considered complicated forms of migraine because of the associated major neurological disturbances with the headache. Hemiplegic migraine is accompanied by hemiparesis. Ophthalmoplegic migraine is accompanied by paresis of ocular nerves. Basilar artery migraine is accompanied by symptoms originating from the brain stem,

Table 1 Headache Classification

Vascular	Muscle contraction	Mixed	Traction
Migraine	Tension	Headaches with features of	Mass lesions
Common	Psychogenic (including anxiety depression)	vascular and muscle contraction	Arteritis
Classic			Neuralgia
Hemiplegic	Myositis		Atypical facial pain
Ophthalmoplegic	Posttraumatic		Temporomandibular joint disorder (TMJ)
Basilar			
Cluster			Disease of sensory organs or teeth
Episodic			
Chronic			
Toxic			
Hypertensive			

such as vertigo, tinnitus, dysarthria, a decreased level of consciousness, or bilateral neurological disturbances.

Cluster Headache

Cluster headache, sometimes called "histamine cephalgia," is characterized by severe unilateral head pain. The pain is usually behind or around one eye with radiation to the jaw, teeth, ear, or occipital area. Other associated symptoms can occur on the affected side of the face. These include lacrimation or injection of the eye, rhinorrhea or congestion of the nostril, drooping of the eye lid, and swelling or sweating of the face. Attacks last an average of 30–60 min and occur from one to ten times a day. The headaches tend to group for weeks to months at a time and mysteriously disappear for months to years. Many attacks occur shortly after 1–2 hr of sleep, possibly coinciding with rapid eye movements [6].

The pain of cluster is extreme and the most severe of the episodic headaches. It often is described by sufferers as boring or burning and like a "hot poker" or "ice pick in the eye." During the pain, patients often move about, pace, or assume unusual positions, unlike the migraineur, who prefers to lie quiet and still.

A less frequently encountered form of cluster headache is chronic cluster. The symptoms are essentially the same; however, the lack of spontaneous remission periods is characteristic of this type. Chronic cluster sufferers rarely experience headache-free periods for more than 2 weeks. This form of cluster can occur de novo (primary chronic cluster) or following an episodic attack (secondary chronic cluster).

Cluster headache occurs in men more frequently than women by a ratio of 5:1 [7]. The symptoms more often begin in the late 20s or 30s and tend to be less frequent after the mid-60s. Children rarely experience cluster headaches, although some chronic cluster sufferers report symptoms beginning in the teens. Many cluster patients have coarse facial skin (peau d'orange), deep nasolabial folds, and an increased frequency of hazel eye color [8].

Toxic Headache

Toxic headaches are usually associated with systemic vasodilatation [3]. The condition can be caused by alcohol, medication, CO_2 retention, elevated temperature, or ingestion of toxic substances. The pain is quite variable, can throb and may be associated with migrainous symptoms.

Hypertensive Headache

Hypertensive headaches are precipitated by a systemic elevation in blood pressure. The diastolic pressure usually will be in excess of 110 mmHg [9]. Symptoms often include severe throbbing pain that is aggravated by exertion or bending.

Muscle Contraction Headache

The muscle contraction-type headache is the most frequently experienced headache and is often referred to as *tension headache*. The pain can be localized, but is often described as a bandlike feeling around the head or across the forehead. The pain varies in intensity and is often provoked by a known stressful situation.

Psychogenic factors, such as depression, chronic anxiety, or unresolved hostilities, are often associated with particularly severe or frequent muscle contraction headache. The headaches associated with these factors are sometimes referred to as *psychogenic* or *functional headaches*.

Other conditions that can contribute to the precipitation of muscle contraction headache are cervical osteoarthritis, chronic myositis, spine abnormalities, and occasionally ocular disease.

Benign posttraumatic headaches are the result of trauma to the head or neck. More frequently these headaches are of the muscle contraction type, but can be vascular or involve scalp nerves. There are reported cases of posttraumatic migraine [10] and cluster [11]. The headaches can begin immediately or lag for weeks after the injury. There appears to be no direct correlation between severity of injury and severity or length of headache.

Mixed Headache

The mixed-type headache has features of both muscle contraction and vascular headaches. The headaches are usually frequent, vary in intensity, and are often continuous. Patients who experience mixed headaches often overuse analgesics [12] and experience medication rebound effects.

Traction and Inflammatory Headache

The traction or inflammatory type of headache is associated with disease or abnormalities of intracranial structures, such as the skull, brain, nerves, meninges, arteries, sensory organs, teeth, or sinuses. The symptoms are elicited by the stretchng or compression of these structures. The headache is extremely variable and can mimic other headache conditions.

Headaches in this category often progress in severity and associated symptoms. The headaches rarely resolve spontaneously and require definitive corrective therapy.

Other Headaches

In addition to the headaches listed in the preceding category, there are numerous other headaches of which some have been named for their particular precipitating cause. The "ice cream headache," "weight lifter's headache," "sexual headache," and "mother-in-law headache" are only a few of the many described in various writings. Most can be classified into one of the already mentioned categories. Some of these headaches will be described in Chapter 4.

REFERENCES

√ 1. Ad Hoc Committee, Classification of Headache. JAMA 1962; 6:717.
√ 2. Headache Classification Committee of the International Headache Society. Cephalagia 1988; 8 (suppl 7):9–96.
3. Diamond S, Dalessio D. Classification and mechanisms of headache. In Diamond S, and Dalesso D, eds, Practicing physician's approach to headache. Baltimore: Williams & Wilkins, 1986: 1–10.
4. Lance JW, Anthony M. Some clinical aspects of migraine. A prospective survey of 500 patients. Arch Neurol 1966; 15:356–361.
5. Bille B. Migraine in school children. Int Arch Allergy 1955; 7:348.
6. Campbell J. Cluster headache. In Rose FC, ed. The management of headache. New York: Raven Press, 1988: 116.
7. Diamond S. Dalessio D, eds. The practicing physician's approach to headache, 4th ed. Baltimore: Williams & Wilkins, 1986: 66–75.
8. Kudrow L. Cluster headache diagnosis and management. Headache 1979; 19:142.

9. Dalessio D. Clinical classification of headache. In Dalessio D, ed. Wolff's headache and other head pain. New York: Oxford University Press, 1988: 9.
10. Raskin N. Post-traumatic headache: the post concessive syndrome. In Headache. New York: Churchill Livingstone, 1988: 272.
11. Friedman A, Mikropoulos H. Cluster headaches. Neurology 1958; 8:653–663.
12. Diamond S, Freitag F. Mixed headache syndrome. Clin J Pain 1988; 4:67–74.

3

Pathophysiology, Genetics, and Epidemiology of Headache

J. Keith Campbell
Mayo Medical School
Rochester, Minnesota

PATHOPHYSIOLOGY OF HEADACHE

The pathophysiology of the primary headache disorders, migraine, cluster headache, and muscle contraction or tension headache, is only partially understood. It was believed for many years that primary headaches could be clearly differentiated into the vascular or vasodilating type, such as migraine and cluster headache, and those headaches in which sustained contraction of the scalp and cervical muscles was responsible for the pain. The beneficial effects of vasoactive drugs, including the ergots and methysergide, on the vascular headaches, and the early demonstration by electromyography of sustained activity in the cervical muscles and scalp muscles in some tension headache sufferers, appeared to confirm the vascular and muscle contraction theories. Stress, dietary factors, and inheritance were thought to be of major importance in the pathogenesis of the two main types of head pain.

In the past 20 years, there has been increasing doubt that the simplistic division of headaches into vascular and tension types is correct [1], and in the past few years evidence that migraine and cluster headache have a neuronal basis, rather than a vascular one, has been increasing [2,3].

15

Migraine and Muscle Contraction Headache—A Continuum?

Migraine is generally an episodic headache, with a defined beginning and resolution in a few hours to several days. Tension or muscle contraction headache has, in the past, been described as a long-lasting headache, with a gradual onset and a gradual resolution. Tension headaches are often diagnosed when the pain occurs daily or is continuous. Migraine has usually been described as a pulsating or throbbing pain, whereas the pain of muscle contraction headache is usually described as steady squeezing, or a constant pressure sensation. Further studies have shown, however, that these distinctions and many other supposed characteristic differences between migraine and tension headaches are far from clear [1,4,5]. Because many of the features that have been used in the past to separate the two forms of headache are similar (Table 1), the relationship between these two forms may be closer than previously realized. Similarly, it has been recognized that migraine is not always episodic and separated by days or weeks of freedom from headache. Mathew and others [6,7] have widely discussed the transformed or evolved headache syndrome in which episodic and clear-cut migraine gradually increases in frequency and eventually results in continuous discomfort—the so-called chronic daily headache. The part played in the transformation by chronic intake or abuse of analgesics and other drugs is unclear, but it is probably of great significance [6,7].

The inability to detect chronic or increased muscle activity by electromyography in many patients suffering from tension or muscle contraction headache or to detect no more activity than in patients with typical migraine attacks [4] is strong evidence that sustained muscle contraction is not responsible for many so-called tension headaches. This is not to deny that holding the head and neck in some strained position is not responsible for a temporary muscle contraction headache. The role of ischemia in the affected muscles and the effect of chronic contraction on the scalp and cervical nerves are presently unclear. Contraction of scalp and cervical muscles in tension headache may be a result of the discomfort, and not the cause [8,9].

Table 1 Biochemical and Pharmacologic Similarities in Migraine and Tension Headache

Agent	Migraine	Tension headache
Amyl nitrite inhalation	Increased	Increased
Histamine injection	Increased	Increased
Platelet serotonin concentration	Decreased	Decreased
EMG activity of scalp muscles	Normal or increased	Normal or increased
Propranolol prophylaxis	Beneficial	Beneficial
Tricyclic prophylaxis	Beneficial	Beneficial
Ergot treatment	Beneficial	Usually ineffective

A common experience in migraine is to develop posterior or posterolateral neck pain in association with the more usual hemicranial pain so typical of this condition. Generally, the neck pain is thought to be due to sustained contraction of the cervical muscles, and it usually develops some hours into the attack; occasionally, however, it may be the harbinger of the hemicranial pain. There is presently no proof that the cervical pain is due to sustained contraction of the muscles, but it does seem to respond to attempts to relax them with heat, ice, or massage. The association of what is presumed to be muscle pain and migraine in this fashion and in patients with features of both vascular and tension headaches has led to use of the term *mixed or combined headache* or to the term *tension-vascular headache*. These terms, however, are not included in the new headache classification proposed by the International Headache Society [10], which suggests that patients having features of both migraine and tension-type headache should be considered to have both conditions.

Migraine: Pathogenesis

Migraine has been classified, for many years, as a vascular headache, because alterations in the caliber of cerebral and cranial blood vessels have been believed to be responsible for both the aura and the pain of classic migraine and for the pain of common migraine. Cerebral vasospasm followed by cerebral and cranial vasodilatation has been invoked in the pathogenesis of the vascular headaches on the basis of clinical observation by Graham and Wolff [11]. Several observations were, however, largely ignored until recently, when the work of Olesen and his coworkers [12,13] began to put the purely vascular pathogenesis of migraine in doubt. There is now a major move toward a central neurogenic theory of migraine and other headaches.

Cerebral Blood Flow Studies in Migraine

By using tomographic techniques capable of recording small changes in regional cerebral blood flow from some 254 areas over each cerebral hemisphere, Olesen [13] studied more than 40 patients with both common and classic migraine. In classic migraine attacks induced by arteriography, the clinical aura has been accompanied, in most cases, by a spreading zone of hypoperfusion, generally beginning in the occipital lobe contralateral to the aura symptoms. The zone or wave of oligemia has been observed to spread forward at 2–3 mm/min, crossing the territory of the cerebral arteries in a way such as to exclude a primary vascular mechanism. The wave of oligemia was generally arrested at the lateral sulcus, but, in some patients, it reached the frontal cortex through the insula. Unlike the aura, which usually resolved in 20–30 min, the cerebral cortical oligemia was observed to last up to 6 hr and, occasionally, persisted even after the pain had resolved. The oligemia zones eventually showed areas of hyperemia. At no

time was subcortical blood flow altered. Cortical hyperperfusion during the
headache phase has also been shown by others [14]. Whether or not the oligemia
observed reached ischemic levels is uncertain. Initial calculations suggested that
it did not, but recent reports indicate that the degree of oligemia may have been
underestimated and that ischemic levels can be reached [15]. The clinical observation of migrainous infarction would support this hypothesis. In common
migraine, Olesen et al. [12] have been unable to detect any changes in cerebral
perfusion.

Spreading Cortical Depression

The spreading oligemia observations in classic migraine have been linked in the
minds and writings of many by two older observations. Lashley [16] reported,
in 1941, on his own migrainous scintillating scotoma. By carefully timing the
spread of the visual hallucination and knowing the size of the visual cortex, Lashley
was able to postulate that a wave of excitation followed by a zone of inhibition
was being propagated across the visual cortex at approximately 3 mm/min.

In 1944, Leão [17], during his experimental work in epilepsy, observed a
wave of electrical excitation spreading across the cortex of lower animals. The
band of increased electrical activity was accompanied by hyperemia and was
followed by electrical depression and pallor of the cortex. The advancing wave
crossed the cortex at 2–3 mm/min.

Thus, in three instances, some alteration in cortical activity has been observed
or calculated to move at 2–3 mm/min and, at least in migraine attacks [13] and
in experimental animals [17], the observations suggest a change in perfusion that
does not follow the distribution of any particular cortical vessel. It should be
stressed, however, that the spreading depression of Leão has never been
demonstrated in humans and has been induced only with difficulty in animals
having a convoluted cortex (gyrencephaly). No study of migrainous subjects has
demonstrated spreading depression, and although the observations on spreading
oligemia [13] and the spreading depression of Leão [17] are often linked in discus-
sions on the pathogenesis of migraine, there is no proof that they are related,
or even significant, in this condition. The observations have, however, led many
investigators to concentrate on a neuronal theory of migraine and to suspect that
the vascular changes may be secondary to alterations in neuronal metabolism.

After the observations of Graham and Wolff [11], few investigators have
disagreed that dilatation of the extracranial vessels is responsible for the pain of
migraine. Increased pulsations of the vessels during the pain, temporary relief
by compression of the arteries, and reproduction of the pain of migraine by experimental distention of the vessels all help support the concept of extracranial
vasodilatation of the vessels being involved in the pain of migraine. Clearly, other
factors must be involved, because vasodilatation that follows exercise, or a hot

bath, or even blushing does not produce pain. The actual mechanism is not yet understood, but it is thought to involve a sterile inflammatory response around the vessels and the trigeminovascular system [2].

"Neurokinin" and Sterile Inflammation

During an attack of migraine, a substance, which has not been fully identified, accumulates in the extracellular space around the scalp vessels [18]. It lowers the pain threshold, increases capillary permeability, and is probably one of the factors in the cascade of events involved in the inflammatory response. The substance, which has been termed *neurokinin*, may be released by an efferent discharge in the trigeminal supply to the vessels.

Trigeminovascular System

On the basis of work using histochemical and immunochemical techniques, Moskowitz [2] showed that the trigeminal nerve is widely distributed to the large pial arteries, the meningeal vessels and sinuses, and the branches of the external carotid artery. Innervation of the vessels is strictly ipsilateral, except for the midline venous sinuses, which are innervated from both trigeminal nerves. The trigeminal nerve sensory fibers, especially the myelinated A delta and the nonmyelinated C fibers, can conduct impulses both centrally and peripherally. When stimulated along their course, the trigeminovascular fibers release substance P peripherally and centrally. Released peripherally along the vessels, substance P initiates the cascade of the inflammatory response. This involves release of bradykinin, histamine, and prostaglandins, degranulation of mast cells, and accumulation of serotonin; vasodilatation and edema result. Experimentally, pretreatment with methysergide and ergot preparations blocks the inflammatory response resulting from trigeminal nerve stimulation. Release of substance P has been stressed, but other neurotransmitters are almost certainly involved, including cholecystokinin, vasoactive intestinal polypeptide, somatostatin, and dynorphin B, which was recently found in nerve fibers surrounding pial vessels [19].

It has been suggested [2] that the trigeminovascular system is responsible for the hemicranial pain of migraine and cluster headache and that the bilateral innervation of midline vessels could help explain migraine attacks that are not lateralized. It has been further postulated that the spreading depression of Leão with its known release of potassium into the extracellular space [20] could depolarize the trigeminovascular system and cause release of substance P peripherally, which initiates the inflammatory response and causes vasodilatation, whereas central release of substance P initiates pain transmission through the descending nucleus of the trigeminal nerve. Thus, the peripheral vascular changes could be triggered by a cerebral neuronal abnormality.

The Role of Serotonin (5-Hydroxytryptamine) in Migraine

Interest in the role of serotonin in the pathophysiology of migraine dates back many years. Sicuteri et al. [21] noted an increase in urinary 5-hydroxyindole-acetic acid, a serotonin metabolite, in some patients during migraine. During attacks of headache, there is a fall in platelet serotonin and a corresponding rise in urinary serotonin in most patients [22,23].

Serotonin is found in the chromaffin cells of the gut, in platelets, and in the cells of the midline raphe nuclei of the medulla, pons, and midbrain. These raphe cells constitute the descending pain-modulating system [24] and also give rise to an ascending system that projects to the thalamus and widely throughout the cerebrum and the pial vessels [25,26]. Raskin [27] postulated that the role of the serotonin neurons is of greater importance in the pathogenesis of headache than platelet or gut serotonin.

Serotonin constricts large arteries and dilates arterioles and capillaries, depending on the resting tonus of the vessels and, therefore, for many years, has been a prime suspect in the pathophysiology of the vascular changes in migraine. Such observations as the induction of headache in migraine sufferers by parenteral reserpine have been considered evidence of the role of serotonin. Reserpine is known to deplete brain serotonin rapidly. The role of circulating platelet serotonin in migraine is hotly debated [28,29].

Role of Other Vasoactive Amines and Phenols in Headache

Histamine.   A potent vasodilator that participates in the inflammatory reaction after being released from perivascular mast cells, histamine has not been incriminated as a prime mover in migraine. There is no increase in the blood histamine values before, during, or after an attack of migraine. The role of histamine in cluster headache is more debatable. During an attack, whole blood histamine increases [30]; however, blockade of H_1- and H_2-receptors with anti-histaminic drugs is without benefit in headache.

Tyramine.   A component of various foods, including cheese, dairy products, some wines, and many other foodstuffs, tyramine causes release of catecholamines from sympathetic nerve endings and serotonin from platelets. The role of tyramine in the pathogenesis of migraine—so-called dietary migraine—is unproved, and yet it is customary to instruct migraineurs to avoid foods rich in tyramine to reduce the frequency of attacks. Strict avoidance of tyramine only rarely results in cessation of headaches.

Phenylethylamine.   A vasoactive amine present in chocolate, many cheeses, and red wines has been identified in the brain [31]. Whether or not this amine has a major role in the causation of migraine is uncertain. Sufferers from migraine that appears to be precipitated by foods containing phenylethylamine are well advised to avoid them, however.

   Phenols.   Attention has been directed recently toward the phenols that are present in wine, cheese, citrus fruits, cocoa, coffee, and some dairy products. Phenolsulfotransferase is responsible for sulfate conjugation of phenols and is necessary in the excretion of these substances. Inactivation of an isoenzyme of phenolsulfotransferase by red wine could allow more vasoactive amines than normal to enter the circulation and, thereby, lead to the widely reported red wine-induced headache.

   Caffeine.   Although caffeine is a component of many headache remedies, its role in the relief of headache and, more importantly, in the precipitation of headache has not been studied widely. Caffeine is a vasoconstrictor, and its benefits in the relief of headache may be due to this property. Improved absorption of analgesics may also be a factor. Excessive amounts of caffeine, usually in the form of coffee, are believed to lead to a caffeine-withdrawal headache as the subject decreases the intake overnight and wakens each morning with a vasodilating headache that responds to further intake of caffeine.

Prostaglandins

Prostaglandins, which are synthesized by many tissues, are potent vasodilators. In primates, intracarotid prostaglandin E_1 produces loss of cerebral vasomotor autoregulation and extracranial vasodilatation [32]. This may explain the observation that a headache follows intravenous administration of this substance to non-migraineurs, often accompanied by nausea and even by a typical migrainous aura [33].
   The role of prostaglandins in migraine has yet to be defined. They are participants in the sterile inflammatory response already mentioned, and the many agents, such as aspirin, that are helpful for alleviation of headache may owe some of their effect to an ability to inactivate these substances.

Sex Hormones and Migraine

Little hard data are available on this subject. The multiple clinical observations on migraine and the effects of the menarche, menstrual cycle, pregnancy, menopause, and oral contraceptives all indicate a definite role, but the exact mechanism whereby fluctuating levels of estrogen and progesterone alter the headache threshold is unclear.

Cluster Headache

Much of the material presented in the preceding section on migraine is relevant to cluster headache. Until recently, cluster headache was classified as a pure vascular headache on the basis of the long-held belief that the pain is due to vasodilatation; however, there is now a move toward a central or brain causation, and the vascular events are becoming of secondary importance [2,27]. The role of the trigeminovascular system is key to the understanding of this syndrome. The suspected presence of a central disturbance of neuronal activity in cluster headache can be delineated by a review of experimental and clinical observations.

Recent Pathophysiological Observations

Horner's Syndrome.   The Horner syndrome seen in cluster headache has not been shown to be due to an abnormality of the first-, second-, or third-order sympathetic neurons. There is evidence of a central lesion that also may be related to the preoptic or hypothalamic abnormality proposed by Sjaastad [34] to explain the facial sweating patterns seen in cluster headache.

Autonomic Asymmetry.   The pupillary response to tyramine eye drops and the electrocardiographic response to hyperventilation were investigated by Boccuni et al. [35] and led them to suspect a central sympathetic abnormality.

Sleep Apnea.   Sleep apnea has been noted in subjects with cluster headache. In most of those studied, the apnea has been of the central type [36].

Auditory- and Visual-Evoked Responses.   Abnormalities of both brain stem auditory-evoked responses and visual-evoked responses in cluster headache point toward a central cause.

Recent Hormonal, Biochemical, and Histologic Observations in Cluster Headache

Prolactin, Melatonin, and Testosterone Levels.   In male patients, the diurnal alterations in serum prolactin levels were abnormal, both during a cluster period and while in remission [37]. Serum prolactin levels increased during attacks, especially nocturnal episodes. Whether the increased secretion is primary or secondary to the pain is unknown. The altered diurnal rhythms, even between attacks, suggest a primary disorder of prolactin control.

The diurnal secretory rhythm of melatonin has shown similar changes in cluster headache. The nocturnal secretion of melatonin is increased, but the effects of sleep disturbances on the secretion patterns are unknown.

Serum levels of testosterone are decreased during cluster periods and return to normal during remissions. Sleep disturbances and stress during the painful stage may be responsible for these variations in hormone production.

5-Hydroxytryptamine Concentration in Platelets.   Even between attacks, levels of whole blood 5-hydroxytryptamine are low in subjects with cluster headache and are similar to levels found in migraineurs. 5-Hydroxytryptamine platelet-uptake kinetics are similar in both migraine and cluster headache and differ from those in normal subjects. Platelet monoamine oxidase activity is also lower in subjects with migraine and cluster headache than it is in normal subjects.

Mast Cell Distribution and Secretion Mechanisms. Studies have demonstrated increased numbers and abnormal distribution of mast cells in biopsy material from the temporal skin ipsilateral to cluster headache [38]. Recent studies [39] on the ultrastructure of mast cells in cluster headache reveal a dissolution pattern of secretion, which is usually associated with a delayed or late tissue reaction, rather than the extrusion-of-granules pattern that is characteristic of an immediate hypersensitivity reaction. These findings support the suggestion that secretion of the mast cells is initiated by antidromic reflex activity in the trigeminal nerve cutaneous branches.

Erythrocyte Choline Levels. Low levels of choline in erythrocytes were reported by De Belleroche et al. [40] in cluster headache. Treatment with lithium resulted in very large increases in choline levels. Similar low choline levels have been observed in bipolar mood disorders. These observations have yet to be verified, but they suggest that the periodicity of cluster headache and bipolar mood disorders may have a common underlying mechanism.

Thus, biochemical, physical, and histological observations all suggest that cluster headache involves a central disturbance of neuronal function that can initiate a disturbance in the trigeminovascular system which, in turn, releases substance P and other vasoactive substances and leads to vasodilatation and the pain of cluster headache. Hardebo [41] postulated that release of substance P by axon reflexes of various lengths in the trigeminovascular network could explain not only the pain of cluster headache but, also, most of the autonomic disturbances.

Surgically produced lesions of the trigeminal pathways in the treatment of cluster headache may give relief by interrupting the substance P-releasing neurons in addition to interrupting the final common pain pathway.

GENETICS OF HEADACHE

That patients with headaches have children with headaches is an almost universal clinical observation. Whether this is due to hereditary or environmental factors is not determined easily. Subjects with clear-cut migraine have a strong family prevalence of headache. Lance and Anthony [42] recorded a positive family history in 46% of patients, compared with a familial occurrence of only 18% in patients with typical tension headache. The current debate over whether or not migraine and tension headache are simply different manifestations of one condition makes these statistics suspect. In one study of migraine [43], a close family member was affected in 65% of cases. Bille [44] reported that children with migraine had a nearly 80% incidence of parental or sibling involvement. Maternal involvement was, by far, the most common pattern. In the rare familial hemiplegic migraine, a dominant pattern of inheritance seems clear; but with this exception, the mode of transmission in other types of migraine is less well defined. Concordance rates in studies of twins have not produced unambiguous results [45,46], but dominant inheritance of a migraine diathesis, with incomplete penetrance, seems most likely.

Cluster headache does not appear to be inherited. It is rare to find more than one affected subject in a family. The prevalence of migraine is the same in cluster headache subjects as in the general population [47]. The lack of a family history in cluster headache, with the high frequency of such a history in migraine, is just one of the factors that makes it unlikely that these two forms of headache are related.

EPIDEMIOLOGY OF HEADACHE

If the incidence, prevalence, and geographic distribution of a condition are to be determined accurately, there must be agreement on the definition of that condition, and diagnostic criteria must be strictly outlined. Because the distinction between two of the most commonly diagnosed primary headache disorders, migraine and tension headache, is unclear and has varied over the past few years, it is probable that accurate statistics have yet to be obtained. The epidemiology of headache, in general, is well documented; it is only when specific primary headaches are considered that relative and absolute statistics are open to different interpretations. Even the statistics of migraine involve problems of definition. If subjects have attacks of both common migraine (without aura) and classic migraine (with aura), are they to be classified as having both types of migraine or are they classified in one category at the expense of the other? For accuracy of reporting the effects of various drugs on migraine, it is vital that the type of migraine be specified, because the response in classic migraine may be quite different from that in common migraine.

Statistics derived from physicians' records, hospitals, and headache clinics are overtly biased toward patients who seek medical care, and they do not take into account the majority of subjects who treat themselves with over-the-counter preparations. Statistical surveys based on questionnaires or on the results of other nonmedical information gathering suffer from many shortcomings, including questionable diagnostic accuracy [48].

Despite these difficulties, statistics based on large-scale population surveys, personal door-to-door surveys, and figures derived from medical facilities and selected closed communities reveal that headache is a very common experience [48]. The numbers of persons suffering headache are staggering. Waters [49] found, in a population in Pontypridd (Wales), that in the year before the survey, 64% of 491 men and 79% of 741 women had suffered headache that they had considered significant. In northern Finland, 58% of men and 73% of women admitted to headache in the year before a similar study [50]. Ziegler et al. [51] estimated that 40% of North Americans have experienced significant headache at some time in their lives.

The high incidence of headaches in adult populations follows a surprisingly high frequency of headaches in children. Bille [44] reported that by the age of 7 years, 2.5% of children had frequent nonmigrainous headaches, 1.4% had migraine, and 35% complained of infrequent, nonspecified types of headache. By age 15 years, the numbers had increased to 15.7% for frequent nonmigrainous headaches, whereas 5.3% had migraine and 54% had experienced occasional nonmigrainous headaches.

The prevalence of migraine in adults has been variously reported to be between 0.5% and 20% of the population in the United States, United Kingdom, and Scandinavia [48]. In children, there is a slight preponderance in boys, but, by the age of puberty, migraine is more common in girls, and it remains more common in females throughout adult life. The relative proportion of headache sufferers having migraine is difficult to assess because of the previously mentioned lack of consensus on the diagnosis. Waters [49] reported that 39% of men and 57% of women who reported headache in the previous year suffered from migraine.

Compared with the prevalence of migraine and tension headache, that of cluster headache is much lower; however, few large-scale surveys have been undertaken. Ekbom et al. [52] found a prevalence rate of only 0.09% for cluster headache compared with a rate of 1.7% for migraine in a survey of male military recruits. In patients attending headache clinics, migraine is 20–50 times more common than cluster headache.

REFERENCES

1. Drummond PD, Lance JW. Clinical diagnosis and computer analysis of headache symptoms. J Neurol Neurosurg Psychiatry 1984; 47:128–133.
2. Moskowitz MA. The neurobiology of vascular head pain. Ann Neurol 1984; 16:157–168.
3. Olesen J. The ischemic hypotheses of migraine. Arch Neurol 1987; 44:321–322.
4. Bakal DA, Kaganov JA. Muscle contraction and migraine headache: psychophysiologic comparison. Headache 1977; 17:208–215.
5. Ziegler DK, Hassanein RS, Couch JR. Headache syndromes suggested by statistical analysis of headache symptoms. Cephalalgia 1982; 2:125–134.
6. Mathew NT, Stubits E, Nigam MP. Transformation of episodic migraine into daily headache: analysis of factors. Headache 1982; 22:66–68.
7. Mathew NT, Reuveni U, Perez F. Transformed or evolutive migraine. Headache 1987; 27:102–106.

8. Kaganov JA, Bakal DA, Dunn BE. The differential contribution of muscle contraction and migraine symptoms to problem headache in the general population. Headache 1981; 21:157–163.

9. Haynes SN, Cuevas J, Gannon LR. The psychophysiological etiology of muscle-contraction headache. Headache 1982; 22:122–132.

10. International Headache Society Headache Classification Committee. Classification and diagnostic criteria for headache disorders, cranial neuralgias, and facial pain. Cephalalgia 1988; 8(suppl 7):10–92.

11. Graham JR, Wolff HG. Mechanism of migraine headache and action of ergotamine tartrate. Arch Neurol Psychiatry 1938; 39:737–763.

12. Olesen J, Larsen B, Lauritzen M. Focal hyperemia followed by spreading oligemia and impaired activation of rCBF in classic migraine. Ann Neurol 1981; 9:344–352.

13. Olesen J. The pathophysiology of migraine. In: Vinken PJ, Bruyn GW, Klawans HL, eds. Handbook of clinical neurology, vol 48. Amsterdam: Elsevier Science Publishers, 1986:59–83.

14. Meyer JS, Zetusky W, Jonsdottir M, Mortel K. Cephalic hyperemia during migraine headaches. A prospective study. Headache 1986; 26:388–397.

15. Olsen TS, Friberg L, Lassen NA. Ischemia may be the primary cause of the neurologic deficits in classic migraine. Arch Neurol 1987; 44:156–161.

16. Lashley KS. Patterns of cerebral integration indicated by the scotomas of migraine. Arch Neurol Psychiatry 1941; 46:331–339.

17. Leão AAP. Spreading depression of activity in the cerebral cortex. J Neurophysiol 1944; 7:359–390.

18. Chapman LF, Ramos AO, Goodell H, Silverman G, Wolff HG. A humoral agent implicated in vascular headache of the migraine type. Arch Neurol 1960; 3:223–229.

19. Moskowitz MA, Brezina LR, Kuo C. Dynorphin β-containing perivascular axons and sensory neurotransmitter mechanisms in brain blood vessels. Cephalalgia 1986; 6:81–86.

20. Hansen AJ Olsen CE. Brain extracellular space during spreading depression and ischemia. Acta Physiol Scand 1980; 108:355–365.

21. Sicuteri F, Testi A, Anselmi B. Biochemical investigations in headache: increase in the hydroxyindoleacetic acid excretion during migraine attacks. Int Arch Allergy Appl Immunol 1961; 19:55–58.

22. Anthony M, Lance JW. The role of serotonin in migraine. In: Pearce J, ed. Modern topics in migraine. London: Heinemann Medical Books, 1975:107–123.

23. Anthony M. The biochemistry of migraine. In: Vinken, PJ, Bruyn GW, Klawans HL, eds. Handbook of clinical neurology, vol 48. Amsterdam: Elsevier Science Publishers, 1986:85–105.

24. Fields HL, Leving JD. Pain—mechanisms and management. West J Med 1984; 141:347–357.

25. MacKenzie ET, Edvinsson L, Scatton B. Functional bases for a central serotonergic involvement in classic migraine: a speculative view. Cephalalgia 1985; 5:69–78.

26. Griffith SG, Burnstock G. Immunohistochemical demonstration of serotonin in nerves supplying human cerebral and mesenteric blood-vessels: some speculations about their involvement in vascular disorders. Lancet 1983; 1:561–562.

27. Raskin NH. On the origin of head pain. Headache 1988; 28:254-257.
28. Hanington E. The platelet and migraine. Headache 1986; 26:411-415.
29. Steiner TJ, Joseph R, Rose FC. Migraine is not a platelet disorder. Headache 1985; 25:434-440.
30. Anthony M, Lance JW. Histamine and serotonin in cluster headache. Arch Neurol 1971; 25:225-231.
31. Sabelli HC, Borison RL, Diamond BI, Havdala HS, Narasimhachari N. Phenylethylamine and brain function. Biochem Pharmacol 1978; 27:1707-1711.
32. Welch KMA, Spira PJ, Knowles L, Lance JW. Effects of prostaglandins on the internal and external carotid blood flow in the monkey. Neurology 1974; 24:705-710.
33. Carlson LA, Ekelund L-G, Oró L. Clinical and metabolic effects of different doses of prostaglandin E_1 in man. Acta Med Scand 1968; 183:423-430.
34. Sjaastad O. The so-called "partial Horner syndrome" in cluster headache. An editorial. Cephalalgia 1985; 5:59-61.
35. Boccuni M, Morace G, Pietrini U, Porciani MC, Fanciullacci M, Sicuteri F. Coexistence of pupillary and heart sympathergic asymmetries in cluster headache. Cephalalgia 1984; 4:9-15.
36. Kudrow L, McGinty DJ, Phillips ER, Stevenson M. Sleep apnea in cluster headache. Cephalalgia 1984; 4:33-38.
37. Waldenlind E, Gustafsson SA. Prolactin in cluster headache: diurnal secretion, response to thyrotropin-releasing hormone, and relation to sex steroids and gonadotropins. Cephalalgia 1987; 7:43-54.
38. Liberski PP, Prusiński A. Further observations on the mast cells over the painful region in cluster headache patients. Headache 1982; 22:115-117.
39. Liberski PP, Mirecka B. Mast cells in cluster headache: ultrastructure, release pattern and possible pathogenetic significance. Cephalalgia 1984; 4:101-106.
40. De Belleroche J, Cook GE, Das I, Joseph R, Tresidder I, Rouse S, Petty R, Rose FC. Erythrocyte choline concentrations and cluster headache. Br Med J 1984; 288:268-270.
41. Hardebo JE. The involvement of trigeminal substance P neurons in cluster headache. An hypothesis. Headache 1984; 24:294-304.
42. Lance JW, Anthony M. Some clinical aspects of migraine: a prospective survey of 500 patients. Arch Neurol 1966; 15:356-361.
43. Friedman AP, von Storch TJC, Merritt HH. Migraine and tension headaches: a clinical study of two thousand cases. Neurology 1954; 4:773-788.
44. Bille BS. Migraine in school children. A study of the incidence and short-term prognosis, and a clinical, psychological and electroencephalographic comparison between children with migraine and matched controls. Acta Paediatr 1962; 51(suppl 136):1-151.
45. Lucas RN. Migraine in twins. J Psychosom Res 1977; 21:147-156.
46. Ziegler DK, Hassanein RS, Harris D, Stewart R. Headache in a non-clinic twin population. Headache 1975; 14:213-218.
47. Ziegler DK. The contribution of epidemiology to the understanding of headache and migraine. In: Hopkins A, ed. Headache: problems in diagnosis and management. London: WB Saunders, 1988:11-35.

48. Andersson PG. Migraine in patients with cluster headache. Cephalalgia 1985; 5:11–16.
49. Waters WE. The Pontypridd headache survey. Headache 1974; 14:81–90.
50. Nikiforow R, Hokkanen E. An epidemiological study of headache in an urban and a rural population in northern Finland. Headache 1978; 18:137–145.
51. Ziegler DK, Hassanein RS, Couch JR. Characteristics of life headache histories in a nonclinic population. Neurology 1977; 27:265–269.
52. Ekbom K, Ahlborg B, Schéle R. Prevalence of migraine and cluster headache in Swedish men of 18. Headache 1978; 18:9–19.

4

Influencing Factors of Headache

R. Michael Gallagher
University Headache Center
Moorestown, New Jersey, and
University of Medicine & Dentistry of New Jersey—
School of Osteopathic Medicine
Stratford, New Jersey

INTRODUCTION

Certain factors or conditions tend to precipitate, or at least contribute to, the frequency or severity of headache attacks. Vascular headache sufferers seem to have an exaggerated reactivity to external and internal stimuli. Muscle contraction headache sufferers overreact to stressful situations. The elimination or reduction of these precipitants will not necessarily prevent headaches completely, but they may cause an overall improvement in attack frequency and severity.

DIET

The role between diet and headache has been discussed and argued by physicians and researchers for many years. Glaudius Galen's early medical writings on headaches suggest a connection. In 1778, John Fothergill [1], a London physician who argued the theory of a headache and food relationship wrote "It is most clear that headache proceeds from the stomach, not the reverse." He believed that headaches resulted from eating foods such as melted butter, fats, spice, and meat pies, and drinking malt liquors. In 1921, T.R. Brown [2] reported a link between migraine attacks and certain foods and suggested their prevention by adopting avoidance diets. Currently, most headache specialists agree that certain dietary factors may contribute to the precipitation of migraine in some patients. With only a few exceptions, dietary factors do not seem to play a crucial role in other headaches, such as cluster or muscle contraction.

Well-controlled double-bind studies are few, but numerous studies and surveys have been conducted by authorities and known headache specialists. Diamond and Blau [3] conducted a survey of 327 physicians who were interested in the headache problem and found that most agreed that migraines can be induced by certain food intake. Van den Bergh [4] reported that 44% of migraine patients surveyed by the Belgian Migraine Society believed that their headaches were triggered by diet. Although many physicians and patients feel that a relationship does exist, an understanding is most difficult and complex, as triggering foods vary from patient to patient.

Complicating the diet–migraine matter is that particular dietary triggers do not always provoke attacks each time they are eaten in given individuals. Migraine attacks can result from a multitude of causative factors, of which diet is only one. Environmental changes, stress, fatigue, and hormonal changes may also play an important role. Some female sufferers report being susceptible to diet-induced migraine only during menses. Others report being susceptible only when fatigued or exposed to strong sunlight.

Some of the foods commonly implicated in diet-related migraine are chocolate, cheese, beans, seafood, nuts, citrus fruits, and onions (Table 1). These foods contain vasoactive amines such as tyramine, phenylethylamine, dopamine, or histamine. The vasoactive amines are physiologically potent and can affect the body vasculature markedly. In susceptible individuals, small amounts can produce headache. Tyramine is found in a substantial number of provocative foods.

Certain food additives such as monosodium glutamate, sodium nitrite, caffeine, and alcohol are also implicated in provoking migraine. The exact mechanism is not completely understood, but it is throught to involve vasoconstriction and dilatation mechanisms.

Tyramine

Tyramine is an amino acid with sympathomimetic properties. It is found in many migraine-provoking foodstuffs and is thought to be nontoxic under usual circumstances. It acts directly on blood vessels and causes the release of endogenous aromatic amines from sympathetic nerve endings and serotonin from platelets [5]. This can result in selective cerebral vasoconstriction and subsequent rebound vasodilatation [6], causing a headache in susceptible persons. It is rapidly metabolized by the liver in normal persons; however, there is evidence to suggest

Table 1 Migraine Precipitating Foods

Beverages	Vegetables
Alcoholic	Fava beans
Caffeine	Lima beans
(limit to 2 C/day)	Navy beans
Chocolate milk	Pea pods
Buttermilk	Sauerkraut
Dairy	Onions
Aged and processed cheese	Desserts
Yogurt	Chocolate
(limit to ½ C/day)	Other
Sour cream	Soy sauce
Meat and Fish	MSG
Pickled herring	Meat tenderizer
Chicken livers	Seasoning salt
Sausage	Canned soups
Salami	TV dinners
Pepperoni	Garlic
Bologna	Yeast extracts
Hot dogs	
Marinated meats	
Aged, canned, or cured meats	
Fruits	
Canned figs	
Raisins	
Papaya	
Passion fruit	
Avocado	
Bananas	
Red plums	
Citrus fruits	
(limit to ½ C/day)	
Baked goods	
Fresh baked breads	
Sourdough	

Source: Extracted from the National Headache Foundation Headache Diet, Chicago, Illinois.

that migraine patients have an altered ability to degredate it to an inactive form [7]. Common tyramine-containing foods are bananas, pods of broad beans, avocado, aged cheese, chicken livers, yogurt, sour cream, and nuts.

Hanington and Harper [6] conducted a blind study involving 17 migraine patients who believed that their headaches were diet related. Capsules containing

100 mg of either tyramine hydrochloride or a lactose placebo were given to patients in 75 different trials. In 26 of the trials, in which patients were given placebos, only two migraine attacks occurred, but in 49 trials, in which patients were given tyramine, 40 migraine attacks occurred within 12 hr. Ryan [8] conducted a more elaborate double-blind study that included 75 patients, in which the results were significantly different. He showed that the power of suggestion played a larger role in causing headache than tyramine did.

Although some controversy still remains on mechanism and the role of tyramine as a migraine precipitant, its avoidance is usually included in a comprehensive migraine treatment program. There does not appear to be a documentable tyramine relationship in the precipitation of muscle contraction or cluster headache. However, there are some patients who report increased susceptibility or provocation of attacks with the ingestion of tyramine-containing foods.

Phenylethylamine

Chocolate, for many years, has been known to precipitate migraine. Although it contains little tyramine, it does contain β-phenylethylamine, which is believed to be the provoking agent. Phenylethylamine, a potent vasoactive amine, is also found in some cheeses and in red wine. Migraine usually occurs within 12 hr after a patient has ingested it. Sandler and colleagues [9] have theorized that phenylethylamine causes vasoactive substances to be released from the lungs, which may have a secondary effect on the cerebral vasculature, which in turn, results in vasodilatation.

Although all clinicians do not accept a chocolate–cluster headache relationship, some sufferers do report the precipitation of attacks shortly after its ingestion.

Sodium Nitrite

Sodium nitrite is a food-coloring and preserving agent found in cured meats, such as hot dogs, bacon, ham, and various processed meats and fish. The amounts added to foods are federally regulated because of possible carcinogenic properties. Small amounts can cause headaches in susceptible individuals by inducing vasodilatation of cerebral blood vessels. The headache usually follows within 1 hr of ingestion.

Similar headaches are sometimes experienced in patients after taking nitrates that are found in many anginal and vascular medications or vitamin supplements containing niacin or nicotinic acid. Occasionally a patient develops a tolerance to nitrates after prolonged use and finds that headache is no longer a problem.

Monosodium Glutamate

Monosodium glutamate (MSG) is a popular flavor enhancer and food preservative. It is commonly found in Chinese food, processed meats, frozen dinners, canned soups, soy sauce, and seasonings. Glutamic acid may have neuroexcititory properties [5] and interferes with glucose transport to the brain, resulting in cerebral vasodilatation and, thereby, vascular headache [10]. Migraineurs who ingest monosodium glutamate often experience a severe attack within hours of ingestion. However, some sufferers can ingest trace amounts with no apparent effect.

Monosodium glutamate can provoke the so-called Chinese food syndrome in nonmigrainous persons if taken in sufficient quantities, as found in Chinese food. Symptoms can include headache, facial flushing, diaphoresis, mood disturbances, gastrointestinal distress, paresthesias, and chest pain. This susceptibility may be due to an inability to metabolize monosodium glutamate properly [11].

Alcohol

Alcohol is a nonspecific vasodilator that can provoke headache attacks in susceptible individuals. It is thought to depress or alter central vasomotor centers, because the direct action of alcohol on blood vessels is insignificant [7]. Of all the precipitating agents, alcohol most consistently provokes headaches in the largest number of patients.

Some migraine sufferers find they can drink certain types of alcohol in small amounts, but not other types. This is probably due to the presence of vasoconstrictive compounds, such as tyramine or histamine, found in certain brands. Those types more likely to induce headaches are red wines, brandy, and gin.

Cluster patients (episodic or chronic) are extremely sensitive to alcohol during active cluster periods. Attacks usually occur within 30 min of intake, regardless of type or brand consumed. Most patients experience these triggered attacks in 70-80% of exposures [12]. During remission periods, when not taking preventative medication, alcohol appears to have no provoking effect.

It is interesting that patients who experience nonvascular headache, will sometimes report that alcohol helps lessen their headaches, rather than precipitate or aggravate them. This is probably due to the sedating qualities of alcohol in some persons.

Overindulgence of alcohol often precipitates a "migrainelike" headache in nonsufferers and a prolonged migraine in sufferers. Interestingly, the drinking of alcohol in a relaxed environment, free of noise, smoke, snacks, and tension, may not trigger the "hangover headache." This is probably due to relaxation and the absence of other triggering and aggravating factors.

Caffeine

Caffeine is a central nervous system stimulant that produces vascular constriction and does not primarily cause headaches. Usually, caffeine is not a problem for most persons. However, excessive consumption of coffee, colas, and caffeine-containing analgesics may lead to a relative rebound vasodilatation and headache, if consumption is suddenly reduced or delayed. Although this phenomenon can occur in many individuals, vascular headache sufferers seem to be particularly susceptible. As the last dose wears off, a headache may result that is relieved by more caffeine or becomes more severe as the caffeine is withheld. Occasionally, individuals who consume substantial amounts during the week may experience weekend headaches if intake is decreased. This caffeine deprivation also accounts for many headaches that are present on awakening.

Occasional patients will report the start of headaches shortly after the ingestion of minimal amounts of caffeine. Whether this is due to a true biological mechanism or to the power of suggestion is difficult to determine. Many persons can consume up to 200 mg of caffeine each day without difficulty. However, one large mug of coffee can contain as much as 250 mg of caffeine (Table 2).

Artificial Sweeteners

Artificial sweeteners, particularly aspartame, have been implicated as migraine precipitants. There have been numerous patients who have reported increased headache, but investigations, on the whole, appear to be inconclusive. In a recent survey, Tipton et al. [13] questioned 190 consecutive headache patients, of whom 8.2% reported aspartame to be a triggering factor in their headaches. In a double-blind study of 40 patients, Schiffman et al. [14] reported a no higher prevalence of aspartame-induced headache than that induced by placebo. Koehlor and Glaros [15], in yet another double-blind study involving 11 patients, reported increased headache as a result of aspartame ingestion.

Fasting

Skipping meals, prolonged fasting, or dieting can provoke headache attacks in susceptible individuals. Five hours of fasting during waking hours and 13 hr of fasting overnight were provocative in a large survey of women sufferers [16]. The mechanism is presumed to involve a relative hypoglycemia, or lowering of blood sugar, which causes vasodilatation. This hypoglycemic mechanism also has been suggested in studies by Dexter and Byer [17] and Blau and Pike [18].

Many migraine sufferers find that morning headaches occur when they sleep late on weekends or holidays. The same patients find that headaches do not occur if they arise at the usual time and eat something before returning to bed for extra sleep.

The fasting headache can be prevented by eating regularly and avoiding any waking fasting for more than 4 hr. Meals should be well balanced, with adequate protein, which digests more slowly than carbohydrates. Some patients who suffer with morning headaches or exercise headaches may benefit from protein snacks before going to bed or exercising.

Table 2 Sources of Caffeine

Source	Amount (mg)
Coffee: 5- to 8-oz cup	
Drip	100–150 mg
Percolated	65–125 mg
Instant	40–110 mg
Decaf, brewed	2–5 mg
Decaf, instant	2 mg
Tea: 5- to 8-oz cup	
Bag, loose	20–75 mg
Canned ice tea	25–35 mg
Soft drinks: 12-oz glass	
Cola	33–60 mg
Mountain Dew	54 mg
Dr. Pepper	38 mg
Chocolate	
Bar, 1 oz	3–6 mg
Cocoa, 8 oz	50 mg
Bittersweet, 1 oz	25–35 mg
O-T-C medication	
Excedrin	66 mg
Vanquish	60 mg
Anacin	32 mg
Midol	32 mg
Cope	32 mg

Other

Head pain of the temple, ear, forehead, or palate can be precipitated in susceptible individuals by ice cream. Cooling of the oral pharynx causes excessive vascular
reaction, and many migraineurs demonstrate unstable vasomotor regulation.
Raskin and Knittle [19] found that 93% of 59 migraineurs and 31% of 49 non-
migraineurs experienced headache after eating ice cream. My own experience
indicates a considerably lower percentage, but a high percentage of migraineurs
do report rapidly developing headache after the ingestion of ice cream or especially
cold foods.

Copper has been implicated in the precipitation of migraine. A recent study
suggested that copper may be the provoking compound in many migraine-
precipitating foods [20]. Chocolate contains little or no tyramine, but is high in
copper content. Citrate and glutamate, both often found in known migraine-
precipitating foods, facilitate copper absorption.

Various other foods or additives that are thought to precipitate migraine attacks are reported by patients physicians. The more commonly reported triggers are fats, milk products, various fruits and vegetables, and salt. Some trace elements are also now being investigated for possible provoking mechanisms. Whether the above-mentioned represent true triggers or idiosyncratic reactions has yet to be determined.

Comment on Diet and Headache Relationship

Although various diet-related vasoactive compounds have been implicated as causes of migraine, further research and investigative studies are needed for a more complete understanding of their role. Many physicians involved in the study of headache believe that dietary factors do play a role in some patients' problems. Although total elimination of headache rarely occurs as the sole result of a food-avoidance diet, many patients do benefit from a comprehensive treatment program that includes dietary restrictions.

HORMONAL INFLUENCES

The influence of hormones on the migrainous patient is substantial. Most migrainous sufferers are women, with increased headache problems occurring with menarche, menses, menopause, gynecological irregularities, and when they are taking hormonal supplements or oral contraceptives. Adult women are subjected to internal fluctuations of sexual hormones during the menstrual cycle, which exert a notable effect on headache frequency and severity in many sufferers.

In support of this relationship are other observations on migraine patients. The incidence of migraine in prepubescent boys and girls is almost equal, suggesting no hereditary sex predisposition. However, as girls undergo the adolescent maturing process, their incidence of migraine increases to more than double that of boys and many migrainous boys experience only rare attacks after puberty.

Sixty percent of women seen by physicians for migraine headache report some relationship of their headaches to the menstrual cycle [21]. Of this group of patients, as many as 25% may suffer with menstrual migraine [21] (headaches that occur exclusively with menses). The physiology of menstrually related migraine is not yet clearly understood; however, it is believed to be related to the natural withdrawal of estrogen in the premenstrual phase of the menstrual cycle [22]. Other mechanisms have been suggested, of which some are prostaglandin changes, fluid and glucose imbalances, and vitamin or immunological deficiencies.

It does not appear that cluster and muscle contraction headaches are significantly influenced by hormonal fluctuation. As with other precipitating factors, some patients do report more headaches during their menses. Headaches can be a part of the premenstrual syndrome (PMS). However, the mechanism by which these headaches are precipitated is not clear.

Oral Contraceptives

Migrainous women who use estrogen oral contraception often experience an increase in headache severity or frequency. This increase may occur immediately or lag for many months after initiation of therapy. Some women without a migrainous history will develop migraine only after the beginning of oral contraception [23]. The cessation of oral contraception may result in a decrease or improvement of attacks in some patients. However, in many patients, attacks may persist for extended periods. The occasional migrainous woman will experience headache improvement with oral contraception.

Higher estrogen dosage birth control pills seem to cause a greater problem than the lower dosage. Nonetheless, even those containing minimal estrogen, can precipitate severe migraine attacks. During the month, the most vulnerable time for headache is the hormone-free period just before menstruation.

The risk of stroke in migrainous women taking oral contraceptives is increased. This is presumed to be due to an increased tendency of platelet aggregation and clot formation [24]. Women who experience complicated migraine, whose attacks change in character, or who develop neurological symptoms when taking oral contraceptives, should discontinue their use.

Pregnancy

Most migrainous women experience notable headache improvement after the third month of pregnancy. The mechanism by which pregnancy causes migraine relief is unclear. The absence of the cyclic rise and fall of estrogen levels, rising estrogenic hormones, changes in platelet aggregation, and protective secretions by the developing baby, all have been suggested.

I have conducted an extensive survey of female migraine sufferers who experience relief during pregnancy. Interviews and questionnaires were completed on sufferers, their mothers, grandmothers, and children, when applicable. The results were inconclusive and did not suggest a consistent pattern of headache relief among the sufferer, parent, or sibling during pregnancy. However, those women who experienced severe headaches with menses and ovulation seemed to fare better during pregnancy.

Little is known about the prevalence of cluster headaches during pregnancy. Although it is thought by many to be improved during pregnancy, as with migraine, cluster attacks can and do occur. Accurate statistical information on this is difficult because of the relatively few female sufferers with childbearing potential. I have seen two cases of sufferers who reported having attacks during pregnancy.

Tension headaches are common during pregnancy and usually continue in women who suffered before they became pregnant. Pregnancy can be a time of contentment in some women, which often will result in fewer headaches. The converse can also occur, with pregnancy being very stressful and the cause of more frequent tension headaches.

Estrogen Replacement

Menopausal women and those having undergone hysterectomies who experience vasomotor symptoms are often treated with replacement estrogen. In general, estrogen therapy intensifies migraine and should be avoided whenever possible. The synthetic form of estrogen may be of more benefit than the conjugated forms [25]. Doses should be kept as low as possible, and continuous therapy is usually more beneficial than interrupted therapy [26].

PSYCHOLOGICAL FACTORS

Personality traits, such as perfectionism or a tendency to make too many self-imposed demands, may increase the frequency of headaches in those already predisposed to migraine. Stressful events, both good and bad, or prolonged periods of stress can have a marked effect on the migrainous sufferer. What actually constitutes stress varies tremendously from patient to patient. Simple changes in routine, changes in one's job, moving, family illness, or feuds are examples of frequently encountered stressful events. Many patients report that headaches occur after the stressful event or in the let down period.

During major crises, such as a child suffering with a critical injury or illness, there is a notable absence of attacks. When the crisis has resolved, significant headaches often occur. Surprisingly, the same patient may find that rather minor stress, such as being late or a slight disagreement, may quickly precipitate severe attacks.

Depression can be a trigger of migraine headache [27]. Many patients suppress anger and do not allow their true feelings to be expressed. This usually emanates from childhood, when controlled good behavior was necessary to gain acceptance or promote family harmony [28]. Migraineurs often rechannel their repressed hostilities into an ambitious quest for success. Continued suppression of true feelings can lead to substantial conflict and depression.

There is much disagreement over the psychological characteristics of cluster headache patients. Graham and associates [29] reported that these patients are "go-getters," Friedman and Mikropoulos [30] reported cluster patients to be ambitious, full of energy, harddriving, and sometimes with aggressive tendencies, and Steinhilber et al. [31] reported hypochondrial and hysterical tendencies. Later studies involving the Minnesota Multiphasic Personality Inventory (MMPI) by Cuypers et al. [32], Kudrow and Sutkus [33], and Androsik et al. [34], did not confirm these findings and were consistent with no psychopathological processes. My experience has been variable. However, there is no doubt that some cluster patients do demonstrate dependency needs and difficulties with suppressed anger. Whether psychological factors are involved in the precipitation of cluster headache is yet to be determined. It is my suspicion that psychological factors do play a role in those patients who experience prolonged cluster periods or whose headaches are unresponsive to medication.

A large number of cluster patients are or have been heavy cigarette smokers. Kudrow [35] reports that these patients smoked more often and smoked more cigarettes than did controls. At our center, a review of 200 consecutive cluster patients showed that 165 were smokers, 31 were exsmokers, and 4 reported no cigarette-smoking history. Most specialists agree that smoke or nicotine, in itself, does not initiate attacks. The heavy smoking may represent a personality characteristic, rather than a provoking factor.

Psychological factors do play a critical role in muscle contraction headache (tension headache). These patients often demonstrate poor coping and adaption to stressful situations. When muscle contraction headaches are frequent or daily, depression may play an important role. However, some clinicians disagree as to whether depression is a provoking factor or a result of chronic pain.

WEATHER

Weather changes seem to be obvious migraine precipitants to some sufferers. However, various studies do not support this theory. Instead, increased headaches tend to be related to the seasons, with spring and fall being the most difficult times for many sufferers.

Low barometric pressure that precedes a storm has long been associated with increased pain and illness. Severe winds throughout the world, such as the Santa Ana of Southern California, the Sharov of Israel, or the Foehn of Switzerland, are reported to cause illness and increased headache [36]. Sulman [37] believed that internal physiological changes occur as a result of high concentrations of atmospheric positive ions associated with such winds. These changes, characterized by increased serotonin levels, could be responsible for the early stages of migraine attacks.

Diamond et al. [38] studied 100 migraine patients over a 21-month period. Nine meteorologic variables were examined: fog, hours of sunshine, thunderstorms, atmospheric pressure, month of the year, change in barometric pressure, daily maximum and minimum temperatures, and deviation of mean daily temperature from normal. No statistically significant deviations were demonstrated for any of the parameters.

In two surveys, Morton [39] discovered that the prevalence of headache was increased in sufferers 48 hr before an earthquake. He postulated that these findings were due to an increased atmospheric positive ion concentration causing a decrease in serotonin levels.

ENVIRONMENT

Many headache sufferers are extremely sensitive to strong sensory stimuli and experience headache from various environmental sources. Bright lights, prolonged sun exposure, glare from water or snow, flickering lights, odors, prolonged noise, and smoke are commonly reported to be participants. Sudden weather changes or prolonged exposure to the cold or heat also seem to increase some patients susceptibility to migraine attacks. These precipitating factors tend to be more important for most patients during periods of stress or fatigue.

In general, many migraineurs adapt to change poorly. They often find it difficult to cope with unfamiliar surroundings or situations. Changes in job, school, residence, or marital status often result in major stress and subsequent headaches.

With the evergrowing popularity of computers and video display terminals (VDT), there has been speculation on their role in precipitating headaches. Some patients report frequent headaches, which they believe to be caused by VDT use. Studies have suggested that these headaches are the result of a multitude of factors [40]. These factors include monotony, job insecurity, poor lighting, visual aspects of the VDT screen, poor posture, noise, ocular problems, and stress. Most of these headaches can be classified as the muscle contraction type.

Cluster headache patients generally do not report environmental factors to be provocative. There are patients, however, who do report being more susceptible when exposed to sudden temperature changes. Episodic cluster patients often experience the onset of attacks in the spring and fall. This interesting periodicity is speculated to result from hypothalamic dysfunction [41,42].,

ALTITUDE CHANGES

Headache is a consistent and prominent symptom of "mountain or altitude sickness." Acute altitude sickness can occur in susceptible individuals exposed to altitudes higher than 8000 ft. It occurs in varying degrees and can include headache several hours after exposure, dyspnea, rapid pulse, anorexia, insomnia, mental disturbances, and pulmonary edema. The headache resembles migraine, is characterized by throbbing, and is aggravated by exertion, cough, movement, and lying down. It is presumed to be caused by relative hypoxia, with reactive vasodilatation or mild cerebral edema [43]. Inhalation of oxygen, gradual return to low altitude, cool fluids, and the cautious use of ergotamine or isometheptene can be helpful in relieving the headache.

Migraine sufferers often report the precipitation of headache while traveling by airplane. Commercial airliners are reported to be pressurized to approximately 8000 ft above sea level; however, the age and mechanical condition of the aircraft greatly affect the actual atmospheric pressure experienced by passengers.

Whether or not exposure to increased altitude with relative hypoxia is the sole precipitating cause of the migraine attack is questionable.

External environmental factors are important when traveling by air. There are substantial preflight stressors, such as traffic, crowded airports, luggage difficulties, lines, and delays. During flight, passengers are exposed to excessive flight noise and dry air, may become dehydrated, and often feel cramped. The combination of these factors and exposure to increased altitude are often enough to provoke a migraine attack in many persons. Adequate hydration, relaxation techniques, exercise and, sometimes, preflight medication, can be preventative.

At our center, in a recent blind study involving six migrainous patients who consistently experienced air travel headache, attacks were decreased equally with diazepam (Valium) 5 mg or the combination of isometheptene 65 mg, dichlorophenazone 100 mg, and acetaminophen 325 mg (Midrin), as compared with placebo (44). Each of the six patients were pretreated with the isometheptene combination for two flights, diazepam for two flights, and placebo for two flights. Pretreatment with isometheptene or diazepam prevented or improved attacks in 80% of exposures.

EXERTION

Physical exercise or exertion, such as sneezing, defecation, prolonged laughing, and sexual activity, may precipitate a migrainous attack in susceptible individuals. The headache starts within minutes of the activity and may become severe immediately or gradually progress. Location of the pain is variable, and attacks can last from minutes to hours. Headaches induced by prolonged exertion are usually longer and more severe. The headaches may be prevented by pretreatment with medication, such as indomethacin, β-blocking agents, ergotamine, or isometheptene, or by quantitative warmup before strenuous exercise [45]. Although uncommon, care should be taken with these patients to ensure that there is no organic problem causing the symptoms.

Exertion or activity does not appear to precipitate cluster headache attacks. Some patients, however, report an amelioration of attacks with rigorous physical exertion [46]. Muscle contraction headache sufferers often experience headaches shortly after strenuous physical activities, especially from those that involve stretching and extreme movements of the neck.

TRAUMA

Trauma to the head, whether trivial or severe, can precipitate headache. The headaches are usually of the muscle contraction variety and are associated with physical signs of muscle spasm. However, trauma can induce or mimic any of the nontraumatic headaches [47]. There appears to be little relationship between the severity of injury and length or severity of head pain. Whiplash injuries, in which there is no direct trauma to the head itself, can also result in post traumatic headaches.

The posttraumatic migraine has increasingly become more evident. It can be precipitated by minor or severe injury to the head [48] or to the neck [49]. However, some clinicians argue that posttraumatic migraine occurs in those individuals who were already predisposed to the migraine condition. Preexisting migraine can be made more frequent or severe by head or neck trauma.

Some clinicians suspect that head trauma can be a factor in precipitating cluster headaches in some patients. A study of 180 sufferers by Manzoni [50] showed that 41 had experienced previous head injury. Our experience has been that many patients identify the start of headaches with trauma or surgery. However, the elapsed time between the presumed precipitating event and the actual start of cluster headaches varies greatly from weeks to years. Whether trauma is a factor or is simply coincidental remains to be determined through investigative studies.

REFERENCES

1. Fothergill J, quoted by Lance JW. In: Headache: understanding and alleviation. New York: Charles Scribner's Sons, 1975:145–146.
2. Brown TR. Role of diet in etiology and treatment of migraine and other types of headache. JAMA 1921; 77:1396–1400.
3. Blau J, Diamond S. Dietary factors in migraine precipitation: the physician's view. Headache 1985; 25:184–187.
4. Van den Bergh V, Amery WK, Waelkens J. Trigger factors in migraine: a study conducted by the Belgian Migraine Society. Headache 1987; 27:191–196.
5. Diamond S, Prager J, Freitag F. Diet and Migraine. Postgrad Med 1986; 79:279–286.
6. Hanington E, Harper A. The role of tyramine in the aetiology of migraine and related studies on the cerebral and extracerebral circulation. Headache 1968; 8:84–96.
7. Diamond S, Dalessio DJ. Practicing physician's approach to headaches, 2nd ed. Baltimore: Williams & Wilkins, 1978:55.
8. Ryan RE Sr, Ryan RE Jr. Headache and head pain. St. Louis: CV Mosby, 1978:78–80.
9. Sandler M, cited by Diamond S, Prager J, Freitag FG. Diet and headache. Postgrad Med 1986; 79:279–286.
10. Krnjevic K. Chemical nature of synoptic transmission in vertebrates. Phys Rev 1974; 54:419.
11. Raskin N. Hot dog, Chinese food, ice cream and cough headaches. Consultant 1978; 32(July):40.
12. Raskin N. In: Headache 2nd ed, New York: Churchill Livingstone, 1988:234.
13. Tipton RB, Newman MD, Cohen JS, Soloman S. Aspartame as a dietary trigger of headache. Headache 1989; 29:90–92.

14. Schiffman SS, Buckley CE, Sampson HA, Massey EW, Baraniuk JN, Follett JV, Warwick ZS. Aspartame and susceptibility to headache. N Engl J Med 1987; 317:1181-1185.
15. Koehlor SM, Glaros A. The effect of aspartame on migraine headache. Headache 1988; 28:10-13.
16. Dalton K. Food intake prior to migraine attacks. Study of 2313 spontaneous attacks. Headache 1975; 15:188-193.
17. Dexter J, Byer J. The evaluation of 118 patients treated with low sucrose, frequent feeding diet. Headache 1981; 21:125.
18. Blau S, Pike D. Effects of diabetes on migraine. Lancet 1970; 2:251-253.
19. Raskin N, Knittle S. Ice cream headache and orthostatic symptoms in patients with migraine. Headache 1976; 16:22-25.
20. Harrison DP. Copper as a factor in the dietary precipitation of migraine. Headache 1986; 26:248-250.
21. Horowski R. Possible role of gonadal hormones as triggering factors in migraine. Funct Neurol 1986; 1:405-414.
22. Somerville B. The role of estradiol withdrawal in the etiology of menstrual migraine headaches. Neurology 1972; 22:355-365.
23. Linet MS, Stewart WF. Epidemiology of migraine. In: Blau JN, ed. Migraine. Baltimore: Johns Hopkins University Press, 1987:467.
24. Irez N, McAllister H, Henry S. Oral contraceptives and stroke in young women; a clinical pathological correlation. Neurology 1978; 28:1216-1219.
25. Raskin N. In Headache, 2nd ed. New York: Churchill Livingstone, 1988:55.
26. Kudrow L. The relationship of headache frequency to hormone use in migraine. Headache 1975; 15:36-40.
27. Diamond S, Diamond-Falk J. In: Advice from the Diamond headache clinic. New York: International Universities Press, 1982:89.
28. Adler C, Adler S, Packard R. In: Psychiatric aspects of headache. Baltimore: Williams & Wilkins, 1987:171.
29. Graham JR, Rogado AZ, Rahman M, Gramer IV. Some physical, physiological, and psychological characteristics of patients with cluster headaches. In: Cochraine AL, ed. Background to migraine. Third migraine symposium 1969. London: Heinemann, 1970.
30. Friedman AP, Mikropoulos HE. Cluster headache. Neurology 1969; 9:27-30.
31. Steinhilber RM, Pearson JE, Rushton JG. Some psychologic consideration of histamine cephalgia. Mayo Clin Proc 1960; 35:691-699.
32. Cuypers J, Altenkirch H, Bunge S. Personality profiles in cluster headache. Headache 1981; 21:228-229.
33. Kudrow L, Sutkus BJ. MMPI patterns specificity in 10 headache disorders. Headache 1979; 19:18-24.
34. Andrasik F, Blanchard EB, Arena JG, Teders SJ, Rodichok LD. Cross validation of the Kudrow-Sutkus MMPI classification system for diagnosing headache type. Headache 1982; 22:2-5.
35. Kudrow L, Cluster headaches. In: Blau JN, ed. Migraine. Baltimore: Johns Hopkins University Press, 1987:123.

36. Raskin N. In: Headache, 2nd ed. New York: Churchill Livingston, 1988:57.
37. Sulman FG, Serotonin-migraine in climatic heat stress, its prophylaxis, and treatment. In: Proceedings of international headache symposium, Elsinore. Headache 1971; 11:205-210.
38. Diamond S, Nursal A, Freitag FG, Gallagher RM. Effects of weather on migraine frequency. Headache 1989; 29:322.
39. Morton LL. Headaches prior to earthquakes. Int J Biometeorol 1988; 32:147-149.
40. Diamond S. Headache from video display terminals. Postgrad Med 1987; 82:184-186.
41. Medina JL, Diamond S, Fareed J. The nature of cluster headache. Headache 1975; 15:309-322.
42. Moore-Ede MC, Czeisler CA, Richardson GS. Circadian timekeeping in health and disease. N Engl J Med 1983; 309:469-479, 530-536.
43. Appenzeller O. Cerebrovascular aspects of headache. Med Clin North Am 1978; 62:474.
44. Gallagher RM. Treatment of air travel induced "altitudinal migraine;" a study of diazepam; the combination of isometheptene, dichlorophenazone and acetaminophen; and placebo. Headache 1989; 29:314.
45. Lambert R, Burnet D. Prevention of exercise induced migraine by quantitative warm-up. Headache 1985; 25:317-319.
46. Atkinson R. Physical fitness and headache. Headache 1977; 17:139-145.
47. Elkind AH. Headache and head trauma. Clin J Pain 1989; 5:77-87.
48. Bennett DR, Fuenning SI, Sullivan G, Weber J. Migraine precipitated by head trauma in athletes. Am J Sports Med 1980; 8:202-205.
49. Winston KR. Whiplash and its relationship to migraine. Headache 1987; 27:452-457.
50. Manzoni GC, Bono G, Lanfranchi M. Cluster headache—clinical findings in 180 patients. Cephalalgia 1983; 3:21-30.

5

Evaluation of the Headache Patient

R. Michael Gallagher
University Headache Center
Moorestown, New Jersey, and
University of Medicine & Dentistry of New Jersey—
School of Osteopathic Medicine
Stratford, New Jersey

INTRODUCTION

An accurate diagnosis is most essential for the effective management of patients with headaches. This is often a difficult and time-consuming task. It is not un-common for headache sufferers to be misdiagnosed and treated with medications that provide no relief. Unfortunately, no accurate diagnostic tests have been discovered that can determine headache types. The diagnosis can be established only by a careful detailed history, followed by a thorough physical examination and appropriate diagnostic tests.

In a quest to find relief, anxious or suffering patients may omit history details that they deem to be unimportant. Busy physicians who are pressed for time may sometimes attempt to make a diagnosis and treat patients without spending ade-quate time. Unfortunately, there are no "short-cuts." Headache patients require sufficient time for a complete evaluation.

HISTORY

Most physicians who have made a study of the headache problem agree that the single most important element of the patient evaluation is the history. It is important to uncover any and all information that may contribute to an understanding of the patient's problem and lead to the establishment of the headache diagnosis. Careful attention must be given to all areas, including personal, social, family, and medical aspects. The most productive time to obtain the history is when the patient is headache-free or not so incapacitated as to interfere with its completeness. This may require an additional appointment.

Headache History

Some headache patients experience more than one type of headache. The sufferers may describe only their most severe headaches and downplay or omit others. It is not unusual for a patient to misinterpret varying degrees of the same headache as completely different headaches or, conversely, different headaches as varying degrees of the same headache. Each headache type must be isolated and identified (Table 1).

Onset

The onset of headaches in one's life can give a clue to the diagnosis. Headaches that begin suddenly, for no apparent reason, in later life can be indicative of serious pathology, whereas headaches that have been occurring for many years without

Table 1 Most Common Chronic Headache Types

Related factors	Migraine	Cluster	Muscle contraction
Sex (M/F)	1:3	5:1	1:1
Onset (avg)	4–30	20–40	Any age
Location	Unilateral or bilateral	Unilateral	Bilateral, occipital, frontal
Pain character	Variable, throbbing	Lancinating, brutal	Dull, tight pressure
Prodrome	Visual aura, vague aura	None	None
Duration	Hours to days	30–90 min	Hours to months
Family history	May be present	None	Frequently present
Accompanying symptoms	Gastrointestinal, neurological	Eye injection, rhinorrhea, lacrimation	Sore neck and muscles

change are less ominous. Migraine often begins in childhood and is manifested by the second or third decade of life. Cluster headache often begins in the third or fourth decade of life. Headaches that begin during stressful life periods or events may be associated with psychogenic causes, such as depression or anxiety.

Many patients will associate the beginning of headaches with some event in their life. Any history of spinal taps, surgeries, illnesses, or accidents should be explored. Trauma to the head or neck, regardless of severity, can precipitate or contribute to a headache problem. Migrainous women will often describe headache onset with menarche, pregnancy, or use of birth control pills.

Location

It is important to ascertain where the pain or symptoms are experienced. Generalized head pain can be indicative of psychogenic headache, pain with a "hatband" or "goggle" distribution can be muscle contraction headache, unilateral pain that switches sides can be migraine. Localized unilateral pain with radiation to the jaw, ear, or base of skull is suggestive of cluster. It must always be kept in mind, however, that there are variations or atypical patterns of all headaches and that any single component of the history is only a part of the total evaluation.

Character and Severity

An accurate description of the character and severity of pain can lead to a more complete understanding of the patient's problem. Headache pain can be described as dull, aching, burning, sharp, boring, squeezing, deep, stabbing, jablike, throbbing, and so on. Pulsating or intense throbbing pain is usually of vascular origin. Cluster patients often describe pain as deep, burning, sharp, and excruciating. Muscle contraction headache patients often describe a constant "bandlike" squeezing pain that is nonincapacitating. The pain of neuralgia is often stabbing, shocklike, an intense.

Frequency and Duration

Many of the chronic syndromes, such as cluster, migraine, and muscle contractiion, are episodic with well-defined pain-free intervals between attacks. Migraine headaches occur from as seldom as several a year to as often as six to eight a month. They last from 6 to 72 hr or longer. Cluster headaches occur from one to ten times daily for periods of weeks to months with pain-free intervals of months to years in most patients. These headaches are relatively short, lasting 30–90 min. Muscle contraction headaches are quite variable and can occur three to four times weekly or only on occasion. They usually last hours to several days.

It is not uncommon for headache specialists to elicit a history of daily continuous headache for months to years. Psychogenic headaches, mixed headaches, neuralgias, and the chronic form of muscle contraction can be continuous, affording the patient little relief. Excessive use of analgesics, ergotamine, or caffeine can be associated with continuous headache. Headaches caused by an organic abnormality are often continuous and progressively worsen over time.

Associated Symptoms

A multitude of symptoms can occur in conjunction with migraine headache. Associated symptoms may include anorexia, nausea, vomiting, constipation, photophobia, alterations in fluid balance, pallor, personality changes, cold extremities, muscle tension of the neck and scalp, vertigo, tremors, diaphoresis, chills, and neurological symptoms, in the complicated form of migraine. After migraine attacks, patients may report lassitude, polyuria, diarrhea, hunger, and body aches.

Cluster headache patients usually experience one or more associated symptoms. These include ipsilateral lacrimation, eye injection, nasal congestion, rhinorrhea, facial droop, perspiration, edema of the eyelid, myosis, or facial flushing. During attacks, patients are often restless and unable to lie still, as opposed to migraineurs, who usually prefer to remain quiet.

There are relatively few associated symptoms with muscle contraction headache, compared with migraine or cluster. Sore and tight muscles of scalp, neck, and shoulder areas are common. Depressive feelings or accompanying irritability are sometimes reported.

Accompanying symptoms that are not typical of the chronic headache syndromes or for the individual being evaluated may be cause for concern. Loss of limb strength, unilateral tinnitus, gait disturbances, diplopia, or other neurological defects may be indicative of organic disease.

Prodrome

Migraine headache is often associated with prodromal symptoms. In classic migraine, the warning symptoms are well-defined and brief. In common migraine, these symptoms are not well-defined and are longer, preceding the headache by as much as 2 days.

The prodromal symptoms in classic migraine are characteristically neurological and are most often visual. The symptoms last from 20 to 40 min, just before the headache begins. Almost any type of visual disturbance may occur, but scotoma (blind spots), fortification spectra (zig-zag lines), photopsia (flashing lights), and diplopia are encountered most frequently. These prodromal symptoms disappear as the headache becomes apparent.

A small percentage of patients experience the complicated form of migraine that is characterized by more severe neurological prodromal symptoms such as slurred speech, confusion, parasthesia, or paresis. These symptoms sometimes continue throughout the headache and, occasionally, remain after the pain has ceased. It is not uncommon for these patients to have an incorrect diagnosis of a stroke or transient ischemic attack (TIA).

Table 2 Headache-Precipitating Factors

Migraine	Cluster
Foods[a]	Alcohol
Excessive sleep	Excessive smoking
Changes of routine	Histamine
Excessive sun	Muscle contraction
Fasting	Stressful situations
Trauma	Fatigue
Weather changes	Trauma
Strong odors	Prolonged unusual positions
Stressful events	
High altitude	
Loud noise	
Bright lights	
Smoke	

[a]See chapter 4.

Common migraine headache sufferers sometimes experience nonspecific prodomal symptoms. These symptoms can manifest up to 48 hr before the pain and may include changes in mood, appetite, energy levels, or sense of well-being. Many sufferers are unaware of these prodromal symptoms, which are often apparent to family members and friends. Writers, artists, and professionals who suffer with common migraine headache, sometimes feel that their most productive work is accomplished during the days preceding an attack.

Precipitating Factors

Certain factors can play a role in the precipitation of headache (Table 2). These may vary from patient to patient, but often include dietary, environmental, psychological, and pharmacological factors. The identification of precipitants can assist the physician in developing a personalized treatment plan (see Chap. 4).

Personality traits are sometimes characteristic of particular headache syndromes (Table 2). Cluster patients may tend to have difficulty dealing with hostility or rage. Muscle contraction headache patients may quickly react to stressful or difficult situations. Migraineurs are often perfectionistic, neat, creative, and resistant to change.

Hormonal Influences

Hormonal fluctuations or changes are associated with increased headache in migraine sufferers. Many sufferers experience severe attacks during menses, ovulation, or while taking supplemental estrogen or birth control pills. Migraine often improves after the third month of pregnancy or after menopause.

Previous Treatment

In some cases, medications previously taken to treat headaches can aid in establishing the diagnosis. A previous good response to ergotamine or isometheptene may indicate vascular headache. However, it should be noted that a previous failure of a medication does not necessarily exclude the headache type for which it was intended. Also, medications taken in the presence of excessive caffeine or analgesic use are often ineffective.

Family History

A review of the family history for headache in antecedent generations, siblings, and children is important. Migraine is familial. The probability that the offspring of two migrainous parents will experience the same is 70%, and it is 45% if only one parent is migrainous [1]. Depression can be familial and may be related to psychogenic or muscle relaxation headache problems. It is not clear whether or not there is a familial link in cluster headache.

Medical History

A general medical history, with system review, should be elicited to determine if any contributing or precipitating medical factors are involved in the patient's headache problem. The possibility of a serious abnormality, such as subdural hematoma, aneurysm, or tumor, must be kept in mind. Previous injuries to the head (trivial or severe), injuries to the neck, arthritis, spinal anesthesia or diagnostic tap, seizures, serious infections, head surgery, severe hypertension, or cancer with possible metastasis can be crucial to the evaluator.

Treatment for concomitant medical conditions could have a bearing on headaches and possibly influence the subsequent treatment plan. Cardiac, renal, or hepatic compromise may significantly limit the medications that can be utilized in treatment.

PHYSICAL EXAMINATION

Headache suffereres, as a whole, enjoy good physical health and rarely exhibit abnormal findings. Nonetheless, the physical examination is extremely important because it will signal any pathologic abnormality, help with the diagnosis, aid in the selection of treatment modality, and establish a baseline such that any future effects of medication may be determined. The thorough examination must include *all* systems and structures, with special attention to the neurological, vascular, and musculoskeletal systems.

Sometimes overlooked during examination is the head. Careful inspection may show the "leonine" facies of cluster, with coarse facial skin (peau d'orange) and deep nasolabial folds [2], or the saddened facies of depression. Palpation may reveal tenderness, masses, evidence of infection or sinusitis, hardened temporal arteries, temporomandibular dysfunction, or trigger points of tic douloureux. Auscultation may reveal the presence of bruits.

The musculoskeletal system can contribute much to the overall evaluation of a patient. Not only can it aid in diagnosis, but it may give clues to precipitating or contributing factors, such as anxiety or tension. Frequently encountered in muscle contraction headache sufferers are significant spasm, tissue changes, and restricted ranges of motion of the cervical and upper thoracic regions. In some cases, migraine sufferers will display dramatic musculoskeletal signs during acute headache and return to the normal state shortly after the attack.

The neurological examination is critical because abnormalities can be obvious or subtle and easily overlooked. It should be thorough and include cerebellar function, the cranial nerves, motor function, sensory discrimination, reflexes, and cognitive abilities. Ophthalmoscopic evaluation of the eye, with direct view of neural and vascular structures, can provide important information. The examiner can determine not only evidence of neurological disease, but also of systemic disease, such as diabetes, malignant hypertension, or inflammatory conditions.

The cardiovascular and peripheral vascular systems are important in determining a treatment program. Many of the medicaments utilized in the treatment of headache affect the heart or vascular systems. Tricyclic antidepressants, β-blockers, calcium channel blockers, or vasoconstrictors can affect the heart rate, rhythm, or function. Methysergide should not be used in the presence of valvular heart disease or impaired peripheral pulses because it can cause a fibrosis with prolonged use. Ergotamine, a vasoconstrictor, should not be used in those patients with peripheral vascular insufficiency.

DIAGNOSTIC TESTING

In the patient with rather typical migriane, cluster, or muscle contraction headache, or a history of long duration, and in the absence of changes in the head pain pattern or abnormal physical findings, little is needed in the way of diagnostic testing. However, should a patient's history reveal an atypical headache pattern, changes in the headache pattern, or abnormal physical findings suggestive of a more serious problem, diagnostic studies and possible consultation should be sought quickly.

Some chronic sufferers may have undergone significant diagnostic workups in a search to resolve or make sense of their headache problem. The timeliness of these tests such as electroencephalogram (EEG), computed tomography (CT), magnetic resonance imaging (MRI), or x-rays is important in determining whether or not it is necessary to repeat these studies. In the absence of physical abnormalities and changes in headache character or pattern, repeat testing is usually not necessary.

Laboratory Studies

Routine laboratory studies to include complete blood count (CBC), urinalysis (UA), and blood chemistry profile can be helpful in determining systemic illness or complications from previous therapy. In addition, these tests can be helpful in monitoring possible future ill effects of prescribed medications. Diagnostically, the sedimentation rate and serum prolactin level can be useful. The sedimentation rate is usually rapid (> 50) with temporal arteritis, and the serum prolactin level may be elevated with pituitary tumors.

Imaging Studies

The skull x-ray is utilized infrequently since the coming of CT and MRI scans. Nonetheless, in some patients, this type of study can be helpful in the diagnosis of pituitary tumor, metastatic disease, fractures, or intracranial calcifications.

Computed tomography enables the clinician to view detailed cross-sectional images of the brain and other structures of the head. It is particularly useful in determining tumor, subdural hematoma, hydrocephalus, cerebral edema, and severe sinus disease. The CT scan can be done in patients with recent onset or changes in headache, or when a central nervous system lesion is suspected.

Magnetic resonance imaging is an excellent, noninvasive diagnostic test that exposes the patient to no radiation. It is the preferred imaging study by many clinicians because of its superior clarity. An MRI study is particularly useful in the examination of soft tissue of the brain and spinal cord. Brain tumors, pituitary adenomas, vascular insults, demyelinizing plaques, and herniated disks are readily visualized. Patients with cardiac pacemakers or surgical clips from previous neurosurgery should not undergo MRI because of the strong magnetic fields involved.

Electroencephalogram

The value of the EEG in the evaluation of the chronic headache patient is unclear and often the subject of considerable debate. However, it is recommended whenever the history is suggestive of seizures. The EEG can be considered in those patients who have been refractory to usual therapy. Anticonvulsant medications, on occasion, have been effective in refractory patients whose EEGs have shown abnormalities [3-5].

Lumbar Puncture

When specifically indicated, the lumbar puncture can provide useful information. It is usually done when there is strong suspicion of intracranial infection, hemorrhage, or psuedotumor cerebri. This procedure is not without risk and is not considered a routine test for headache evaluation.

REFERENCES

1. Diamond S, Dalessio DJ. Taking a headache history. In: Diamond S, Dalessio DJ, eds. The practicing physician's approach to headache, 4th ed. Baltimore: Williams & Wilkins, 1986:11–26.
2. Graham JR. Cluster headache. Headache 1972; 11:175–185.
3. Jay GW. Migraine and epilepsy. Keeping current in treatment of headache 1983; 2(4):3–11.
4. Rapoport AM, Sheftell FD, Gordon B. Successful treatment of migraine with anticonvulsant medication in patients with abnormal EEG. Headache 1989; 29:309.
5. Jay GW. Epilepsy, migraine, and EEG abnormalities in children: a review and hypothesis. Headache 1982; 22:110–114.

6

Rationale of Headache Therapy

Arthur H. Elkind
Elkind Headache Center
Mt. Vernon, New York and
New York Medical College
Valhalla, New York

INTRODUCTION

During the past 30 years, there have been considerable advances in our understanding of headache mechanisms and therapy. Some advances in headache therapy have come about as a consequence of progress in understanding the pathophysiology of head pain, and others have been related to developments in neuropharmacology and vascular pharmacology.

Some drugs available today were first introduced only in the early 1960s, and several classes of drugs were not available for use at that time. The range of medications available today is extensive and offers the primary care physician, as well as the specialist, numerous avenues of approach to headache therapy. Several newer classes of drugs are quite specific, and if the therapist focuses treatment on the appropriate diagnostic category, the chance of success is good. An appropriate cliche would be "to tailor the treatment to the disorder."

Treatment must relate to a specific diagnosis or, at times, to a combination of headache diagnoses. Patients often self-treat, particularly in muscle contraction or tension headaches. Over-the-counter drugs are consumed in enormous quantities by the public. The headaches treated are frequently of the tension type, although lay individuals may designate them sinus headache or use other inappropriate terms. Migraine attacks also are treated with over-the-counter drugs, but if the treatment is unsuccessful or the symptoms disturbing, the patient will often visit the physician. The physician must then select one of several treatment approaches.

The state-of-the-art approach to the patient in the late 1980s is to formulate an impression of the diagnosis or multiple diagnoses. A correct diagnosis can be formulated only by a detailed medical and personal history. Questioning should be directed toward specifics of the sufferer's headaches, to determine headache frequency and duration, constancy, accompanying symptoms, effects of the sufferer's life-style, onset, and contributing factors of the headaches. Complicating illness or conditions can preclude certain effective drugs. An example of this would be ergotamine administration in individuals with arterial or venous vascular disease. If headaches are preventable by avoiding certain activities or substances that trigger an attack, the therapy would be aimed at avoiding such situations. Details of substances that are ingested that can act as migraine precipitants may be pertinent [1], as well as any additional triggers that can be determined [2]. In effort-induced headache, the prescriber may suggest administration of a drug before beginning the activity, in an attempt to prevent the attack [3]. The rationale of therapy is to prevent headache attacks and associated symptoms. The physician must also be confident that the treatment will not harm the individual.

Pregnancy is occasionally associated with severe and frequent headaches, although most migraineurs experience fewer attacks during the second and third trimesters of pregnancy. In pregnant women, therapy should be selected, if definitely necessary, that will have the least adverse effects of mother and fetus [4,5]. Biofeedback and other behavior modification techniques are nonpharmacologic forms of treatment. They may be effective in migraine, tension, and mixed headaches, and permit the avoidance of drugs in pregnancy for the acute attack. Pharmacologic treatment is best avoided during pregnancy.

HEADACHE AND SYSTEMIC DISEASE

Headaches that are associated with systemic disease often require treatment of a symptomatic nature because of the severity of the pain. Therapy must also be directed at the primary disorder for several reasons. The primary disease may be serious enough to warrant continuous and prophylactic treatment. Usually, the headaches are secondary and, with resolution of the primary disorder, the headaches will improve. Hypertension comes to mind as a common medical problem with serious sequelae if left untreated or insufficiently treated. The headaches usually promptly resolve with the appropriately effective treatment. The pharmacologic armamentarium is extensive and highly effective in treating hypertension. Several drugs are available that are effective in migraine and hypertension. The use of β-adrenergic-blocking agents, either selective, such as metoprolol, or nonselective, such as propranolol, would be desirable for treatment in patients with hypertension and migraine. Temporal arteritis or giant cell arteritis of the temporal arteries is another systemic disorder in the elderly for which treatment is mandatory for the primary disorder, and the head pain will resolve shortly after institution of treatment [6,7]. Treatment should be instituted promptly to prevent blindness.

Emergency treatment or urgent treatment is necessary at times in hypertension with headaches to prevent intracerebral injury. Pheochromocytoma may present with headache, as well as other symptoms, including tachycardia, tremor, sweating, and warrants urgent treatment.

STATUS MIGRAINOSUS

Severe intractable migraine, also known as status migrainosus, may require emergency treatment to prevent dehydration if vomiting is protracted and overuse of ergot-type drugs has occurred. The severe distress accompanying status migrainosus warrants emergency treatment, and the hopelessness of the patient is only one of the reasons besides the fluid loss and overuse of drug [8]. The latter problem is serious, at times, and patients may be dependent on narcotics, ergot, and sedatives, such as barbiturates, or on tranquilizers, such as benzodiazepines. Occasionally, chronic daily headache may be associated with significant depression. Patients are desperate with exhausting use of medications and no response. The use of monamine oxidase (MAO) inhibitors at such times may be extremely helpful in returning the individual to a more normal life-style. The physician can interrupt the downward spiral by halting the use of numerous ineffective dependency-producing agents. Use of MAO inhibitors in such circumstances can be most helpful, but they require careful administration to compliant individuals.

PATIENT/PHYSICIAN INTERACTION IN THERAPY

The disorder to which the headaches are related should be explained to the patient if it is a systemic or structural disorder. In migraine, tension, or mixed headaches (features of muscle contraction and migraine) the physician should also explain a planned therapy and the rationale for its use. Frequency, severity, length of attack, accompanying symptoms, all have a role in the plan of treatment, and the patient should play an active role in this treatment. Explanations, in lay terms, of mechanisms of drug action and the physician's goals in management may be helpful. A proper understanding on the part of the patient will increase compliance in medication use as well as the use of nonpharmacologic modalities.

Physicians often have negative feelings in treating patients with chronic headache disorders, particularly those in whom symptoms persist in spite of attempts at treatment. Chronic headache patients often require a sympathetic, understanding approach by the physician. The plan of therapy should include a gradual introduction of medications. An accepted phase of headache management is the substitution of additional medications if they cause side effects or if they prove ineffective. Occasional patients may require repeated trials with different drugs, both for acute and prophylactic management, before a satisfactory response is obtained. Despite reports of success in the medical and lay literature, individual patients will often fail to respond. A change in class of drug utilized, adding a combination of drugs, varying the dose, or adding a nonpharmacologic technique may suddenly produce a gratifying response in a previously refractory patient.

During the recent decade, with the advent of potent vasoactive compounds in treating migraine, the physician's ability to attenuate migraine attacks has increased, and use of these agents has become more readily accepted. Interestingly, the exact mechanism of action in preventing migraine may not be as it was thought to be. The β-adrenergic class of compounds and the calcium entry blockers may be active in reducing migraine frequency for reasons other than their reported and accepted pharmacologic action.

ACUTE VERSUS PROPHYLACTIC THERAPY

Acute Therapy

Often, patients present with occasional severe migraine attacks, and the physician must decide if acute or prophylactic therapy (also known as interval therapy) is indicated. A useful guide is the patient's own inclination to daily use of medication and the likelihood of compliance. If the symptoms warrant preventive therapy, it is the preferable course. However, some patients will refuse daily preventive drug usage, and acute therapy for their severe attacks may be necessary. When patients are first seen, it is sometimes difficult to estimate their headache frequency an intensity. It may be helpful to start these patients on some form of abortive therapy until a clearer picture can be obtained of their headache freqency (Table 1). Abortive therapy should depend on the rapidity with which relief must be obtained. Migrainous individuals will require prompt-acting or rapidly absorbed agents, whereas tension headache sufferers may respond to slower-acting drugs and the oral drug route. The route of administration will often be determined by the migraine sufferers ability to take oral medication, or is there a need for parenteral or rectal administration because of nausea and vomiting, which suggests poor gastric absorption through the oral route. Inhalation and sublingual administration is also available for patients requiring ergotamine tartrate, but unable to utilize the oral route. The degree of success with ergotamine agents

Table 1 Rationale of Abortive Therapy

Migraine
  Modify or alleviate the headache and associated symptoms
  Individual agent [e.g., ergotamine tartrate or dihydroergotamine mesylate)
  Combination agents for preventing associated symptoms such as nausea (e.g., NSAID
    and metaclopramide)
  Avoid drug overuse; if it occurs more than twice a month consider prophylaxis

Tension headache
  Analgesic for pain relief
  Short-acting barbiturate for relief of anxiety and associated muscle contraction
  Keep the frequency to two attacks or less per week

Systemic or structural diseases
  Treat the primary disorder
  Consider analgesic use

is variable by the inhalation and sublingual routes of administration. Unfortunately, many patients with migraine and gastrointestinal symptoms are never given effective migraine medications and sometimes are given tension headache medications with obvious less-than-satisfactory results. The use of agents that affect gastric emptying, such as metaclopramide, and permit rapid absorption of an effective agent can make a dramatic difference to the migraine sufferer. The use of rectal suppositories, which are not dependent on gastric emptying, can make a great difference for the migraine sufferer.

Many patients with an occasional migraine attack, although it may be severe and accompanied by gastrointestinal and visual symptoms, may respond satisfactorily to an appropriate abortive medication. If attacks occur once a month or fewer, abortive therapy is indicated. If episodes occur twice a month, with prompt resolution of symptoms with treatment without adverse effects, prophylactic therapy would not be indicated. Attacks occurring more often than twice a month, or if a less-than-satisfactory response is realized from abortive medication, preventive therapy should be considered.

Many other forms of acute headache, including the headache after head trauma, warrant symptomatic treatment. The goal is to reduce the intensity and length of pain and to use clinical judgment in the necessity for prophylactic therapy. As the patient begins to use abortive therapy more often, particularly with barbiturates, ergotamine, or narcotic agents, consider prophylaxis. A limit should be set on the number of tablets or capsules of any preparation containing butalbital, ergotamine tartrate, or narcotic-containing agents. If the number of units exceeds 8 or 10/week, consider initiating another mode of therapy, particularly a prophylactic drug or combination of agents.

Prophylactic Therapy

Migraine

Prophylactic therapy in migraine is indicated when the frequency of attacks is greater than two or three a month (Table 2). Also, it is preferred when the migrainous attacks are extremely severe and incapacitate the patient. Many afflicted individuals are unable to work or continue their usual activities. Patients at times anticipate their next headache and limit their personal and family activities. Prophylactic agents used in these instances may be helpful in reducing the severity, frequency, and duration of attacks.

Visual and neurological symptoms may be frightening and disabling to the patient. In these cases, prophylactic therapy is indicated. Reassurance to the patient may improve his or her well-being and actually reduce headache occurrence.

Some patients with migraine find that the usually effective abortive compounds, such as ergot or isometheptene, produce unacceptable side effects or may be contraindicated. In these instances, prophylactic treatment is indicated.

Menstrual Headaches

Headaches related to the menstrual cycle, including the muscle contraction and migraine types, may benefit from a combined abortive regimen and short-term

Table 2 Rationale of Prophylactic Therapy

Migraine
  Indicated if frequency exceeds two or three attacks a month
  Disorder is disabling and disrupts life-style of the individual at a frequency of one attack per month or if premonitory symptoms are alarming
  The use of appropriate and effective abortive agents is contraindicated or cannot be tolerated because of side effets
  Abortive agents are not effective or the use of parenteral agents is required for relief; headache onset is too rapid for effective abortive therapy

Menstrual migraine
  Consider preventive therapy starting before the onset of menses with a prophylactic drug and continue until the menstruation is over

Tension headache or mixed headache
  Prophylactic therapy indicated if analgesics are used more than two days a week
  Abortive therapy is ineffective
  Depression is present with increasing frequency of headaches
  Tendency to drug abuse, includes analgesics, barbiturates, and narcotics

Cluster headache
  Abortive therapy should be attempted including high concentration oxygen therapy
  Prophylaxis is usually necessary because of abrupt headache onset

propylactic therapy. Patients can be given medications several days before the onset of menses and continuing through the menses on a daily preventive basis. Some of the effective medications include nonsteroidal anti-inflammatory agents, β-blockers, and vasoconstrictors. Many individuals are severely disabled by these attacks and anticipate a monthly bout with extreme distress. A backup abortive medication is usually necessary for headaches that do occur. Response to medication can vary from patient to patient and, often, trials with several different compounds are necessary. An occasional patient on a continuous prophylactic regimen will find an exacerbation of headaches at the time of or near the menses. Increase in dosage of their prophylactic regimen at such times may prevent the reappearance of headache.

Muscle Contraction or Tension Headache

One would use similar guidelines for the treatment of muscle contraction or tension headache when intermittent. When attacks are frequent or disabling, preventive therapy is warranted. Abortive therapy may be added for those attacks that do occur. The excessive use of analgesics would suggest the use of preventive therapy, although the pain may have been controlled.

Several recent reports have suggested frequent analgesic use in headache patients may be associated with a tendency to a chronic daily headache [9,10]. However, the use of chronic analgesics for other disorders, such as in arthritis, is not associated with chronic daily headache [11]. The headache therapist should direct attention to interrupting the individual's frequent drug use of analgesics. Nonpharmacologic means including biofeedback, other behavior modification techniques, psychotherapy, and diet therapy are at times helpful. Inpatient hospital treatment may be necessary to assist those who are subject to significant drug withdrawal. Pharmacologic therapy often will include agents used for headache prevention, and a noticeable decrease in headache attacks may be observed.

Daily Headache

Chronic daily headache or daily mixed headaches warrant prophylactic treatment. The daily use of analgesics must be avoided as habituation, tolerance, and possible analgesic rebound headaches can occur. At times, hospitalization may be helpful in interrupting continuous headache, permitting a period of concentrated therapy of both drug and nondrug therapies. The removal of the suffering patient from their stressful surroundings and close observation by the physician can ensure patient compliance and provide often-needed reassurance. The use of different drug combinations that may affect vital signs, heart rate, and equilibrium may be best started in a hospital environment. Prophylactic management may warrant classes of drugs, such as MAO inhibitors or various combinations of β-adrenergic blockers, calcium entry blockers, antidepressants, phenothiazines, or nonsteroidal anti-inflammatory agents.

Cluster Headache

Cluster headache, usually severe and with a rapid onset of pain, warrants abortive therapy. Unfortunately, attacks are relatively short-lived (15–45 min) and often occur nocturnally. Abortive therapy plays a relatively minor role, because the headache usually resolves before effective blood levels of a drug are reached. In most cases of cluster headache, prophylactic therapy is necessary.

CONCLUSION

Physicians treating many headache patients are often impressed by the disruptive effects of the headache disorder on the individual's life-style. Their spouses, families, coworkers, and friends are often aware of the headaches' effect. The ability to work, engage in social and community activities is frequently disturbed. Patients will often withdraw, perhaps leading to feelings of guilt, depression, and hostility turned inward. The net effect is an exaggerated response to the headache and an even greater need for effective therapy. Prompt intervention by the physician with the use of all the pharmacologic and nonpharmacologic means available are often necessary to return the patient to a productive and pain-free state. Early treatment in many instances will interrupt the downward progression of many headache sufferers, before the disorder has progressed to a chronic daily problem. Some patients with intermittent headache may progress after several years to a constant headache disorder. Individuals with recurrent migraine also may progress to a chronic headache.

The approval of propranolol HCl by the Food and Drug Administration (FDA) for the treatment of common migraine headache has been noteworthy in altering the natural history of frequently occurring migraine. Propranolol has been shown not only to be effective, but has an acceptable side effect profile. Since 1978, other agents have been introduced, such as calcium entry blockers and potent nonsteroidal anti-inflammatory agents, which increase our selection of acceptable agents for headache treatment. Drug combinations that may include the older tricyclic antidepressants as well as nonpharmacologic techniques, such as behavior modification, diet, and short-term psychotherapy, contribute to an overall feeling of optimism in the treatment of headache patients.

The rationale in treating headache patients is prevention, whenever possible, and the relief or modification of symptoms of those attacks that do occur. The physician's interest in the patient with expressions of understanding in conjunction with the skillful use of the various treatment modalities often will produce an improved life for headache sufferers.

REFERENCES

1. Kohlenberg RJ. Tyramine sensitivity in dietary migraine: a critical review. Headache 1982; 22:30–34.
2. Elkind AH. Provoking influences of migraine: the controversies. In: Saper JR, ed. Controversies and clinical variants of migraine. New York: Pergamon Press, 1987:87–96.
3. Mathew NT. Indomethacin responsive headache syndromes. Headache 1981; 21:147–150.
4. Dalessio DJ. Classification and treatment of headache during pregnancy. Clin Neuropharmacol 1986; 9:121–131.
5. Rayburn WF, Lavin JP Jr. Drug prescribing for chronic medical disorders during pregnancy: an overview. Am J Obstet Gynecol 1986; 155:565–569.
6. Healey LA, Wilske KR. The systemic manifestations of temporal arteritis. New York: Grune & Stratton, 1978.
7. Rosenfeld SI, Kosmorsky GS, Klingele TG Burde RM, Cohn EM. Treatment of temporal arteritis with ocular involvement. Am J Med 1986; 80:143–145.
8. Couch JR, Diamond S. Status migrainosus causative and therapeutic aspects. Headache 1983; 23:94–101.
9. Granella F, Farina S, Malferrari G, Manzoni GC. Drug abuse in chronic headache: a clinico-epidemiologic study. Cephalalgia 1987; 7:15–19.
10. Kudrow L. Paradoxical effects of frequent analgesic use. Adv Neurol 1982; 33:335–241.
11. Does analgesic abuse cause headaches de novo? [letter to Editor]. Headache 1988; 28:61.

7

Prophylactic Treatment of Migraine

R. Michael Gallagher
University Headache Center
Moorestown, New Jersey, and
University of Medicine & Dentistry of New Jersey—
School of Osteopathic Medicine
Stratford, New Jersey

John Stirling Meyer, Makoto Ichijo and Masahiro Kobari
Veterans Administration Medical Center
and Baylor College of Medicine
Houston, Texas

Jamshid Lofti
Baylor College of Medicine,
and St. Luke's Episcopal Hospital
Houston, Texas

F. Clifford Rose and P. T. G. Davies
Princess Margaret Migraine Clinic
Charing Cross Hospital
London, England

Glen D. Solomon
Cleveland Clinic Foundation
Cleveland, Ohio, and
Pennsylvania State University College of Medicine
Hershey, Pennsylvania

INTRODUCTION

Migraine is a common disorder. Between 10 and 15% of the United States population suffer from migraine headaches sometime in their life [1–3]. This type of headache usually is not associated with demonstrable structural disease of the brain. In a series of 725 consecutive patients referred to a London headache clinic with

65

a diagnosis of migraine, only 16 had a more serious cause for their headache, such a brain tumor or ateriovenous malformation [2]. Although the vast majority of migraine sufferers never seek professional care for their headaches, migraine remains a common reason to seek medical advice and treatment.

First, and primary, in the treatment of the headache patient is the demonstration of concern and support for their chronic condition. It is not only crucial that the physician conduct an in-depth patient interview relative to the types of headache, precipitating factors, and previous therapies, but also to explore the social and emotional consequences that the headaches have had on the patient's life. It is valuable to understand why the patient has chosen this particular time to seek medical care and to review previous experiences with headache practitioners, both satisfactory and unsatisfactory. This should enable the physician to tailor therapy to the patient's specific needs.

Most headache patients seek reassurance from their physician. Patients with head pain, especially when accompanied by neurological symptoms, are frequently concerned about brain tumors or aneurysms. A careful physical and neurological examination, and often radiographic-imaging studies and laboratory evaluation, are required to allay these fears. These demonstrations of concern, support, and reassurance may be largely responsible for the placebo response rate that approaches 40% in many studies of headache therapies.

NONPHARMACOLOGIC MIGRAINE PROPHYLAXIS

Before pharmacologic therapy is instituted, nonpharmacologic measures should be taken to reduce migraine trigger factors. Counseling should include recommendations in the areas of diet, sleep patterns, and medication use. Additionally, patients habituated to daily analgesics containing caffeine, butalbital, narcotics, or benzodiazepines, generally will not respond to prophylactic therapy until the habituation ends and drug withdrawal is completed. This may require hospitalization for detoxification.

Elimination of foods and beverages with vasoactive qualities may reduce the frequency of migraine attacks. About one-quarter of patients believe their attacks are provoked by eating certain foods [4]. Many headache specialists recommend avoidance of alcoholic beverages, particularly red wines, aged cheeses, chocolate, peanuts, large amounts of monosodium glutamate (MSG), and foods rich in nitrates or nitrites (hot dogs, luncheon meals) [5]. The limitation of caffeine consumption to two or three beverages daily may reduce the risk of caffeine rebound headaches. The role of the artificial sweetener aspartame as a trigger for migraine is controversial. Two studies [6,7] of aspartame as a precipitant of migraine have had conflicting results, leading to the advice that patients who believe their headaches are precipitated or worsened by aspartame should avoid its ingestion, whereas most migraine sufferers do not need to avoid this sugar substitute. The role of foods in provoking migraine is controversial, with some studies supporting [8] the value of elimination diets and others [9] showing limited benefits.

Hypoglycemic states are often characterized by headache, and small drops in blood glucose levels can trigger migraine in susceptible persons [10]. The eating of meals on a regular schedule and avoiding prolonged fasting (skipping meals or sleeping late) may reduce the frequency of migraine attacks. The addition to the diet of high-protein foods and complex carbohydrates may prevent large fluctuations in blood sugar.

Changes in sleep patterns, including oversleeping, undersleeping, or napping, can trigger migraine. Excessive sleep may induce relative hypoglycemia and precipitate headaches. Therefore, regular sleeping patterns are suggested.

Certain medications, including oral contraceptives [11], estrogens [12], and vasodilators [13], can precipitate migraine. In addition, oral contraceptives may increase the risk of stroke in the migraine patient [14]. When possible, oral contraceptives are discontinued and estrogens are eliminated, or prescribed at a low dose in an uninterrupted regimen. The potential risk of uterine cancer should be considered whenever uninterrupted estrogens are prescribed, and regular gynecological evaluation is required.

An additional nonpharmacologic therapy for migraine is biofeedback, with use of both thermal training (hand warming) and muscle relaxation techniques. Sargent and associates [15] reported improvement in about two-thirds of 62 migraine patients with this technique. Biofeedback is particularly useful in young patients, pregnant or lactating women, and in patients who fear medications or cannot tolerate drug therapy.

PHARMACOLOGIC MIGRAINE PROPHYLAXIS

Advances in the prophylactic treatment of migraine have, until recently, come largely by chance and trial and error. Because knowledge of the pathophysiology of migraine is too rudimentary to enable a truly rational approach to drug development, it is upon the knowledge of the properties of effective drug treatments that recent ideas concerning the pharmacology of migraine have been founded. These drugs have not only improved our ability to prevent migraine attacks, but have allowed further hypotheses about the mechanisms involved in migraine.

The pharmacologic treatment of migraine may be either prophylactic or symptomatic (abortive). The decision to use daily medications as prevention should be based upon the frequency of attacks, ability to tolerate symptomatic medications, effectiveness of symptomatic medications and, most importantly, the effects of migraine on the quality of life of the patient. Although some experts suggest that patients with two or more migraines each month should receive prophylactic therapy, some patients with less frequent attacks may benefit from preventive therapy if migraine leads to frequent absence from work or interruption of family life. Also, some patients with more frequent attacks, who respond promptly to abortive drugs, can be spared the expense and potential side effects of daily medication.

Saper [16] lists five guidelines for the use of prophylactic medications, rather than symptomatic treatment. These include (a) migraine frequency of more than one to two headaches each week, (2) medical contraindications for symptomatic therapies, (c) failure of symptomatic therapies, (d) occurrence of attacks with predictable regularity (i.e., menstrual migraine), and (e) known substance abuse tendencies.

For the prophylaxis of migraine, several therapies are available, including antiserotonin–antihistaminic agents, β-blockers, calcium channel blockers, antidepressants, anticonvulsants, and nonsteroidal anti-inflammatory drugs [10]. Several newer drug therapies are in development or testing, with promising early results, including angiotensin converting enzyme (ACE) inhibitors, 5-HT$_1$-like receptor agonists, estrogen and antiestrogen drugs, alprazolam, methyl donors, and opiate antagonists.

β-Adrenoceptor Antagonists in the Treatment of Migraine

In 1948, Ahlquist first introduced the classification of adrenoceptors into α and β. α-Adrenoceptor stimulation produces mainly excitatory effects (e.g., vasoconstriction), whereas that of the β-adrenoceptor is mainly inhibition (e.g., vasodilatation). These two major groups have since been subdivided into α_1, α_2, and β_1, β_2. β_1-Adrenoceptors bind epinephrine and norepinephrine with approximately equal affinities, whereas β_2-adrenoceptors bind epinephrine with an approximately 30-fold greater affinity than it does norepinephrine. β-Adrenoceptors are widely distributed throughout the body, β_1 occurring primarily in the heart and adipose tissue, β_2 in the smooth muscle of bronchioles and arterioles. They are present also on neurons and blood vessels in the central nervous system, the highest β_1-adrenoceptor concentrations being in the pineal gland, cerebral cortex, and striatum, whereas β_2-adrenoceptors are present in low concentrations in many areas of the brain. Little is known of central β-adrenoceptor function.

Drugs that competitively antagonize the action of catecholamines and other agonists at β-adrenoceptors form the large family commonly known as β-blockers. Propranolol (Inderal) was the first β-blocker to be used in clinical medicine. Given its ability to attenuate sympathetic stimulation, propranolol was initially used for the treatment of angina pectoris, when it was found serendipitously to have migraine prophylactic properties. Since then, many new β-blockers have been synthesized, developed, evaluated, and marketed, but only some possess migraine prophylaxis ability, and their pharmacologic differences may be of clinical relevance. As a group they may be considered first-line agents for migraine prophylaxis, with individual choice depending upon clinical requirements. Propranolol remains the best-studied and most widely used member of this group for migraine prophylaxis but, for clinical and theoretical reasons, newer compounds are beginning to replace it.

Mechanism of Action

Despite much research, there is, as yet, no answer to how certain β-blockers prevent migraine. This is perhaps not surprising, considering each β-blocker acts on a wide range of different tissues, has a variety of actions, that are to varying degrees different from other members of the family, and our understanding of the pathophysiology of migraine is so poor. In discussing the pharmacologic properties of those β-blockers that are effective prophylactic agents, we must consider certain clinical findings. They work in only about 70% of patients, but whether this reflects varying mechanisms for the migraine attack or different drug actions is unknown. It is not possible to predict who will respond to this treatment, and both common and classic migraine appear to be equally responsive. Beneficial action may take time to become apparent and outlasts the period of drug treatment. Propranolol and metoprolol have active metabolites, whereas atenolol and pindolol do not.

Action at the β-Adrenoceptor. Two observations make it most unlikely that β-blockade per se is the mode of action in migraine prophylaxis. Firstly, potent β-blockers that possess intrinsic sympathomimetic activity (ISA) do not appear to be effective, and second the non–β-blocking dextro isomer of propranolol appears, from one small trial, to be as effective as the racemic mixture available commercially. The fact that cardioselective drugs appear to be as effective as nonselective drugs suggests that β_2-receptor blockade is unimportant for efficacy in migraine prophylaxis. It will be of interest to know whether β_2-selective agents are effective in migraine prophylaxis; if β-adrenoceptor blockade is not an essential property for migraine prophylaxis: this new approach offers a promising line for drug development.

Pure antagonists at β-adrenoceptors are much more likely to increase receptor numbers than are partial agonists (those with ISA) and, hence, the activity of a variety of endogenous agents acting at β-adrenoceptors may be enhanced by this "up-regulation." If this is the mode of action in migraine prophylaxis, then it could be hypothesized that migraine is related to a generalized β-adrenoceptor defect. Whether this is in the central nervous system (CNS) (see next section) or in the periphery is speculative. Up-regulation of other receptors by pure β-antagonist ("heterologous" up-regulation) is another possibility.

The presence of ISA may act adversely to counteract any possible beneficial effect that β-blockers may have in migraine prophylactic treatment [17]; and animal work has indicated that ISA may differ quantitatively and qualitatively in different β-blockers. With practolol, Wale et al. [18] showed that, in dogs, the ISA effects upon heart rate were present throughout the whole dose range studied, in contrast with pindolol, the ISA of which was manifest only at higher doses, as is oxprenolol and acebutalol, findings that support the idea [19] that all β-blockers would ameliorate migraine, if given in sufficient quantity.

Central Nervous System Action.   The central noradrenergic and adrenergic
pathways arise from nuclei in the midbrain, pons (locus coeruleus), and medulla,
and project, in a widely diverging manner, to most parts of the limbic system
and to almost all areas of the cerebral (neo) cortex. Experimental evidence suggests that activation of this system leads to an enhanced responsiveness in those
systems that handle higher functions, whereas serotonergic transmission
counteracts this response [20]. In this setting, an interplay between (nor) adrenergic
and serotonergic systems could cause migraine as a result of an imbalance in these
systems. The imbalance could be rectified through receptor up-regulation or
through an effect on serotonin receptors upon which some β-blockers work through
their antianxiety action, since anxiolytic drugs, such as diazepam, are not regarded
as effective migraine prophylactic agents. A reduction in CNS sympathetic outflow
could be considered a theoretical mode of action, but there is little evidence that
β-blockers do inhibit sympathetic outflow. No clues come from lipid solubility,
as levels of β-blockers in human brain and in cerebral spinal fluid (CSF) do not
relate to migraine prophylactic efficacy. Cruickshank and Neil-Dwyer [21] showed
that CSF levels, after long-term dosing, were higher for water-soluble atenolol
than for lipophilic propranolol, whereas brain concentrations were 10–20 times
less. Furthermore, plasma levels of effective β-blockers do not relate to individual
responsiveness.

Vascular Action.   It is not known precisely what the respective roles of α-,
β-, and β_2-receptors are in the various regions of the cranial vasculature, or
whether this is disturbed in migraine. β-Blockade may reduce vasodilatation and,
if this is important in the symptomatology of migraine, be expected to reduce
the headache. Xenon-133 cerebral blood flow studies have shown that propranolol
does not alter cerebral blood flow.
To what extent the presence of ISA would influence vascular behavior is
uncertain and, hence, little can be concluded about a vascular basis for migraine
from a consideration of ISA.

Platelet Action.   According to the platelet theory of migraine, drugs that
inhibit platelet activity would be expected to be of benefit in the prophylaxis of
migraine. Propranolol inhibits platelet aggregation and adhesion. Uptake of
serotonin into platelets is reduced and release from platelets has also been reported
to be reduced. These effects are thought to be possibly related to membrane-
stabilizing action and to involve interference with calcium mobilization in the
platelet, but any effect β-blockers have on platelet behavior may be of little
relevance to migraine.

Membrane Stabilizing Activity. (Local Anesthetic Effect, "Quinidinelike"
Action).   Membrane stabilizing activity (MSA) is probably not clinically relevant, since it is only expressed at plasma levels 50- to 100-fold higher than that

necessary to effect optimal β-blockade. There is no relation between β-blockers possessing MSA and migraine prophylaxis.

Serotonin Antagonism.   Although little is known about the function of CNS β-receptors, and the effects of antagonists at these receptors, there is more extensive evidence that some β-blockers interact with central serotonin (5-HT) receptors [22]. Microiontophoretic application of $(-)$-, but not $(+)$-propranolol rapidly and reversibly blocked the suppressant effects of the 5-HT_{1a}-selective agonists ipsapirone (BAY q 7821) and 8-hydroxy-2-(di-n-propylamino)tetralin (8-OH-DPAT) on the firing rate of the serotonergic dorsal raphe neurons [23]. However, clinical responsiveness does not appear to correlate with interaction at 5-HT_1 or 5-HT_2 receptors [24,25]. Furthermore, atenolol has no action at 5-HT receptors.

Despite intense investigation there appears to be no single property of β-blockers that explains their mode of action. Perhaps a combination of properties is required or else some other unknown actions. It is some consolation that after over 20 years of use in the treatment of hypertension, it is still not known whether they act in this condition centrally or peripherally.

β-Blockers in Migraine Prophylaxis

The choice of β-blocker selection in the treatment of migraine lies with atenolol (Tenormin), metoprolol (Lopressor), nadolol (Corgard), propranolol (Inderal),* or timolol (Blocadren)† (Table 1). All lack partial agonist activity (intrinsic sympathomimetic activity; ISA). The clinically important properties that vary among these compounds are (a) cardioselectivity (β_1-selectivity) and (b) lipid solubility, since this determines CNS penetration and, hence, CNS side effects. The pharmacologic differences between the β-blockers have led to differences in absolute contraindications, and a given agent may cause fewer side effects in certain patients. Because, in individual patients, use of an inappropriate β-blocker can have important clinical implications, careful choice of a β-blocker allows the clinician to optimize therapy.

Cardioselectivity may be an important consideration in obstructive airway disease, in conditions affecting peripheral blood flow, and in exercise tolerance. When β_2-blockade is clearly undesirable, selective β_1-blockers may be safer in low doses.

In patients with asthma or obstructive pulmonary disease, β_2-receptors must remain available to mediate adrenergic bronchodilatation. In such patients, β_1-selective drugs in low doses have been shown to cause a lower frequency of

*Propranolol is approved by the Federal Drug Administration (FDA) in the United States for the prevention of common migraine headache.
†Timolol is approved by the Federal Drug Administration (FDA) in the United States for the prevention of migraine headache.

Table 1 β-Blockers In Migraine Prophylaxis

Generic name	Trade name	Daily dosage (mg)	Cardioselectivity
Atenolol	Tenomin	50–100	Yes
Metroprolol	Lopressor, Betolac	50–200	Yes
Nadolol	Corgard	40–160	No
Propranolol	Inderal[a]; Inderal LA	80–320	No
Timolol	Blocadren[b]	10–60	No

[a]Approved by FDA in the United States for common migraine.
[b]Approved by FDA in the United States for migraine.

side effects than similar doses of a nonselective drug [26]. Even β_1-selective agents must be used cautiously if there is a history of obstructive airways disease because these agents are only relatively selective and will have effects on the β_2-receptor, particularly at higher doses. Because β_2-receptors mediate dilation of arterioles, selective β_1-blockers are less likely to impair peripheral blood flow, important when peripheral blood flow is compromised (e.g., Raynaud's syndrome, a condition associated with an increased prevalence of migraine [27]. A selective β_1-agent may show advantages in terms of less impairment of exercise tolerance. In untrained individuals, β-blockers have little effect on exercise tolerance, but in trained subjects, exercise tolerance is affected more by unselective than by selective β-blockers, perhaps because of β_2-blocking effects upon muscle glycolytic processes and, possibly, upon blood glucose and potassium levels during exercise [28].

Migraine is associated with enhanced platelet activity and, in some patients, is a risk factor for stroke. Platelet activation generates platelet aggregates and leads to the release of vasoconstricting agents, such as serotonin and thromboxanes. Therefore, it has been suggested that agents that reduce, or at least fail to promote, platelet activation should be preferred for migraine prophylaxis [29]. Human platelet β-adrenoceptors are mainly of the β_2-subtype, and their blockade would be expected to release aggregation mediated by platelet α_2-receptors. Nonselective β-blockade not only increases platelet aggregability, but also decreases fibrinolytic activity compared with the β_1-selective blocker metoprolol [20]. Atenolol and metoprolol are cardioselective, whereas nadolol, propranolol, and timolol are not.

β-Blockers may produce a variety of CNS side effects, such as drowsiness, fatigue, lethargy, sleep disorders, nightmares, depressive moods, and hallucinations. In general, these side effects are related to the lipid solubility of the β-blockers, those with lipid solubility having the most effect [30]. The distribution coefficients of β-blockers between n-octanol and buffer were good predictors of brain concentrations after long-term oral dosing, but not of CSF concentration.

Atenolol is the least lipid-soluble, metoprolol is less lipid-soluble than propranolol, but more so than atenolol.

Clinical Trial of β-Blockers

Propranolol Versus Placebo.   In 1972, Weber and Reinmuth carried out the first controlled trial of propranolol (80 mg/day) against placebo in 19 patients [31] and found that 79% responded better to propranolol than to placebo. Since then, many other trials of propranolol versus placebo have been undertaken. Efficacy has varied in these trials from 55 to 84%, with doses ranging from 80 to 240 mg/day. In 1982, Diamond et al [32] described a single-blind, placebo-controlled trial with propranolol (80–160 mg/day) and found that 72% of 245 patients responded to propranolol with no decline in drug efficacy in 80 patients who remained on propranolol therapy for at least 6 months. Following cessation of propranolol therapy, 40% of patients found that the benefit continued so that their headaches did not rebound to prior treatment levels. Similarly, in a retrospective analysis of 1036 patients treated for migraine between 1972 and 1980, Rosen found that 84% of 865 patients treated for at least 1 year with propranolol (up to 320 mg/day) reported continuing benefit compared with 32% of 171 patients in the (probably inadequate) control group who were treated differently [33].

Other β-Blockers Versus Placebo or Propranolol.   There have been trials of many other β-blockers, but only atenolol, metoprolol, nadolol, and timolol have been shown to possess migraine prophylactic properties. From these studies, it would appear that there is perhaps little to choose among these agents in terms of efficacy in migraine prophylaxis. At β-blocking doses equivalent to those of propranolol, pindolol (Visken), alprenolol, and oxprenolol have little or no beneficial activity. Of relevance to the mechanism of action of β-blockers is one study that suggested that practolol (no longer available for routine clinical use) has migraine prophylactic properties [34].

Dosage

Individual variation in requirements mean that low doses, which may be effective in some migraine sufferers, will be taken in many without benefit. Therefore, it is reasonable to start with a moderate dose, so that efficacy can be expected in a high percentage. Atenolol (100 mg/day), metoprolol (100 mg/day), nadolol (40 mg/day), propranolol (80 mg/day), and timolol (10 mg/day) could be starting doses. Only atenolol and nadolol may be given once daily; there are convenient long-acting preparations of metoprolol and propranolol (Inderal LA). There is probably little to be gained by starting at smaller doses and increasing after a few days. Although benefit may be seen immediately, lack of efficacy cannot be assumed for about 2 months. At this time, if no benefit is seen, a doubling of dosage may be considered, provided the patient's cardiovascular status is satisfactory. Although a fall in pulse rate and blood pressure can be expected, absolute levels will depend, to some extent, on pretreatment levels. A pulse of fewer than 50 beats/min and systolic blood pressure less than 100 mmHg may suggest that the dosage is maximal for that patient if full β-blockade has not occurred. If the patient is fully β-blocked, then increasing the dose will obviously have no further effect on β-adrenoceptors. In the absence of both side effects and benefit, high doses may be tried within a relatively short time. If benefit is then apparent, reduction in dosage may then be made. For propranolol, nonresponders on a high dose regimen may gain from the addition of amitriptyline, although the mechanism of this augmentation is unknown because amitriptyline is also an effective agent by itself.

Once maximal doses have been reached without short-term success, a desire to change to alternative prophylactic agents is almost inevitable, but there is some evidence that drug efficacy may increase progressively during prolonged therapy [25]. If efficacy is achieved, drug therapy can, in theory, be continued indefinitely. In some sufferers, 3–6 month period of treatment may be sufficient. A fall-off in efficacy can occasionally be seen over time, but this may be remedied by an increase in dosage. In the special case of menstrual migraine, treatment for a week or 2 before menstruation and, for the few days during, is worth trying. Whether an alternative β-blocker will be effective when the initial one was not is a question no study has addressed. Clinical impression is that some patients may find one type of β-blocker more effective than another.

Side Effects

As a group, β-blockers have a considerable safety margin; side effects are more common with higher doses and tend to be more frequent in the elderly, but diminish with time. The side effects that can occur with all β-blockers used in migraine prophylaxis relate to β_1-blockade. Fatigue, bradycardia, cold extremities, and postural dizziness are the principal side effects caused by β-blockers. Fatigue is probably the most common side effect of treatment with these agents, occurring in about 20% on direct questioning. It occurs with all β-blockers, is unrelated to ISA, and tends to wear off after a few weeks. It is not clear how β-blockers induce fatigue.

Coldness of extremities is probably related to diminished cardiac output. When the incidence of cold extremities, fatigue, and postural dizziness was examined against heart rate in hypertensive patients receiving long-term oral treatment with atenolol, the incidence of side effects was no higher in the low heart rate groups, with the possible exception of dizziness. Cruickshank concluded that bradycardia should rarely be a reason for stopping β-blocker therapy, even in the elderly [28].

Fortunately, migraine is uncommon during pregnancy, but occasionally some patients suffer severely, whereas others may relapse after delivery. Although migraine prophylaxis is not recommended during pregnancy, particularly during the first trimeser, β-blockers are probably less safe than pizotyline. With breast feeding, the quantity of β-blocker in the milk is unlikely to be clinically significant.

Calcium Channel Blockers in the Treatment of Migraine

Mechanism of Action

Calcium is involved in a wide variety of biological processes, including blood clotting, neuromuscular transmission, regulation of enzyme activity, bone metabolism, and cell death. Almost all of body calcium is present in bone. Less than 1% of total body calcium is in the extracellular fluid, of which 50% is ionized. In the intracellular fluid, the concentration of calcium, most of which is ionized, is about 10,000 times less than in the extracellular fluid. The cells are extremely sensitive to minute changes in intracellular calcium concentrations.

For calcium ions to enter cells, they must pass through protein molecules embedded in the lipid bilayered cell membrane. These protein molecules are the so-called pores or channels that selectively gate the passage of calcium ions. There are similar selective channels for other ions such as sodium (Na^+) and potassium (K^+). The ion channels can be opened either by changes in the membrane potential (voltage-operated channels) or by release of neurotransmitters and their subsequent interaction with receptors (receptor-dependent channels) [35].

Mechanism responsible for muscle contraction differ slightly for smooth, cardiac, and striated muscle fibers [36]. Cardiac and smooth-muscle fibers rely mainly on extracellular sources of calcium for contraction. In the skeletal muscle, the redistribution of intracellular calcium is the primary mechanism for raising concentrations of intracytoplasmic calcium. In either situation, this increase in the intracellular concentration of calcium starts a chain of events that ultimately produce contraction of muscle fibers [37]. Therefore, calcium is considered to be the messenger for exitation–contraction coupling and the final common pathway for muscle contraction. In the smooth muscle of the vessel walls, initiation of the contractile process is by action potentials involving the association of calcium with the calcium-dependent regulatory protein called calmodulin [38]. The calcium–calmodulin complex then activates myosin light-chain kinase, which, in turn, catalyzes phosphorylation of myosin. Actin, in combination with phosphorylated myosin, brings about smooth-muscle contraction, as shown in Figure 1. Likewise, the entry of calcium into nerve cells influences their functional activity.

Several pharmacologic agents are available that are capable of limiting or blocking the passage of calcium through cellular membrane channels. These

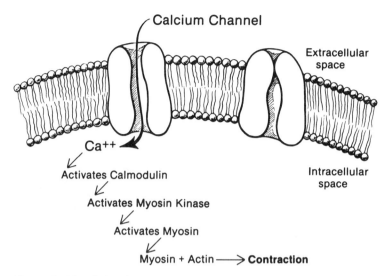

Figure 1 The chain of events from the entry of calcium through the calcium channel from the extracellular space to the activation of smooth-muscle contraction.

drugs are called *calcium antagonists* or *calcium channel* (or *calcium entry*) *blockers*. Each cell membrane has several different calcium channels that may be selectively altered by calcium channel blockers [39]. Because the cellular entry of calcium initiates contraction of vascular smooth muscle, calcium channel blockers exert both antispasmodic and slight vasodilator actions [40].

The calcium channel blockers, verapamil, diltiazem, nifedipine, nimodipine, and flunarizine, have been effective in the prophylaxis of migraine (Table 2) [41].

Calcium Channel Blockers in Migraine Prophylaxis

Verapamil (Calan, Isoptin) was one of the first calcium channel blockers (CCB) to be investigated for possible benefit in the prophylaxis of migraine in the United States. This drug was first proved effective as a coronary artery vasodilator in essential or Prinzmetal's angina [42]. The coronary vasodilator action is accompanied by a fall in oxygen consumption of the heart muscle. In animal experiments, it also lowered the tone of the cerebral vessels and lowered systemic arterial pressure [43]. Verapamil also appears to inhibit arterial vasospasm, to inhibit platelet aggregation, and to block platelet serotonin release [44].

Table 2 Calcium Channel Blockers In Migraine Prophylaxis

Generic name	Trade name	Average daily dose (mg)	Frequency
Diltiazem	Cardizem	60–120	Divided
Flunarizine	Sibellium	5–10	Once or divided
Nifedipine	Procardia	10–30	Divided
Nimodipine	Nimotop	90–120	Divided
Verapamil	Calan (-SR); Isoptin (-SR)	240–480	Once (SR) or divided

Flunarizine (Sibellium), was one of the first, and most extensively, investigated calcium channel blockers reported from Europe. It appears to be less selective for blood vessels than more recent CCBs [45]. Flunarizine has a membrane-stabilizing effect and protects laboratory rats from brain hypoxia [46]. It also appears to protect against calcium overload and cell death. Apparently, it does not affect resting vascular smooth muscle and myogenic activity, but renders smooth-muscle cells less responsive to vasoconstrictor stimuli. In animal models, it has been argued by Wauquier et al. [47] that flunarizine is unique for its protection against hypoxic-induced brain damage. Because brain hypoxia and ischemia probably play a part in the pathogenesis of migraine, such a protective effect is important.

Nifedipine (Procardia, Adalat) and nimodipine (Nimotop) have also been evaluated for their prophylaxis of migraine. Experiments on canine basilar and femoral arteries [48] have shown that nifedipine is a sensitive inhibitor of contraction of the basilar artery (induced by serotonin, phenylephrine, and potassium), with little or no effect on the femoral artery; consequently, it has a more selective action for cerebral blood vessels. Nimodipine also shares this property.

Diltiazem (Cardizem) is a calcium channel blocker with marked antiplatelet aggregation effect. However, it is a relatively weak calcium channel-blocking agent, with poor selectivity for vascular smooth muscle [49,50].

Clinical Trials of Calcium Channel Blockers

Flunarizine. Louis, in 1981 [51], was the first to evaluate flunarizine in a double-blind, placebo-controlled parallel group study. Twenty-nine patients were treated with flunarizine (10 mg) for 3 months, and the results were compared with 29 patients receiving placebo. Migraine frequency was reduced by 57% in the flunarizine group, compared with 14% in the control group. A 2-month therapeutic delay period was observed.

In 1983, Diamond studied migraine patients taking flunarizine (10 mg/day) [52]. After a 1- to 3-month placebo stabilization period, a single-blind crossover study was begun in which 17 patients experienced a statistically significant reduction in headache frequency or severity, or both (average 53%).

Verapamil.   Solomon et al. in 1983 [53], gave verapamil in doses of 80 mg four times daily to 12 patients who showed an overall reduction in migraine frequency of 49%, whereas 8 of the 12 (67%) noted 50% or greater improvement in migraine frequency.

In 1984, Markley [54] carried out a double-blind, crossover study of the prophylactic efficacy of verapamil in patients with migraine. The number of patients was also small and only 14 out of 28 completed the study. The dose of verapamil was 80 mg three times a day, and the duration of the investigation was 4 months. It was concluded that verapamil was significantly superior to placebo in prophylaxis of chronic migraine headaches. Mean migraine frequency decreased from 6.7 migraine attacks per patient per month during placebo treatment to 3.8 migraines per patient per month in the treated group. Constipation was the only important side effect of this drug, and the headaches returned after cessation of treatment.

Nimodipine.   Nimodipine therapy was investigated by Gelmer, in 1983 [55], in a double-blind, placebo-controlled parallel design study in 60 patients, of whom 50 completed the trial. Patients had classic or common migraine and at least two to three attacks a month. The dose of nimodipine was 40 mg three times daily. The percentage improvement (69%) showed that after week 8 through week 12 of treatment, therapeutic benefits were significantly higher during nimodipine therapy than during placebo treatment ($p < 0.01$). During nimodipine treatment, headaches were less frequent and severe, and their duration was shortened.

Diltiazem.   There are few reports of diltiazem use in the prophylaxis of migraine. In a pilot study by Riopelle and McCans [56], in 1982 90 mg/day was used in 15 patients with frequent migraine attacks (more than two a week). They recorded an 86% reduction in frequency and 55% in severity.

Nifedipine.   In 1987, Jonsdottir et al. [57] studied 66 patients with different types of vascular headache treatment with nifedipine (Procardia) for a mean interval of 4.5 months (range, 1–26 months). The group treated included 13 classic migraine, 13 common migraine, 17 cluster, and 17 combined headaches. A 65% decrease in frequency and severity occurred with a total daily dosage of 30–120 mg of nifedipine. Best results were obtained in classic migraine (77%) and the least response in combined headache (41%). There was a 65% decrease in frequency of common migraine.

Verapamil, Nifedipine, Nimodipine.   Meyer et al., in 1984 [58] carried out an open trial of long-term prophylactic therapy with verapamil (240 mg/day) in 44 patients with different types of headache (classic migraine, 15; common migraine, 11; cluster, 14; and muscle contraction, 4). Results were compared with a similiar trial using the calcium channel blockers nifedipine and nimodipine. All three drugs were effective in controlling migraine and cluster, but not in muscle contraction headache.

Jonsdottier et al., in 1987 [57], reported combined long-term (5 years) results of prophylactic trials with verapamil, nimodipine, and nifedipine. One hundred eifhteen patients were treated with verapamil (160–480 mg/day) for a mean interval of 5.6 months (range: 1–28 months). The diagnostic categories in these patients were classic migraine, 25; common migraine, 26; chronic cluster, 34; and combined headaches, 33. Verapamil was efficacious in treatment of 81% of patients with common and 72% of those with classic migraine.

Nimodipine versus Flunarizine.   Busone, in 1987 [59], compared nimodipine and flunarizine treatment among 30 patients with common migraine. Nimodipine was equally effective with flunarizine in reducing the frequency of attacks.

Dosage

Dosage of the calcium channel blockers is quite variable and is dependent upon individual tolerance and cardiovascular status. Flunarizine is given 5–10 mg/day once or twice each day. Verapamil is given 80–120 mg three to four times a day or in 180–240-mg sustained-release form twice a day. Nimodipine dosage is variable, ranging from 90 to 240 mg/day divided into three or four daily doses. Nifedipine 10–20 mg is given three to four times a day.

Side Effects

The side effects of CCBs are dose-dependent and are mainly due to undesirable extensions of their calcium-blocking effects on the CNS, the smooth muscle of the heart, peripheral blood vessels, and bowel. The prevalence of side effects in various studies has been between 20 and 60%, but all of these side effects are usually transient, clinically unimportant, and seldom require dicontinuation of therapy.

The most important side effects reported with flunarizine were daytime sedation and weight gain. Mild vertigo, dry mouth, anxiety, and some nonspecific gastrointestinal symptoms were uncommon.

The most commonly reported side effects of verapamil are constipation and cardiac abnormalities, including bradycardia, hypotension, and atrioventricular conduction defects. Vascular changes, such as edema of the hands and feet, flushing, and lightheadedness, are less common. Side effects are usually mild and transient and severe enough to warrant discontinuance in few patients. Verapamil increases blood levels of digoxin and quinidine [60] and potentiates the negative ionatropic effects of β-blockers.

The frequency of side effects with nifedipine has varied among different reports. Most authorities agree that this drug has little or no effect on the atrioventricular conduction systems. Flushing, headache, tachycardia, and diarrhea are often mentioned. Other side effects include edema, skin rash, and peripheral vascular symptoms.

Nimodipine appears to be the calcium channel blocker having the fewest reported adverse effects. These are usually CNS or gastrointestinal complaints. Muscular complaints and menstrual discomfort, behavioral changes (e.g., irritability, fatigue), and light-headedness were the most frequently reported side effects.

No reliable information is available on specific side effects during the treatment with diltiazem for migraine prophylaxis. However, it shares some of the reported adverse reactions of verapamil, including a drug interaction with digoxin.

Comment

It is not certain why and how calcium channel blockers achieve these impressive results in the prophylactic treatment of migraine. It is probable that they prevent vasoconstriction at the onset of classic migraine attacks, in keeping with the vascular theory. However, it should be borne in mind that they may also block entry of calcium into nerve and glial cells, which may alter the blood–brain barrier and change the balance of neurotransmitter systems, as well as altering the behavior of the cerebral vasculature [61].

In controlled studies, efficacy of calcium channel blockers compare favorably with all the other traditional forms of antimigraine treatment. In view of individual variations in therapeutic response and the incidence of side effects, several different calcium channel blockers should be evaluated in difficult cases.

Nonsteroidal Anti-Inflammatory Drugs in the Treatment of Migraine

Platelet activity in migraineurs differs from controls, with chronic aggregation and significant increases in platelet adhesiveness during the headache phase of migraine. The aggregated platelets release vasoactive prostaglandins and serotonin [62,63]. These changes are responsible for the increased level of plasma serotonin during the headache prodome and the subsequent decrease during the headache phase. Prostaglandin E_1 causes dilatation of the external carotid arteries, whereas prostaglandin F_2 induces intracerebral vasoconstriction [64]. Nonsteroidal anti-inflammatory drugs act to inhibit inflammation through their effects on chemotaxis, phagocytosis, lysosomal enzyme release, kinin generation, and formation of prostaglandins [65].

Several nonsteroidal anti-inflammatory drugs have been reported to have prophylactic activity in migraine. Among these are aspirin [66], naproxen [65,67], ketoprofen [68], flufenamic acid [68], tolfenamic acid [70], and fenoprofen calcium [71]. Others, such as ibuprofen (Motrin, Rufin), diclofenac (Voltaren), tolmetin (Tolectin), and piroxicam (Feldene), may be of benefit to some persons.

Naproxen (Naprosyn) is a propionic acid derivative, with analgesic, anti-inflammatory, and antipyretic properties. It is completely absorbed after oral administration and achieves therapeutic serum concentrations after 20–30 min, and maximum concentration after 2 hr. Its biological half-life is 12–15 hr [72]. The sodium salt of naproxen, naproxen sodium (Anaprox), is more rapidly absorbed than naproxen, producing earlier and higher plasma levels [73]. Because of these differences, naproxen is often chosen for prophylactic use, whereas naproxen sodium has been used as both an abortive [74,75] and a prophylactic agent [65].

The usual dosage for migraine prophylaxis of naproxen is 500 mg twice daily and, for naproxen sodium, 550 mg twice daily. The usual dosage of naproxen sodium for aborting a migraine attack is 825 mg initially, followed by 275 mg in 30 min, if needed [74].

Similar to naproxen, fenoprofen calcium (Nalfon) is also a propionic acid derivative, with analgesic, anti-inflammatory, and antipyretic properties. This nonsteroidal agent has also been effective in the prophylaxis of migraine [71]. When compared with placebo, fenoprofen significantly reduced migraine frequency. Additionally, mefanamic acid (Ponstel), 250 mg twice or three times daily, is used to prevent menstrual migraine, taken three days before onset of menses and continued through menses [76].

One of the important advantages of nonsteroidal anti-inflammatory drugs is the absence of cardiovascular effects. These drugs may be used safely in patients with underlying cardiac disease, whereas β-blockers or calcium channel blockers might be contraindicated. Additionally, unlike β-blockers and some calcium channel blockers, nonsteroidal anti-inflammatory drugs to not lower blood pressure. These qualities allow this class of drugs to be used in combination with most other migraine prophylactic agents.

The most common adverse effect of the nonsteroidal anti-inflammatory drugs is gastric upset. Other side effects may include light-headedness, fatigue, and edema. Concomitant use of H_2-antagonists, such as cimetidine (Tagamet), ranitidine hydrochloride (Zantac), famotidine (Pepcid), or nizatidine (Axid), may minimize gastric irritation. Misoprostol (Cytotec), an antisecretory and mucosal-protecting agent, has prevented mucosal injury in some patients taking nonsteroidal anti-inflammatory drugs [77].

Antidepressants in the Treatment of Migraine

The antidepressants, particularly tricyclic agents such as amitriptyline, have been used in the prevention of migraine for several years (Table 3) [78]. These drugs are most useful in patients with the mixed headache syndrome or in migraine patients with depressive features. Tricyclic, tricycliclike, and monoamine oxidase inhibitor drugs [79] have been effective, with the former two groups being preferred because of the lower frequency of side effects and potentially serious

Table 3 Tricyclic and Tricycliclike Antidepressants in Migraine Prophylaxis

Generic name	Trade name	Daily average dose (mg)
Amitriptyline	Elavil; Endep	50–150, divided or at bedtime
Nortriptyline	Aventyl; Pamelor	50–150, divided or at bedtime
Imipramine	Tofranil	50–150, divided or at bedtime
Trimipramine	Surmontil	50–150, divided or at bedtime
Doxepin	Adapin; Sinequan	50–150, divided or at bedtime
Desipramine	Norpramin; Pertofane	50–150, divided or at bedtime
Protriptyline	Vivactil	10–40, divided
Amoxapine	Asendin	50–250, divided or at bedtime
Maprotiline	Ludiomil	75–225, divided or at bedtime
Trazodone	Desyrel	50–300, divided or at bedtime
Fluoxetine	Prozac	10–30, divided
Buproprion	Wellbutrin	75–300, divided

drug interactions. This group includes amitriptyline (Elavil, Endep), nortriptyline (Pamelor, Aventyl), imipramine (Tofranil), trimipramine (Surmontil), doxepin (Sinequan, Adapin), desipramine (Norpramin, Pertofrane), protriptyline (Vivactil), amoxapine (Asendin), and the tricycliclike drugs maprotyline (Ludiomil), trazodone (Desyrel), fluoxetine (Prozac), and buproprion (Wellbutrin). The efficacy of these drugs has been shown in several studies [78–80].

The mechanism of action of the antidepressants in headache is uncertain. Raskin [81] states that the cardinal abnormality of migraine is the defective modulation of serotonin (5-HT) release, with intermittently reduced synaptic serotonin levels and secondarily increased dorsal raphe neuronal-firing rates. Some of these drugs (trazodone, fluoxetine), selectively inhibit serotonin uptake in both brain and human platelets [80,82], which may mediate both platelet activation and vasomotor regulation [81]. Extended treatment with antidepressants decreases the density and changes the affinity of 5-HT_1-receptor binding and reduces the number of 5-HT_2-receptors [82]. Certain tricyclic antidepressants, such as amitriptyline, have calcium channel blocking properties [83] that may prevent vasoconstriction and cerebral hypoxemia.

The choice of tricyclic drug is dependent on the unique characteristics of each agent. Drugs such as desipramine, protriptyline, and fluoxetine are nonsedating and, therefore, are the preferred choice for patients without a sleep disorder. Additionally, fluoxetine and buproprion have minimal anticholinergic effects and may cause weight reduction. Of the sedating tricyclic drugs, trazadone has minimal anticholinergic effects and does not commonly cause weight gain. These drugs are reviewed in another chapter.

Alprazolam (Xanax), a benzodiazepine with antidepressant effects, may have efficacy in migraine headaches. Othmer and colleagues [84] reported on one patient with refractory migraine and depression who was studied in a placebo-controlled, double-blind trial with alprazolam. This patient responded to alprazolam, 5 mg/day, with complete headache relief, but had no response to placebo. Additional studies with many patients will be needed to confirm this work.

Other Drugs Used in the Migraine Prophylaxis

Methysergide

Methysergide (Sansert),* a lysergic acid derivative closely related to the ergot alkaloids, has been used in migraine prophylaxis since the work of Sicuteri [85], in 1959, and Freidman and Elkind [86] in the early 1960s. It inhibits the vasoconstrictor effects of norepinephrine [87]. Unlike LSD, methysergide has little action on the nervous system [88].

The mechanism of action of methysergide is uncertain. It may act by reducing the pain-producing effect of serotonin that has been released from platelets and absorbed to the vessel walls, by reducing the vasocontrictor activity of serotonin in small arteries, by maintaining tonic vasoconstriction of large arteries once the serotonin level has fallen, or by some unknown mode of action [87].

Lance and colleagues [89,90] state that methysergide is the most useful prophylactic agent in migraine, suppressing migraine completely in 26% of patients and giving substantive improvement to an additional 40%, at a dose of 2–6 mg/day. Side effects were reported in about 40% of patients, predominately abdominal discomfort and muscle cramps, but were usually transient.

---

*Methysergide is approved by the Federal Drug Administration in the United States for the prevention of vascular headache.

The major limitation to the use of methysergide is the potential side effect of retroperitoneal, cardiac, or pulmonary fibrosis. This is a rare side effect, with the highest reported incidence being 1% (in patients treated continuously) [91]. The fibrosis usually regresses after discontinuation of the drug, but permanent fibrotic changes have been reported [90]. To reduce the likelihood of this potentially serious side effect, methysergide should be discontinued for at least 4 weeks every 6 months [92], and patients should be evaluated by intravenous pyelography, chest x-ray, and electrocardiogram regularly during treatment. Peripheral vasoconstriction and limb claudication can occur if the daily dose exceeds 8 mg [93]. Because of the serious potential problems with this agent, the marked increase in migraine frequency during the "drug holiday," and the availability of other agents, methysergide should be used infrequently in migraine prophylaxis.

Cyproheptadine

Cyproheptadine (Periactin) has serotonin antagonist effects similar to methysergide, but it is also an active histamine H_1-antagonist. In addition, it has a weak anticholinergic activity and mild central depressant properties [88]. Although there have been few controlled trials of this drug in headache [10], it is considered to be the drug of choice in children by some clinicians. In adults, the usual dosage is 12–32 mg daily, in divided doses.

The major side effects of cyproheptadine are sedation, appetite stimulation, weight gain, dry mouth, and constipation. Because these side effects tend to be troublesome to adults, and because the drug has only modest success in this aged group, cyproheptadine is not commonly prescribed for this population.

Pizotyline

Pizotyline (Sandomigran) is a smooth-muscle serotonin receptor antagonist, similar to cyproheptadine. It has an antiamine effect against serotonin and histamine, as well as against acetylcholine, tryptamine, and catecholamines [94]. This drug is not now available in the United States. Several studies have shown the efficacy of pizotyline in migraine, with between 40% and 79% of patients reporting benefit [93]. The usual dosage is 1.5 mg/day in three divided doses. Side effects include weight gain, drowsiness, and dizziness.

Ergotamine and Dihydroergotamine

Ergotamine has long been considered the drug of choice in the abortive treatment of migraine headache. Ergotism, although rare, is a condition of peripheral vasospasm, gastrointestinal upset, and autonomic disturbances, which can occur with ergot overuse [95]. Additionally, long-term use of ergotamine is associated with fibrotic processes (retroperitoneal, pulmonary, or pericardial fibrosis) [96].

The combination of ergotamine 0.6 mg, phenobarbital 40 mg, and belladonna 0.2 mg is found in sustained-release form (Bellergal-S). It can reduce the frequency and duration of attacks in some individuals [97]. Drowsiness, lightheadedness, and dry mouth are the most commonly reported side effects. The usual ergotamine precautions should be taken, and it should not be used in the presence of elevated temperature or active infection. Rebound headaches can occur upon withdrawal of the drug.

Oral dihydroergotamine was evaluated by Newman and colleagues [98]. In a study of 40 patients, 5 mg twice daily was administered. Attack frequency fell from 3.3 attacks a month to 1.3 attacks a month with active drug, but only to 3.0 attacks a month with placebo (p < 0.001). Ninety-five percent of patients noted some improvement with dihydroergotamine therapy. No side effects were reported with this study. Currently, in the United States, dihydroergotamine is available only in injectable form (DHE-45).

Clonidine

Clonidine chloride (Catapres, Dixarit), a widely used antihypertensive drug, has been used extensively in Europe for migraine prophylaxis. Reduced frequency and severity of attacks, especially in patients sensitive to tyramine, were oberved in 25–65% of patients, depending upon the methods and lengths of follow-up [34]. Several double-blind studies have failed to show significant benefit, and its use in the United States remains in question [93].

Dosage is quite variable. In Europe doses ranging from 75 to 150 μg/day. In the United States 0.1 mg is the smallest dosage available and 0.1–0.2 mg/day is generally used. Clonidine is tolerated well by most individuals. The most commonly reported side effects include fatigue, nausea, and vertigo.

Angiotensin-Converting Enzyme Inhibitors

A new class of antihypertensive drugs, the angiotensin-converting enzyme (ACE) inhibitors, may also have value in migraine prophylaxis. Captopril (Capoten) has been reported to inhibit the enzyme enkephalinase, thereby blocking the breakdown of the naturally occurring opiate, enkephalin. Opiates inhibit the release of substance P from primary sensory neurons. Substance P induces vasodilatation, plasma extravasation, nasal and conjunctival congestion, and may take part in the nociceptive transmission within the trigeminal system.

Although there are no large studies of ACE inhibitors in migraine, preliminary experience with these drugs is encouraging. Minervini et al. [99] studied 12 patients with both classic migraine and endogenous depression. After treatment with captopril, 50 mg three times daily, all 12 patients had over 50% improvement in migraine index, 8 were headache-free, and 9 had significant attenuation of depressive symptoms. The only side effect reported was hypotension. Sicuteri

[100] evaluated 35 patients in an uncontrolled trial and found that 23 of 35 patients (11 with hypertension and migraine) had significant benefit.

Anticonvulsant Drugs

Because of a slightly higher incidence of seizure disorders in the migraine population compared with the general population, anticonvulsant agents have been advocated in the management of migraine. Carbamazepine (Tegretol) was more effective than placebo in one trial of 48 patients with classic migraine [101] but this work could not be substantiated by Anthony and Lance [102]. Most authors [10,87,93] find no use for anticonvulsants for the prophylaxis of migraine in the adult population. However, some clinicians argue that phenytoin (Dilantin) is useful in the treatment of selected patients.

Estrogens and Estrogen Antagonists

Menstrual migraine remains one of the most refractory to treatment of all headaches. The physiological withdrawal of estrogens during the premenstrual phase has been suggested as the precipitating event leading to migraine [103]. Eighteen women with menstrual migraine and regular menstrual cycles were treated with percutaneous estradiol, 1.5 mg/day, for 7 days each month, started 48 hr before the expected onset of migraine [104]. When compared with placebo, menstrual attacks occurred significantly less often (31% of cycles versus 96% of cycles), and those that did occur were milder and shorter in duration. Only one patient developed a migraine after stopping the estradiol, but a few patients noted amenorrhea or changes in cycle duration. This report contrasts with the poor results seen with oral estrogen therapy [11].

Tamoxifen (Nolvadex), an antiestrogen, may also be effective for some women with migraine. Powles [105] reported on six women whose migraines were significantly improved while they were taking tamoxifen, 20 mg daily. All of these patients were taking tamoxifen for benign mammary dysplasia. In three patients, who discontinued tamoxifen, the headaches recurred within a few weeks. This work needs to be confirmed by a placebo-controlled study before tamoxifen is considered as a primary therapy for migraine.

5-HT$_1$-Like Receptor Agonists

Serotonin (5-HT) is thought to play a key role in the pathophysiology of migraine [81]. The platelet content of serotonin diminishes during a migraine attack, and the excretion of the main breakdown product of serotonin, 5-hydroxyindoleacetic acid (5-HIAA) increases during an attack. Additionally, a serotonin-releasing factor is present in the plasma during a migraine, but not at other times [106]. Medications that block the reuptake of serotonin (i.e., tricyclic antidepressants) and others that act on the 5-HT$_2$-receptor (i.e., methysergide, pizotyline) are effective in the prophylaxis of migraine. A new compound under studied, sumatriptan, is a

5-HT$_1$ agonist reported to alleviate the pain and nausea of migraine with parenteral or oral use. Although early data suggest that this drug may become a useful abortive agent, data on prophylactic use are lacking.

Opiate Antagonists

Naltrexone (Trexan), a long-acting oral congener of naloxone, was reported to yield marked improvement in two patients with postconcussional syndrome marked by severe headache, blackouts, and amnesia [107]. Although this paper did not describe the headaches in detail, many patients report the onset of migraine after head trauma. Naloxone (Narcan) may offer an additional treatment option for the refractory, posttraumatic headache sufferer.

Calcitonin

A comparatively recent report from Italy [108] found that salmon calcitonin, in a daily dosage of 100 units intramuscularly, was more effective than placebo in reducing migraine frequency, intensity, and duration. Although this work needs to be confirmed in larger studies, it offers the possibility of a new modality of treatment. The problem of daily intramuscular injections may eventually be overcome by the development of intranasal calcitonin products [109].

Methyl Donors

The role of serotonin in migraine has been discussed previously. S-Adenosylmethionine (SAM) is a methyl donor that acts as a cosubstrate in the metabolism of serotonin and norepinephrine. SAM activates cerebral serotonin turnover and causes an increase in 5-HIAA concentrations in CF and plasma. In an Italian pilot study [110], 124 patients were treated with a 2-hr intravenous infusion of 400 mg of SAM every morning for 30 days. The headache index was reduced significantly ($p < 0.01$), as was the use of pain relievers. The daily use of an intravenous prophylactic agent makes this therapy untenable at present; however, if oral dosage forms become available, methyl donor therapy may have value.

Fish Oil

Omega-3 fatty acids in high doses can inhibit prostaglandin synthesis and reduce platelet serotonin release [111]. Glueck and colleagues [111] studied 15 migraine patients in a double-blind, placebo-controlled trial of omega-3 fatty acid (max EPA), 15 g/day. They reported a statistically significant improvement in headache intensity, but they did not report on headache frequency. Because this work was published only in abstract form, it is difficult to evaluate the overall efficacy of this treatment. Because the dosing of fish oil requires 15 capsules/day, this therapy remains both expensive and impractical.

Conclusion

In reviewing the various therapies available for the prophylaxis of migraine, two points should always be considered: placebo effect and direct comparison of therapies. Placebo effect is well known in most studies of migraine drugs. Couch [112] found that more than 50% improvement in headache parameters was reported by 10–36% of patients. He also noted that during a 4-week placebo trial, 35% of patients reported a 75% improvement, 28% reported 50–74% improvement, and only 20% noted no improvement or worsening. This suggests that initial physician contact is beneficial for most patients, regardless of the therapy initiated. It is also suggested that physician counseling on nonpharmacological therapy, such as diet and sleep modification, is beneficial.

While there are several prophylactic agents that have been shown superior to placebo in multiple clinical trials, no one agent has been proven superior to the other drugs in direct clinical trials. There are no published guidelines to determine the "correct" prophylactic drug for a given patient. The physician must individualize therapy based on a number of patient characteristics—concomitant illness, other medications, blood pressure, evidence of depression or sleep disorder, and prior medication experiences.

Patients with migraine and concomitant hypertension will benefit from treatment with a β-blocker, calcium channel blocker, or ACE-inhibitor, while those patients with low blood pressure readings may be better candidates for therapy with nonsteroidal anti-inflammatory drugs [13]. Patients with concomitant depression should not be given beta blockers but should benefit from antidepressants or ACE-inhibitors [13]. Drug interactions may be particularly dangerous in patients taking monoamine oxidase inhibitors, but should be considered with any patient taking multiple medications.

Because of the large amount of clinical experience with β-blockers, these drugs are generally considered the first-line prophylactic drugs. Calcium channel blockers, particularly varapamil in the United States and flunarizine and nimodipine in Europe, are widely regarded as useful alternatives to the beta blockers. These drugs would be selected in patients who either had contraindications to beta blockers, were intolerant of beta blocker side effects, or who failed to respond to therapy with beta blockers. The nonsteroidal anti-inflammatory drugs are valuable, either as first-line therapy or in combination with a β-blocker or calcium channel blocker for difficult-to-manage patients. Although there are no studies to determine whether combinations of agents are more effective than single-agent therapy, combination therapy is often applied in clinical practice. The antidepressants are frequently chosen for patients with the mixed headache syndrome or for patients with both migraine and depression or sleep disorder. The antiserotonin drug methysergide, although clearly one of the most effective prophylactic agents, is generally selected for patients in whom all other therapies have failed, because of the risk of serious adverse effects. Additional experience is needed with drugs such as the angiotensin-converting enzyme inhibitors and calcitonin to determine their role in migraine prophylaxis.

In conclusion, migraine is both a common and often difficult-to-treat illness. With the proper combination of nonpharmacologic, abortive, and prophylactic therapies, most patients will have a beneficial response.

REFERENCES

1. Waters WE, O'Connor PJ. The epidemiology of migraine. Boehringer Ingelheim, Bracknell: Berks, 1975.
2. Lance JW. Mechanism and management of headache, 4th ed. London: Butterworth, 1982:130.
3. Bruyn GW. Epidemiology of migraine: "a personal view." Headache 1983; 23:127–133.
4. Selby G, Lance JW. Observations on 500 cases of migraine and allied vascular headache. J Neurol Neurosurg Psychiatry, 1960; 23:23.
5. Diamond S, Dalessio DJ. Migraine headache. In: Diamond S, Dalessio DJ, eds. The practicing physician's approach to headache, 4th ed. Baltimore: Williams & Wilkins, 1986:44–65.
6. Schiffman S, Buckley CE, Sampson HA, Massey EW, Baraniuk JN, Follett JV, Warwick ZS. Aspartame and susceptibility to headache. N Engl J Med 1987; 317:1181–1185.
7. Koehler SM, Glaros A. The effect of aspartame on migraine headache. Headache 1988; 28:10–13.
8. Monro J, Brostoff J, Carini C, Zilkha K. Food allergy in migraine: study of food allergy and RAST. Lancet 1980; 2:1.
9. Medina JL, Diamond S. The role of diet in migraine. Headache 1978; 18:31.
10. Ziegler DK. The treatment of migraine. In: Dalessio DJ, ed. Wolff's headache and other head pain, 5th ed. New York: Oxford University Press, 1987:87–111.
11. Dennerstein L, Laby B, Burrows GD, Hyman GJ. Headache and sex hormone therapy. Headache 1978; 18:146–153.
12. Kudrow L. The relationship of headache frequency to hormonal use in migraine. Headache 1975; 15:36–40.
13. Solomon GD. Management of the headache patient with medical illness. Clin J Pain 1989; 5:95–99.
14. Collaborative Group for the Study of Stroke in Young Women. Oral contraception and increased risk of cerebral ischemia or thrombosis. N Engl J Med 1973; 288:871–878.
15. Sargent JD, Green EE, Walters ED. The use of autogenic feedback training in a pilot study of migraine and tension headaches. Headache 1972; 12:120–124.
16. Saper JR. Treatment of migraine. In: Saper JR, ed. Headache disorders. Boston: John Wright, 1983:61–87.
17. Shanks RG. In: Proceedings Astra symposium, migriane and beta-blockade, Munich. May, 1984.

18. Wale JL, Conway AJ, Reeves M. The influence of the intrinsic sympathomimetic activity of beta-adrenoceptor antagonists on haemodynamic effects in anaethetized dogs. Clin Exp Pharmacol Physiol 1979; 6:11-19.

19. Steiner TJ, Joseph R. Practical experience of beta-blockage in migraine: a personal view. Postgrad Med J 1984; 60(suppl 2):56-60.

20. Winther K. Hedman C. beta-Adrenoceptor blockade, platelets and rheologic factors. Cephalalgia 1986; 6(suppl 5):33-39.

21. Cruickshank JM, Neil-Dwyer G. Beta-blocker brain concentrations in man. Eur J Clin Pharmacol 1985; 28 (suppl):21-23.

22. Middlemiss DN. Blockade of the central 5-HT autoreceptor by beta-adrenoceptor antagonists. Eur J Clin Pharmacol 1986; 120:51-56.

23. Sprouse JS, Aghajanian GK. Propranolol blocks the inhibition of serotonergic dorsal raphe cell firing by 5-HT$_1$ selective agents. Eur J Pharmacol 1986; 128:295-298.

24. Peatfield R. Drugs and the treatment of migraine. Trends Pharmacol Sci 1988; 9:141-145.

25. Behan PO, Reid M. Propranolol in the treatment of migraine. Practitioner 1980; 224:201-204.

26. Prichard BN. Pharmacologic aspects of intrinsic sympathomimetic activity in beta-blocking drugs. Am J Cardiol 1987; 59:13F-17F.

27. Zahavi I, Chagnac A, Hering R, et al. Prevalence of Raynaud's phenomenon in patients with migraine. Arch Intern Med 1984; 144:4:742-744.

28. Crickshank JM, Prichard BN. In: beta-Blockers in clinical practice. Edinburgh: Churchill-Livingstone, 1988.

29. Joseph R, Steiner T, Schultz L, Rose CF. Platelet activity and selective beta-blockade in migraine prophylaxis: a case for preferring beta$_1$ adrenoceptor blockers. Stroke 1988; 19:704-708.

30. Koella WP. CNS-related side effects of beta-blockers with special reference to mechanisms of action. Eur J Clin Pharmacol 1985; 28:55-63.

31. Weber RB, Reinmuth OM. The treatment of migraine with propranolol. Neurology 1972; 22:366-369.

32. Diamond S, Kindrow L, Stevens J, Shapiro DB. Long-term study of propranolol in the treatment of migraine. Headache 1982; 22:268.

33. Rosen JA. Observations in the efficacy of propranolol for the prophylaxis of migraine. Ann Neurol 1983; 13:9.

34. Kallamanta T, Hakkarainen H, Hokkanen E, Tuovinen T. Clonidine in migraine prophylaxis. Headache 1977; 17:169-172.

35. Hagiwara S, Byerly L. Calcium channel. Annu Rev Neurosci 1981; 4:69-125.

36. Walsh MP. Calcium regulation of smooth muscle contraction. In: Marme D, ed. Calcium and cell physiology. Berlin: Springer-Verlag, 1985:170-203.

37. Sturek M, Hermsmeyer K. Calcium and sodium channels in spontaneously contracting vascular muscle cells. Science 1986; 233:475-478.

38. Cheung WY. Calmodulin: an overview. Fed Proc 1982; 41:2253-2257.

39. Peroukta CJ. The pharmacology of calcium channel antagonists: a novel class of anti-migraine agents? Headache 1983; 23:278-283.

40. Cauvin C, Loutzenhiser R, Van Breeman C. Mechanism of calcium antagonist induced vasodilatation. Annu Rev Pharmacol Toxicol 1983; 23:373-396.

41. Solomon GD. Comparative review of calcium channel blocking drugs in migraine. Headache 1985; 25:368-371.

42. Solberg LE, Nissen RG, Vliestra RE, Callahan A. Prinzmetal's variant angina-response to verapamil. Mayo Clin Proc 1978; 53:256-259.

43. Gaevyl MD, Pavlova LI. Effects of verapamil on the cerebral circulations. Bull Exp Biol Med 1978; 85:472-474.

44. McGoon M, Vlietstra R, Holmes D, Osborn JE. The clinical use of verapamil. Mayo Clin Proc 1982; 57:495-510.

45. Perutka SJ, Banghart SB, Allen GS. Relative potency and selectivity of calcium channel antagonists used in the treatment of migraine. Headache 1984; 24:55-58.

46. Amery WK, Wauquier A, Va Nueten JM, DeClerck F, Van Reempts JV, Janssen PAJ. The anti-migrainous pharmacology of flunarizine (R 14 950), a calcium antagonist. Drugs Exp Clin Res 1981; 7:1-10.

47. Wauquier A, Ashton D, Marronnes R. The effects of flunarizine in experimental models related to the pathogenesis study of flunarizine (Sibelium) in migraine. Headache 1981; 21:235-239.

48. Allen GS, Banghart BS. Cerebral arterial spasm: part 9. In vitro effects of nifedipine on serotonin, phenylephrine and potassium-induced contractions of canine basilar and femoral arteries. Neurosurgery 1979; 4:37-42.

49. Greenberg DA. Calcium channel antagonists and the treatment of migraine. Clin Neuropharmacol 1986; 9:311-328.

50. Greenberg DA. Calcium channel and calcium channel antagonists. Ann Neurol 1987; 21:317-330.

51. Louis P. A double-blind placebo-controlled prophylactic study of flunarizine (Sibelium R) in migraine. Headache 1981; 21:235-239.

52. Diamond S, Schenbaum H. Flunarizine, a calcium channel blocker, in the prophylactic treatment of migraine. Headache 1983; 23:39-42.

53. Solomon GD, Griffith Steel MC, Spaccavento LJ. Verapamil prophylaxis of migraine. JAMA 1983; 250:2500-2502.

54. Markley HG, Cheronis JCD, Piepho RW. Verapamil in prophylactic therapy of migraine. Neurology 1984; 34:963-976.

55. Gelmers HJ. Nimodipine, a new calcium antagonist in the prophylactic treatment of migraine. Headache 1983; 23:106-109.

56. Riopelle RJ, McCans JL. A pilot study of the calcium antagonist diltiazem in migraine syndrome prophylaxis. Can J Neurol Sci 1982; 9:269.

57. Jonsdottir M, Meyer JS, Rogers RL. Efficacy, side effects and tolerance compared during headache treatment with three different calcium blockers. Headache 1987; 27:364-369.

58. Meyer JS, Dowell R, Mathew N, Hardenburg J. Clinical and hemodynamic treatment of vascular headaches with verapamil. Headache 1984; 24:313-321.

59. Bussone G, Baldini S, D'Andrea G, Cananzi A, Frediani F, Caresia L, Milone F, Boiardi A. Nimodipine vs flunarizine in common migraine. A ocntrolled pilot trial. Headache 1987; 27:76-79.

60. Klein HO, Lang R, Weiss E, Desegni E, Libhaber C, Kapilansky E. The influence of verapamil on serum digoxin concentration. Circulation 1982; 65:998-1003.

61. Govoni S, Battaini F, Magnoni MS, Trabucchi M. Non-vascular central nervous system effects of calcium entry blockers. Cephalalgia 1985; 5(suppl 2):115–118.
62. Couch JR, Hassanein RS. Platelet aggregability in migraine. Neurology 1977; 27:843–848.
63. Deshmukh SV, Meyer JS. Cyclic changes in platelet dynamics and the pathogenesis and prophylaxis of migraine. Headache 1977; 17:101–108.
64. Simon LS, Mills JA. Non-steroidal anti-inflammatory drugs. N Engl J Med 1980; 302:1179–1185.
65. Ziegler DK, Ellis DJ. Naproxen in prophylaxis of migraine. Arch Neurol 1985; 42:582–584.
66. O'Neill BP, Mann JD. Aspirin prophylaxis in migraine. Lancet 1978; 2:1179–1181.
67. Lindegaard KF, Ovrelid L, Sjaastad O. Naproxen in the prevention of migraine attacks. A double-blind placebo-controlled crossover study. Headache 1980; 20:96–98.
68. Stensrud P, Sjaastad O. Clinical trial of a new antibradykinin, anti-inflammatory drug, ketoprofen, in migraine prophylaxis. Headache 1974; 14:96–100.
69. Vardi Y, Rabey JM, Streifler M. Migraine attacks: alleviation by an inhibitor of prostaglandin synthesis and action. Neurology 1976; 26:447–450.
70. Hakkarainen H, Vapaatolo H, Gothoni G. Tolfenamic acid is as effective as ergotamine during migraine attacks. Lancet 1979; 2:326–327.
71. Diamond S, Solomon GD, Freitag FG, Mehta N. Fenoprofen in the prophylaxis of migraine: a double-blind, placebo controlled study. Headache 1987; 27:246–249.
72. Dahl H. Naproxen (Naprosyn). Pharmacokinetics: therapeutical relevance and tolerance profile. Cephalagia 1986; 6(suppl 4):69–75.
73. Moyer S. Pharmacokinetics of naproxen sodium. Cephalalgia 1986; 6(suppl 4):78–80.
74. Sargent JD, Baumel B, Peters K, Diamond S, Saper JR, Eisner LS, Solbach P. Aborting a migraine attack: naproxen sodium vs ergotamine plus caffeine. Headache 1988; 28:263–266.
75. Johnson ES, Ratcliffe DM, Wilkinson M. Naproxen sodium in the treatment of migraine. Cephalalgia 1985; 5:5–10.
76. Diamond S, Solomon GD. Pharmacologic treatment of migraine. Rat Drug Ther 1988; 22:1–5.
77. Lanza FL, Aspinall RC, Swabb EA, Davis RE, Rack MF, Rubin A. Double-blind, placebo-controlled endoscopy comparison of mucosal protective effects of misoprostol vs cimetidine on tolmetin-induced mucosal injury to the stomach and duodenum. Gastroenterology 1988; 95:289–294.
78. Couch JR, Hassanein RS. Amitriptyline in migraine prophylaxis Arch Neurol 1979; 36:695–699.
79. Anthony M, Lance JW. Monoamine oxidase inhibition in the treatment of migraine. Arch Neurol 1969; 21:263–268.
80. Pies R. Trazodone and intractable headaches. J Clin Psychiatry 1983; 44:317.
81. Raskin NH. Pharmacology of migraine. Annu Rev Pharmacol Toxicol 1981; 21:463–478.
82. Ogren SO, Ross S, Hall H. Archer T. Biochemical and behavioural effects of antidepressant drugs. In: Burrows GD, Norman TR, Davies B, eds. Antidepressants. Amsterdam: Elsevier Scientific, 1983; 15–29.

83. Peroutka S, Allen GS. The calcium antagonist properties of cyproheptadine: implications for antimigraine action. Neurology 1984; 34:304–309.

84. Othmer SG, Othmer E, Varanka TM, Strong DM. Refractory migraine headache controlled with alprazolam: case report. J Clin Psychiatry 1985; 46:494–495.

85. Sicuteri F. Prophylactic and therapeutic properties of 1-methyl-lysergic acid butanolamide in migraine. Int Arch Allergy Appl Immunol 1959; 15:300–307.

86. Freidman AB, Elkind AH. Appraisal of methysergide in treatment of vascular headaches of migraine type. JAMA 1963; 184:125–128.

87. Lance JW. In: Mechanism and management of headache, 4th ed. London: Butterworth, 1982:178–204.

88. Douglas WW. Histamine and antihistamines; 5-hydroxytryptamine and antagonists. In: Goodman LS, Gilman A, (eds). The pharmacological basis of therapeutics, 5th ed. New York: Macmillan, 1975:622.

89. Curran DA, Hinterberger H, Lance JW. Methysergide. Res. Clin Stud Headache 1967; 1:74.

90. Curran DA, Lance JW. Clinical trial of methysergide and other preparations in the management of migraine. J Neurol Neurosurg Psychiatry 1964; 27:463.

91. Graham JR. Cardiac and pulmonary fibrosis during methysergide therapy for headache. Am J Med Sci 1967; 254:23–24.

92. Bana DS, MacNeal PS, Le Compte PM. Cardiac murmurs and endocardial fibrosis associated with methysergide therapy. Am Heart J 1974; 88:640–655.

93. Peatfield R. Headache. Berlin: Springer-Verlag, 1986:125–142.

94. Diamond S, Medina J. Newer drug therapies for headache. Postgrad Med 1980; 68:125–138.

95. Hokkanen E, Waltimo O, Kallantra T. Toxic effects of ergotamine used for migraine. Headache 1978; 18:95–98.

96. Robert M, Derbaudrenghien JP, Blampain JP, Lamy F, Meyer PH. Fibrotic processes associated with long-term ergotamine therapy. N Engl J Med 1984; 311:601.

97. Elkind A. Primary headache rx: how to pick from a growing array of drugs. Mod Med 1983; Sept:118–145.

98. Neuman M, Demarez JP, Harmey JL, Le Bastard B, Cauquil J. Prevention of migraine attacks through the use of dihydroergotamine. Int J Clin Pharmacol Res 1986; 6:11–13.

99. Minervini MG, Pinto K. Captopril relieves pain and improves mood depression in depressed patients with classical migraine. Cephalalgia 1987; 7(suppl 6):485–486.

100. Sicuteri F. Enkephalinase inhibition relieves pain syndromes of central dysnociception (migraine and related headache). Cephalalgia 1981; 1:229–232.

101. Rompel H, Bauermeister PW. Aetiology of migraine and prevention with carbamazepine (Tegretol). Results of a double-blind cross-over study. S Afr Med J 1970; 44:75–80.

102. Anthony M, Lance JW, Somerville B. A comparative trial of prindolol, clonidine, and carbamazapine in the interval therapy of migraine. Med J Aust 1972; 1:1343–1346.

103. Sommerville BW. Estrogen withdrawal migraine. 1. Duration of exposure and attempted prophylaxis by premenstrual estrogen administration. Neurology 1975; 25:239–244.

104. De Lignieres B, Vincens M, Mauvais-Jarvis P, Mas JL, Touboul PJ, Bousser MG. Prevention of menstrual migraine by percutaneous oestradiol. Br Med J 1986; 293:1540.

105. Powles TJ. Prevention of migrainous headaches by tamoxifen. Lancet 1986; 2:1344.

106. Anthony M, Hinterberger H, Lancce JW. The possible relationship of serotonin to the migraine syndrome. In: Friedman AP, ed. Res Clin Stud Headache 1969; 2:29-59.

107. Tennant FS, Wild J. Naltrexone treatment for postconcussional syndrome. Am J Psychiatry 1987; 144:813-814.

108. Gennari C, Chierichetti MS, Gonelli S, Vibelli C, Montagnani M, Piolini M. Migraine prophylaxis with salmon calcitonin: a cross-over, double-blind placebo controlled study. Headache 1986; 26:13-16.

109. Micieli G, Cavallini A, Martgnoni E, Covelli V, Facchinetti F, Nappi G. Effectiveness of salmon calcitonin nasal spray preparation in migraine treatment. Headache 1988; 28:196-200.

110. Gatto G, Caleri D, Michelacci S, Sicuteri F. Analgesizing effect of a methyl donor (S-adenosylmethionine) in migraine: an open clinical trial. Int J Clin Pharmacol Res 1986; 6:15-17.

111. Glueck CJ, McCarren T, Hitzemann R, Allen C, Hogg E, Kloss R, Thompson B, Yunker R, Gartside P, Lazkarzewski PM. Amelioration of severe migraine with omega-3 fatty acids: a double-blind, placebo-controlled trial. Am J Clin Nutr 1986; 43:710.

112. Couch JR. Placebo effect and clinical trials in migraine therapy. Neuroepidemiology 1987; 6:178-185.

8

The Abortive Treatment of Migraine

Ninan T. Mathew
Houston Headache Clinic
Veterans Administration Medical Center
Houston, Texas

INTRODUCTION

The frequency of migraine attacks vary from patient to patient. Most patients, whether taking prophylactic medication or not, will require some form of abortive treatment. *Abortive* or *symptomatic treatment* is the treatment of headaches once they have begun. The goal of this treatment is to lessen the severity and duration of attacks. In some patients, the headaches can be completely aborted, whereas in others, they are only made more tolerable.

There are many components to most migraine attacks. In addition to pain, these can include nausea, vomiting, photophobia, sonophobia, and anxiety. All of the components may require treatment. In many cases, attacks of mild to moderate intensity can be managed by sleep, antinausea agents, simple analgesics, and the application of cold to the head.

Sleep is a usual part of the natural recovery process of migraine. Patients who can sleep generally will recover faster than those who only rest or doze [1]. Most patients can sleep during an attack, but some cannot because of apprehension, anxiety, or the pain. These patients may require medication. The use of diphenhydramine (Benadryl) or a short-acting benzodiazepine will often help. Other measures include a quiet darkened room (because of sonophobia and photophobia) and the avoidance of any stimulants such as caffeine.

Sleep and rest can be impractical for some patients, especially if the attacks of migraine occur during working hours. In fact, in those patients, treatment that does not produce drowsiness is most appropriate.

Cold packs applied to the forehead or temples may relieve some symptoms in a number of patients. Lance [2], in a study using controlled application of cold and heat, found cold to be useful in 15 out of 20 patients.

DRUG THERAPY DURING ACUTE MIGRAINE ATTACKS

General

Impaired Drug Absorption

Absorption of salicylates [3], ergotamine, and tolfenamate [4] is impaired during migraine attacks. Delayed absorption is correlated with the severity of headache and gastrointestinal symptoms, rather than duration of the attack and the type of migraine. Reduced gastrointestinal motility is probably the most important mechanism for this impaired drug absorption. Barium studies performed during the past have demonstrated gastric stasis and prolonged gastric-emptying time, compared with the time in the same patients when they are headache-free [5–7]. Metoclopramide (Reglan) injected 10 min before the ingestion of aspirin normalized its absorption in patients with migraine, but not in control subjects [8]. Metoclopramide is known to accelerate gastrointestinal motility and gastric emptying in humans [9]. Several reports have shown that administration of oral metoclopramide (10 mg) together with the treatment of choice is more effective than the latter alone [4,10–12].

Timing of Abortive Medications

The importance of early treatment must be stressed in the initial discussion with each patient. Patients are reluctant to take medications before the pain becomes severe. At that stage of the migraine attack, oral medications are absorbed poorly because of the delayed gastric emptying, and the patients may be prone to take large doses of strong analgesics and narcotics without benefit. In addition, severe nausea and vomiting may make it impossible to take medications orally. The dilating extracranial arteries rapidly become rigid and resistant to vasoconstrictive agents as the attack progresses. If the migraine headache is present on awaking, drugs taken by mouth are unlikely to give substantial relief. Rectal, inhalation, or parenteral routes of administration have to be used for adequate relief.

Antiemetics

Gastrointestinal symptoms are common accompaniments of migraine attacks, occurring in almost 95% of patients [13]. In Volan's series [13], 26% had nausea only, 48% nausea and vomiting, and 21% nausea, vomiting, and diarrhea. Metoclopramide (Reglan) is the preferred antiemetic during an acute migraine attack because it is a dopamine D_2 antagonist, which promotes normal gastrointestinal activity, rather than depressing it, as phenothiazines tend to do. Metoclopramide can be administered orally or as an intramuscular injection. The antinausea effect of metaclopramide is due to its dopamine D_2-receptor blockage action, whereas the gastrokinetic effect may be due to its action through cholinergic activity at muscarinic sites, both at central and peripheral locations [14].

Metoclopramide usually is well tolerated. However, it may occasionally produce severe extrapyramidal reactions, including muscle spasms and oculogyric crises, and should be used with caution, particularly in children. These reactions occur within 36 hr of starting treatment and usually disappear within 24 hr after withdrawing the drug. All patients should be warned of the possibility of these side effects. Metoclopramide alone is ineffective as a pain reliever during migraine attacks [15].

Simple Analgesics

Aspirin, 650–1000 mg (10–15 gr), taken orally, especially with 10 mg of oral metoclopramide, may be all that is necessary to abort an attack. Aspirin [16], acetaminophen [17], codeine [18], and propoxyphene (Darvon) [19] are superior to placebo in the treatment of acute attacks of migraine. Analgesic effects of aspirin and other agents are augmented by caffeine [20]. Although aspirin is extensively used in the treatment of migraine, recent data suggest less impressive clinical response under carefully monitored conditions. Soluble aspirin was found to be "highly effective" in only 44% of 61 patients treated by Ross-Lee and associates [16]. In a double-blind, placebo-controlled study, Tfelt-Hansen and Olesen [10] found effervescent aspirin alleviated the headaches in only 37% of 94 patients. The reasons for generally less-than-satisfactory response to aspirin are due partly to the gastric stasis and impaired absorption of aspirin during the acute attack and also because the prostaglandin mechanisms are only one among a whole range of chemical mechanisms active in the pathogenesis of migraine.

Nonsteroidal Anti-Inflammatory Drugs In Treatment of Acute Migraine

In addition to the reduction or suppression of inflammatory reaction, certain nonsteroidal anti-inflammatory agents (NSAID) have been shown to have other properties, such as the central analgesic activity of ketoprofen (Orudis); platelet antiaggregant action of aspirin, tolfenamic acid, and naproxen (Naprosyn); and cerebral vasoconstrictive action of indomethacin. The analgesic property has been shown to be independent of prostaglandin inhibition [21,22]. Beneficial effect of NSAIDs in migraine may be due to more than one reason including inhibition of prostaglandin synthesis, platelet aggregation, release of serotonin from platelets, and release of bradykinin. In addition, there is a decrease in the capillary permeability and inflammatory reaction counteracting sterile inflammation. In treating acute migraine, it is essential for the drug to have high bioavailability, with an early and high peak in serum level and absence of serious side effects. In a recent review of literature, Pradalier et al. [23] showed that, in most double-blind trials, NSAIDs have been superior to placebo and equal to the reference drugs, such as ergotamine, in the treatment of acute migraine attacks. Both the severity of the attacks and duration of the attacks are beneficially affected by NSAIDs.

Naproxen

Naproxen (Naprosyn) and its sodium salt (Anaprox) are effective and safe in the treatment of acute migraine [24,25]. Naproxen is regularly and completely absorbed after oral or rectal administration, and peak plasma levels are reached 1 hr after naproxen sodium and up to 2 hr after naproxen administration [26]. Rapid absorption of naproxen sodium results in increases in its effects during headache attacks [27]. The biological half-life of naproxen is 12–15 hr. Doses for an acute attack are approximately 750–1000 mg.

Meclofenamate Sodium

The anthralinic acid derivative, tolfenamic acid, has been studied and compared with placebo and ergotamine in the treatment of acute migraine. Tolfenamic acid was reported to be better than placebo and as effective as ergotamine in the treatment of acute migraine [28]. Personally, I find a combination of 1 mg of oral ergotamine with 200 mg of meclofenamate sodium (Meclomen), which is also an anthralinic acid derivative, very effective as an abortive treatment for acute migraine. It can be repeated after 1 hr. Meclofenamate alone is as effective as naproxen sodium, but the addition of ergotamine results in significant improvement in the effectiveness.

Isometheptene Mucate

Isometheptene is a sympathomimetic agent, with vasoconstrictive properties. It is available in combination with acetaminophen 325 mg and dichloralphenazone 100 mg (Midrin, Isocom), or caffeine 100 mg and acetaminophen 325 mg (Migralam). Isometheptene is a very useful agent in the abortive treatment of mild to moderate migriane attacks [29–31]. Two capsules are taken initially at the onset of headache, followed by one capsule at 1-hr intervals until the headache is relieved or until a total of six capsules have been taken. Drowsiness and nausea are possible side effects. Midrin is contraindicated in patients with extreme hypertension, hepatic and renal disease, as well as patients taking monoamine oxidase inhibitors. It is a satisfactory, well-tolerated, and effective agent for attacks of mild to moderate severity.

Ergotamine

Fluid extracts of ergot were used for the treatment of migraine as early as the end of the 19th century. Ergotamine tartrate was isolated in 1918, and its use for migraine began in the 1920s. Since that time, this drug has remained the most consistently effective agent for the treatment of acute migraine attack.

Mode of Action

Graham and Wolff [32], in 1938, showed for the first time that intravenously administered ergotamine reduced the pulsations of the temporal and occipital arteries, with a close temporal relationship to the decline in the intensity of headache in most patients during migraine attacks. Later experiments by Saxena et al. [33] and Lance et al. [34] established the powerful and selective vasoconstrictive action of ergotamine on the external carotid arterial system. It also has a peripheral vasoconstrictive effect. The vasoconstrictive effect may be mediated partly through the α-adrenergi blockade and, to a greater degree, by the direct effect on the arterial serotonin (5-HT) receptors [35,36]. Ergotamine has no significant vasoconstrictive effect on the intracranial circulation [37] and, therefore, can be safely used in patients with classic migraine who are in the aura phase of the attack. It has been shown that the effect of ergotamine on arterial tone depends on the preexisting resistance of the vascular bed. When the vascular resistance is low, ergotamine acts as a constrictor, but when the vascular resistance is increased, it may produce vasodilatation [38]. This, in turn, will explain how ergotamine will prevent both the vasoconstrictive and vasodilatory phase of the migraine attack.

The arterial constriction caused by parenteral or rectal ergotamine in migraine usually lasts at least 24 hr [39,40]. The therapeutic half-life of ergotamine is 2.5 hr and, therefore, there is a marked discrepancy between the time of sustained peripheral vasoconstrictor activity and the plasma ergotamine concentration. The disassociation between plasma blood levels and vasoconstrictive activity is difficult to explain. By means of radioimmunoassay techniques, it has been established that metabolic breakdown of ergotamine may occur in two phases: one with a half-life of 2.5 hr and another with a half-life of 20 hr [41–43]. One of the possible explanations is that biological activity of ergotamine may be due to one or more of its metabolites, and the elimination of the half-life of metabolites conforms closely to the duration of peripheral vasoconstriction after administration.

Although constriction of cranial noncerebral blood vessels seems to be an important effect of ergotamine in terminating a migraine attack, there are other actions of egotamine that may be equally important. The closure of the cephalic arteriovenous shunts that open during the migrainous attacks, may be an important mode of action of ergotamine [44]. Wolff [45] throughout his writing, emphasized the importance of neurogenic inflammation as part of the acute migraine attack, and it was felt the vasoactive polypeptides [neurokinins) [46] played a key role in the neurogenic inflammation. Ergotamine may act by suppression of the release of these neurokinins. In fact, recently, Saito and colleagues [47] have shown that ergotamine blocked the experientially induced neurogenic inflammation in the dura mater. In summary, in migraine the noncerebral cranial vasculature is dilated and sensitized by mediators of a sterile inflammatory response. Mediators (vasoactive polypeptides, including substance P) of the sterile inflammatory response would reduce the nociceptive response. Ergotamine causes sustained vasoconstriction of these blood vessels and reduces the sterile inflammation. The vasoconstrictive response is elicited in the peripheral blood vessels also, and this is, in practice, the most undesirable side effect of ergotamine. In addition to the peripheral effects, ergotamine has significant effects on serotonin turnover in the brain [48]. Ergot alkaloids depress the firing rate of serontoninergic neurons in the brain stem raphe nucleus [49]. Imperfect correlation between the scalp arterial constriction and headache relief could probably be explained by the variety of other actions of ergotamine, including possible central serotoninergic actions.

Administration of Ergotamine

Ergotamine is currently the most effective medication available for the treatment of acute attacks of migraine. Its use is limited, to some degree, by its poor and erratic absorption [50], potential side effects, and ease of overuse, with subsequent toxicity or rebound headache phenomena [51–53]. Ergotamine is available in oral, sublingual, aerosol, and rectal suppository forms (Table 1). The general principles of administration of ergotamine are that an adequate dose should be administered, as soon as possible, and that an subnauseating dose should be found in individual patients. The sensitivity to ergotamine varies from person to person, and nausea is a common side effect. A dose that produces substantial nausea and vomiting may be too high and can actually intensify the migraine attack in some patients. The nausea-provoking effect may be centrally mediated [54]. Arterial serotonin receptors are blocked with high doses of ergotamine, resulting in vasodilatation, rather than constriction, and this will explain the paradoxic effect of aggravation of the intensity of headache with high doses of ergotamine [55,56]. Ala-Hurula et al. [57] found that ergotamine tartrate was rapidly absorbed, the half-time absorption rate being 30 min, with peak plasma concentrations being reached 2 hr after ingestion. Concentrations of ergotamine after

Table 1 Ergot Preparations

Route of administration and brand name	Composition			
	Ergot alkaloid (mg)	Caffeine (mg)	Belladonna (mg)	Barbiturate (mg)
Oral				
Caffergot	Ergotamine 1	100	0.12	Pentobarbital 30
Wigraine	Ergotamine 1	100		
Ergotrate	Ergonovine 0.2			
Bellergal-S	Ergotamine 0.6		0.2	Phenobarbital 40
Rectal				
Caffergot suppository	Ergotamine 2	100		
Wigraine suppository	Ergotamine 2	100		
Inhalation				
Medihaler	Ergotamine 0.36			
Sublingual				
Ergomar	Ergotamine 2			
Ergostat	Ergotamine 2			
Injectable				
DHE-45	Dihydroergotamine 1			

rectal administration were significantly higher than those after the oral route at all points up to 3 hr, and serum levels after a dose given by inhalation were higher than that given by mouth at most points, even though the aerosol dose was only half that given by mouth [58]. Therefore, ergotamine is most effective when given either by suppository or in aerosol form.

The rectal suppository form of ergotamine (Cafergot, Wigraine) is the preparation of choice because the absorption and the serum levels are much higher than by oral administration, which has a bioavailability of only 5%. The dose of ergotamine by suppository is 1 mg (one-half suppository) or 2 mg (whole suppository). However, some patients require only 0.5 or 0.25 mg, which requires cutting the suppository into smaller sections. Subnauseating doses can be found in individual patients by asking them to use small portions of suppository, one-fourth each, when they are headache-free and arrive at an appropriate sub-nauseating dose. Wilkinson et al. [1] analyzed a group of 310 patients, who received ergotamine suppository treatment for acute attacks of migraine, to assess the efficacy. Most patients were better after 180 min: 40% of the patients were headache-free, 51% had slight residual headaches, and 9% were slightly improved. The most important finding was that none of the patients worsened. They felt that significant factors affecting the rate and extent of recovery from the acute attack were the duration of headache before the patient came for treatment with ergotamine, the kind of medications taken before the initiation of treatment, and whether or not the patient slept. Patients who were able to sleep after ergotamine was taken were better than those who only rested or dozed [1].

There is an aerosol preparation of ergotamine (Medihaler Ergotamine), with 0.36 mg/inhalation. Each cartridge contains 50 doses and is composed of a fine powder of ergotamine. It is not in solution with the vehicle contained in the canister; therefore, patients must be instructed to shake the canister very well before each inhalation. They should first exhale completely and then direct the spray into the posterior wall of the mouth and take a complete inhalation, which should be continued to maximum capacity and held as long as possible. The breath may then be released through semiclosed lips. One to three puffs (0.36–1.08 mg) can be taken, and it has been shown that the serum levels obtained are comparable with those of subcutaneous ergotamine injections [58]. Disadvantages of aerosol inhalation are the bulkiness of the canister and difficulty on the part of some patients to follow the instructions to get an adequate inhalation.

Sublingual ergotamine (Ergomar, Ergostat) is available in an uncoated, pulverized formulation as 2-mg tablets. They are reported to be more effective than the coated tablets used orally. Sublingual preparation generates low blood levels, as only a small fraction of the medication is absorbed in 5 min [60]. Even though it has been reported to be pharmacologically active [61,62], its clinical effectiveness is not always reliable. The usual dose is one tablet (2 mg). Oral ergotamine tablets (Cafergot, Wigraine) are available in the coated form, and its bioavailability is about 5%. The recommended oral dose is 1–2 mg, the maximum amount being 8–10 mg/week to avoid ergotamine rebound phenomenon. It is better to restrict the use of ergotamine to twice a week. The oral form is most effective in patients with a clear-cut aura that appears several minutes before the headache begins.

Ergotamine in combination with phenobarbital and belladonna (Bellergal-S) can be used in the acute treatment of migraine. Its absorption is somewhat slower than other preparations, but the incidence of associated nausea is low. One tablet is taken at the onset of the headache and can be repeated in 6–8 hr (see also chaps. 7 and 10).

Ergonovine is an ergot alkaloid with a structure similar to methysergide. It is available in 0.2-mg tablets (Ergotrate) and is well tolerated by most migraineurs. Two tablets are taken at the onset of the headache and repeated in 2 hr, if necessary. It should not be used in patients with Prinzmetyl's angina, vascular insufficiency, asthma, or pregnancy (see Chap. 10).

Side Effects of Ergotamine

The vast majority of patients tolerate ergotamine well, and its benefit far outweighs the side effects and risk of possible complications. In about 5–10% of patients, there are side effects such as abdominal cramps, dizziness, muscle cramps in the thigh and calf muscles, paresthesias involving the distal extremities, and diarrhea. Less commonly, there are other side effects, including syncopal episodes and tremor. When preparations that contain caffeine are used, patients may complain of a restless feeling and palpitation for a period after ingestion. Nausea and vomiting are the most common side effects of ergotamine. Drowsiness may occur in some patients. Out of 256 patients referred to the National Poisons Information Service in London between 1977 and 1981, with signs of ergotamine poisoning, nausea and vomiting occurred in 47, drowsiness in 22, mild peripheral ischemia in 20, muscle paresis in 12, convulsions in 4, and renal impairment in 1 [63]. There was one death.

There is a wide variability in sensitivity to ergotamine from individual to individual, particularly if it is given by mouth. In a group of 25 patients taking between 7 and 60 mg of ergotamine a week, the adverse effects were not always proportional to the dose of ergotamine [58]. There are many patients who have consumed excessive amounts of ergotamine for years without any ill effects [64]. Serious side effects occur in fewer than 0.01% of patients [65]. The serious side effects can occur occasionally after relatively brief exposures to modest doses of the drug. These complications include myocardial infarction [66], renal arterial stenosis [67], cerebral infarction, cerebral arteriopathy, and cerebral atrophy [68,69]. The serious complications with the use of ergotamine occur usually in patients who use the medication daily and continuously in doses that exceed 3 mg, especially in suppository form [70].

There are certain risk factors that predispose to the development of ergotamine toxicity. These include hyperthyroidism, malnutrition, pregnancy, renal and hepatic disease, sepsis, and very importantly, preexisting coronary artery and peripheral vascular disease. It is very important to obtain a detailed history of any cardiac symptoms, especially angina or previous history of myocardial infarction, and symptoms of peripheral vascular disease. Patients who smoke heavily must be specifically evaluated to rule out coronary artery disease and peripheral vascular disease before ergotamine is prescribed. Angina pectoris or intermittent claudication of the lower extremities may occur in some patients and should be an indication to stop ergotamine. Antibiotics, such as erythromycin or troleandomycin (formerly triacetyloleandomycin) may precipitate peripheral vascular constriction when used concomitantly with ergotamine [71,72]. Overall, it is our practice to not use ergotamine when there is an intercurrent infection.

Even though convulsions are reported as a part of clinical manifestations of ergotamine toxicity, they are relatively rare [73]. The most serious complication of ergotamine intoxication is the occurrence of peripheral ischemia, resulting in gangrene and development of dementia. The peripheral ischemia effects are predominately in the lower extremities, although they can affect the upper extremities. The signs and symptoms are bilateral and symmetric and appear in the distal areas of the limbs. Initially, the problem starts out as distal paresthesia and is often intermittent, later becoming constant. Coldness of the extremities and pain on exertion of the limbs, such as walking or using the arms, become increasingly obvious. It is most important that patients who use ergotamine are warned of such symptoms and that follow-up examinations should include examination of the extremities for peripheral pulses and ischemic symptoms. Ergotamine characteristically affects the muscular arteries in the lower extremities. The vasospastic segment is usually at the lower third of the leg, with collateral circulation around it [74]. With prolonged vasospasm, intimal changes occur that result in thrombosis and subsequent ischemic gangrene. Ergotamine not only affects the peripheral blood vessels, but also mesenteric, cerebral, coronary, renal, and ophthalmic circulation [75,76]. Thrombophlebitis involving varicose veins that sometimes become painful [77], peroneal palsy [78,79], and occasional fibrotic reactions involving pleura, pericardium, and retroperitoneal areas, have been reported [80–82]. Anorectal ulcers may develop in some patients who frequently use ergotamine suppositories [83].

Dihydroergotamine

Dihydroergotamine (DHE-45) became available for use in the 1940s and was reported in several uncontrolled series to be effective in the abortive treatment of migraine headaches [84–86]. Although it is a venoconstrictor, useful in the treatment of orthostatic hypotension [87], its vasoconstrictor effect on arteries is only modest [88,89]. Other advantages of dihydroergotamine over ergotamine are that it causes less nausea and that there is very little physical dependency [90,91]. Overall, it is safer than ergotamine, although, like ergotamine, idiosyncratic reactions occur occasionally, and rare incidents of severe peripheral arterial [92] and coronary spasm [93] have been reported. Dihydroergotamine is currently available only in parenteral form. Intranasal preparations are being evaluated, with some success, but they are not now available for common use. Callaham and Raskin [90] published the results of a double-blind, crossover study of intravenous dihydroergotamine against placebo for acute migraine. Dihydroergotamine had a beneficial effect, especially when administered first. Overall, 85% of patients responded. In the same year, Raskin published another study of repetitive intravenous dihydroergotamine for intractable migraine [90], comparing it plus metoclopramide against intravenous diazepam. Dihydroergotamine was more effective; it provided more rapid and more complete pain relief, nearly always within 48 hr of hospitalization. A follow-up program with dihydroergotamine rectal suppositories or subcutaneous injections was also effective in this randomized and open study. In a recent study by Belgrade et al. [94], 64 patients with acute migraine were treated in the emergency room with dihydroergotamine, meperidine, or butorphanol. Posttreatment pain scores were lowest in the dihydroergotamine group. Eight of the 21 patients who received dihydroergotamine had greater than 90% reduction in pain, compared with 3 of 19 patients who received butorphanol, and none of 22 who received meperidine.

Peak plasma levels of dihydroergotamine are rapidly achieved after parenteral administration in an ascending order as follows: 15–45 min after subcutaneous injection [95], 30 min after intramuscular injection [96], and 2–11 min after intravenous injection [97]. Subcutaneous injection gave the lowest plasma level, being about 40% lower than that of intramuscular injection. Horton [84] recommended that if the attack has not already peaked, subcutaneous or intramuscular injection of 1 mg of dihydroergotamine will be sufficient for 90% of patients; a few may require 2 mg. It is our practice to prescribe dihydroergotamine to be given as an intramuscular injection at home as a self-injection. The great advantage of this practice is the opportunity for the patient to receive the medication early in the headache phase, without having to go to the emergency room or the physician's office to obtain injections.

The emergency room treatment of acute migraine has been revolutionized by the use of intravenous dihydroergotamine. Many cases can be managed without using narcotic analgesics. The protocol varies from center to center. It is our practice to give 10 mg of metoclorpramide intravenously slowly, followed by 0.5 mg of dihydroergotamine slowly by the same route 2–3 min. If the attack has not began to subside in 30 min, another 0.5 mg of dihydroergotamine is given, without metoclorpramide. In some centers 5 mg of prochlorperazine (Compazine) [90] or 25 mg of promethazine (Phenergan) is used preceding the first dose of dihydroergotamine intravenously. The experience of headache clinicians who use dihydroergotamine extensively is that it is an effective treatment, with minimal incidence of vasospasms, chest pain, or other reactions. This is consistent with the large experience of Raskin [98].

Other Medications Used in Acute Migraine

Chlorpromazine

As an alternative to the use of narcotic injections, chlorpromazine (Thorazine) has been tried. Intramuscular chlorpromazine was reported to be useful for acute migraine by Iserson et al. [99]. However, the relief occurred only after an average of 55 min. Lane and Ross [100] used intravenous chlorpromazine in doses of 5–50 mg and reported that in 38 out of 52 occasions, the therapy was completely effective, and the headache was relieved in 5–20 min in most patients. Mild residual headache occurred in 11 of 52 occasions, and three patients received very mild relief. The adverse effects were minimum, with most patients reporting drowsiness and 10 out of 52 reporting symptoms of hypotension. The hypotensive symptoms cleared with bed rest and a short bolus of IV fluids. They concluded that the administration of chlorpromazine intravenously was superior to alternative modes of therapy, especially narcotic medications. In some emergency departments, it is routine to give 7.5–30 mg of chlorpromazine intravenously, repeated as 7.5 mg boluses, slowly through the intravenous tube of a normal saline drip [101]. Chlorpromazine is useful, not only in relieving pain, but the anxiety and vomiting also is helped quite dramatically. The main disadvantage is the occurrence of hypotension. Because these patients are usually supine because of the severity of symptoms, hypotension seldom produces any symptoms. Clearly, it is prudent to keep all patients who have received parenteral chlorpromazine supine for 4 hr and to follow their blood pressure every 30 min throughout the interval.

Narcotics in Acute Migraine

Some clinicians feel that in many patients with migraine, parenteral narcotics are not helpful or, at best, produce only transient benefit. Also they can increase nausea and vomiting. There are theoretical considerations that support the idea that narcotic analgesics are not the most effective medications for acute migraine. One view is that because the narcotic analgesic effect may be dependent upon the integrity of serotoninergic projections from raphe nuclei [102], and that migraine may be a state characterized by depletion of central nervous system serotonin, narcotics are incapable of producing effective analgesia for acute attacks of migraine. However, it is the experience of most clinicians that at least some patients do obtain adequate relief from the pain of migraine with parenteral narcotics, provided the dose is adequate. Overall, because of the addictive potential with frequent use, we discourage the use of narcotic injections in the emergency room as the sole treatment for acute migraine. However, the careful, discriminate use of narcotics has a place in the management of acute migraine in some patients. A recent comparative study [94] of a single dose of meperidine (Demerol, Mepergan), butorphanol (Stadol), and dihydroergotamine further supports the idea that dihydroergotamine is a better choice as an injectable medicine for acute attacks of migraine.

DRUG THERAPY FOR STATUS MIGRAINOSUS

Many patients with migraine present to the emergeny room with prolonged migraine attacks lasting for 48 hr or more. At that stage, the headache is resistant to self-administered medications and produces sufficient disability or debilitation to make presentation to the hospital justifiable. They are not only in severe pain, but are often under emotional distress and suffer from nausea and vomiting, which can produce dehydration and electrolyte imbalance. These symptoms are true indications for hospitalization. Patients should be put to rest in a quiet semidarkened environment. Dehydration and electrolyte imbalance from vomiting or from profuse sweating require intravenous fluid and medication. Most patients who are admitted to the hospital with status migrainosus have already taken narcotic medications orally or parenterally, and there is no purpose in administering additional narcotics.

Dihydroergotamine

The repetitive injection of dihydroergotamine (DHE-45) intravenously every 8 hr by Raskin [91] has revolutionized the therapeutic approach to the treatment of status migrainosus. Metoclopramide is preferred to phenothiazines for suppression of nausea, because it is better tolerated than repetitively giving proclopamine or promethazine. It also suppresses the withdrawal symptoms from narcotic medications [102]. Our practice is to insert a heparin lock into an arm vein and to slowly give metoclopramide, 10 mg, intravenously, followed by 0.5 ml of DHE-45. If the patient does not become nauseated, the dose of DHE is increased to 1 ml and repeated every 8 hr. Metoclopramide need not be repeated for more than three or four doses, especially if the patient remains free of nausea. The usual practical problems are pain and swelling at the site of heparin lock, which may extend into a larger area in the arm. Occasionally, superficial phlebitis may develop as a result of repeated dihydroergotamine injections. Many patients will complain of severe pain when injections are given, and this possibility, along with swelling and redness, should be explained to the patient before the dihydroergotamine is implemented. The extrapyramidal side effects of metoclorpramide also must be explained to patients. Apart from the local discomfort and pain at the site of injection, other side effects include muscular pains, often involving the leg, and nausea. Occasionally, a patient may complain of chest pain, especially those who have undiagnosed coronary artery disease. It is a good policy to obtain a thorough history of coronary symptoms and an electrocardiogram before the dihydroergotamine is started. Most patients become headache-free over a period of 48 hr, with some showing the beneficial effect in 8–16 hr. In those, who are prone to very severe episodes of headache, prescriptions are given to use dihydroergotamine at home as a self-administered intramuscular injection. Patients who are prone to frequent episodes of severe headache and status migrainosus are candidates for prophylactic therapy. The contraindications for use of dihydroergotamine include history of angina, myocardial infarction, vascular insufficiency, pregnancy, infection, and ergot hypersensitivity.

Corticosteroids in Status Migrainosus

To terminate status migrainosus, a parenteral corticosteroid in the form of dexamethasone (Decadron) is sometimes used [104,105]. This treatment is rather empirical and probably derives from the traditional role of corticosteroids as a last resort in neurological diseases. They may exert their action by reducing inflammation of the blood vessels or by sensitizing the blood vessels to vasoconstricting effects of circulating vasoactive substances. Gallagher [106] treated 162 patients, with and without steroids, for status migrainosus in the emergency department of a large community hospital. This was a randomized comparative study of three groups of patients. Seventy-two percent of those treated with meperidine, promethazine, and dexamethasone felt more relief compared with 29% of those treated with meperidine and promethazine, and 37% of those treated with meperidine and dihydroergotamine. From this limited study, he concluded that dexamethasone is a useful agent for emergency treatment of continuous intractable migraine attacks. Some clinicians use hydrocortisone 100–200 mg every 8 hr intravenously for 24 hr. Corticosteroid treatment for longer periods should be undertaken with great care. In general, if corticosteroids have not terminated the status migrainosus in 24 hr, they are unlikely to do so later.

REFERENCES

1. Wilkinson M, Williams K, Leyton M. Observation on the treatment of an acute attack of migraine. In: Friedman A, Critchley M, eds. Research and clinical studies in headaches, vol 6. Basal: S Karger PP 1978:141–146.
2. Lance JW. The controlled application of cold and heat by a new device (Migra-Lief apparatus) in the treatment of headache. Headache 1988; 28:458–461.
3. Volans GN. Migraine and drug absorption. Clin Pharmocokinet 1978 3:313–318.
4. Tokola RA, Neuvonen PJ. Effects of migraine attack and metoclopramide on the absorption tolfenamic acid. Br J Clin Pharmacol 1984; 17:67–75.
5. Carstairs LS. Headache and gastric emptying time. Proc R Soc Med 1958; 51:790–791.
6. Kreel L. The use of metoclopramide in radiology. Postgrad Med J 1973; 49(suppl):42–45.
7. Kaufman J, Levine I. Acute gastric dilatation of the stomach during attack of migraine. Radiology 1936; 27:301–302.
8. Volans GN. The effect of metoclopramide on the absorption of effervescent aspirin in migraine. Br J Clin Pharmacol 1975; 2:57–63.
9. Albibi R, McCallum RW. Metoclopramide: pharmacology and clinical application. Ann Intern Med 1983; 98:86–95.
10. Tfelt-Hansen P, Olesen J. Effervescent metoclopramide and aspirin (Migravess) versus effervescent aspirin or placebo for migraine attacks: a double blind study. Cephalalgia 1984; 4:107–111.
11. Hakkarainen H, Allonen H. Ergotamine vs metoclopramide vs their combination in acute migraine attacks. Headache 1982; 22:10–12.
12. Ross-Lee L, Heazlewood V, Tyrer JH, Eadie MJ. Aspirin treatment of migraine attacks: plasma drug level data. Cephalalgia 1982; 2:9–14.

13. Volans GN. Absorption of effervescent aspirin during migraine. Br Med J 1974; 2:256–258.

14. Costall B, Gunning SJ, Naylor RJ. An analysis of the hypothalamic sites at which substituted benzamide drugs act to facilitate gastric emptying in the guinea-pig. Neuropharmacology 1985; 24:869–875.

15. Tfelt-Hansen P, Olesen J, Aebelholt-Krabbe A, et al. A double blind study of metoclopramide in the treatment of migraine attacks. J Neurol Neurosurg Psychiatry 1980; 43:369–371.

16. Ross-Lee L, Eadie MJ, Tyrer JH. Aspirin treatment of migraine attacks: clinical observations. Cephalalgia 1982; 2:71–76.

17. Peatfield RC, Petty RG, Rose FC. Double blind comparison of mefenamic acid and acetaminophen (paracetamol) in migraine. Cephalalgia 1983; 3:129–134.

18. Somerville VW. Treatment of migraine attacks with an analgesic combination (Mersyndol). Med J Aust 1976; 1:865–866.

19. Hakkarainen H, Gustafsson B, Stockman O. A comparative trial of ergotamine tartrate, acetyl salicylic acid and a dextropropoxyphene compound in acute migraine attacks. Headache 1978; 18:35–39.

20. Laska EM, Sunshine A, Mueller F, et al. Caffeine as an analgesic adjuvant. JAMA 1984; 251:1711–1718.

21. Berge OG. Regulation of pain sensitivity, influence of prostaglandins. Cephalalgia 1986; 6(suppl 4):21–23.

22. Abramson S, Korchak H, Ludewig R, et al. Modes of action of aspirin-like drugs. Proc Natl Acad Sci USA 1985; 82:7227–7231.

23. Pradalier A, Clapin A, Dry J. Treatment review: non-steriodal anti-inflammatory drugs in the treatment and long term prevention of migraine attacks. Headache 1988; 28:550–557.

24. Nestvold K, Kloster R, Partinen M, Sulkava R. Treatment of acute migraine attack: naproxen and placebo compared. Cephalalgia 1985; 5:115–119.

25. Johnson ES, Ratcliffe DM, Wilkinson M. Naproxen sodium in the treatment of migraine. Cephalalgia 1985; 5:5–10.

26. Moyer S. Pharmacokinetics of naproxen sodium. Cephalalgia 1986; 6(suppl 4):77–80.

27. Nestvold K. Naproxen and naproxen sodium in acute migraine. Cephalalgia 1986; 6(suppl 4):81–84.

28. Hakkarainen H, Vapaatalo H, Gothoni G, Parantainen J. Tolfenamic acid is as effective as ergotamine during migraine attacks. Lancet 1979; 2:326–328.

29. Yrill GM, Swinburn WR, Liversedge LA. A double-blind crossover trial of isometheptene mucate compound and ergotamine in migraine. Br J Clin Pract 1972; 26:76–79.

30. Diamond S. Treatment of migraine with isometheptene, acetaminophen, and dichloralphenazone combination: a double-blind, crossover trial. Headache 1976; 15:282–287.

31. MacNeal P, Davis D. Use of methyl-iso-octenylamine in migraine, Ann Intern Med 1947; 26:526–528.

32. Graham JR, Wolff HG. Mechanism of migraine headache and action of ergotamine tartrate. Arch Neurol Psychiatry 1938; 39:737–763.

33. Saxena PR. Selective vasoconstriction in carotid vascular bed by methysergide: possible relevance to its antimigraine effect. Eur J Pharmacol 1974; 27:99–105.

34. Lance JW, Spira PJ, Mylecharane EJ, Lord GDA, Duckworth JW. Evaluation of drugs applicable to treatment of migraine in the cranial circulation of the monkey. Res Clin Stud Headache 1978; 6:13–18.

35. Fozard JR. The animal pharmacology of drugs used in the treatment of migraine. J Pharm Pharmacol 1975; 27:297–321.

36. Muller-Schweinitzer E. Evidence for stimulation of 5-HT receptors in canine saphenous arteries by ergotamine. Naunvn-Schmiedebergs Arch Pharmacol 1976; 295:41–44.

37. Edmeads J. Cerebral blood flow in migraine. Headache 1977; 17:148–152.

38. Aellig WH, Berde B. Studies of the effect of natural and synthetic polypeptide type of ergot compounds on a peripheral vascular bed. Br J Pharmacol 1963; 36:561–570.

39. Tfelt-Hansen P, Paalzow L. Intramuscular ergotamine: plasma levels and dynamic activity. Clin Pharmacol Ther 1985; 37:29–35.

40. Tfelt-Hansen P, Eickhoff JH, Olesen J. The effects of single dose ergotamine tartrate on peripheral arteries in migraine patients: Methodological aspects and time effect curve. Acta Pharmacol Toxicol 1980; 47:151–156.

41. Rosenthaler J, Munzer H. 9-10-Dihydroergotamine production of antibodies and radio-immunoassay. Experientia 1976; 32:234–235.

42. Orton DA, Richardson RJ. Ergotamine absorption and toxicity. Postgrad Med J 1982; 58:6–11.

43. Aellig WH, Nuesch E. Comparative pharmacokinetic investigations with tritium-labelled ergot alkaloids after oral and intravenous administration in man. Int J Clin Pharmacol 1977; 15:106–112.

44. Saxena PR, Koedam NA, Hof RP. Ergotamine induced constriction of cranial arteriovenous anastomoses in dogs pretreated with phentolamine and pizotifen. Cephalalgia 1983; 3:71–81.

45. Wolff HG. Wolff's headache and other head pain, 3rd ed. revised by DJ Dalessio. New York: Oxford University Press, 1972:257–268.

46. Chapman LF, Ramos AD, Goodell H, Silverman G, Wolff HG. A humoral agent implicated in vascular headache of migraine type. Arch Neurol 1960; 3:223–229.

47. Saito K, Markowitz S, Moskowitz MA. Ergot alkaloids block neurogenic extravasation in dura mater, proposed action in vascular headaches. Ann Neurol 1988; 24:732–737.

48. Sofia RD, Vassar HB. The effect of ergotamine and methysergide on serotonin metabolism in the rat brain. Arch Int Pharmacodyn Ther 1975; 216:40–50.

49. Aghajanian GK. The modulatory role of serotonin at multiple receptors in the brain. In: Serotonin neurotransmission and behavior. Jacobs BL, Gelperin A, eds. Cambridge: MIT Press, 1981:156–185.

50. Eadie MJ. Ergotamine pharmacokinetics in man. Cephalalgia 1983; 3:135–138.

51. Rose FC, Wilkinson M. Ergotamine tartrate overdose. Br Med J 1976; 1:525.

52. Tfelt-Hansen P, Krabbe AE. Ergotamine abuse. Do patients benefit from withdrawal? Cephalalgia 1981; 1:29–32.

53. Saper JR, Jones JM. Ergotamine tartrate dependency: features and possible mechanism. Clin Neuropharmacol 1986; 9:244–256.

54. Loew DM, van Deusen EB, Meier-Ruge W. Effects on the central nervous systems. In: Ergot alkaloids and related compounds, vol 49,Handblood of Experimental Pharmacology. Berde B, Schild HO, eds. New York: Springer-Verlag, 1978:421–531.

55. Hardebo JE, Edvinsson L, Owman C, Svendgaard N-A. Potentiation and antagonism of serotonin effects on intracranial and extracranial vessels. Neurology 1978; 28:64–70.

56. Ostergaard JR, Mikkelsen E, Voldby B. Effects of 5-hydroxytryptamine and ergotamine on human superficial temporal artery. Cephalalgia 1981; 1:223–228.

57. Ala-Hurula V, Myllyla VV, Arvela P, Heikkilla J, Hokkanen E. Systemic availability or ergotamine tartrate after oral rectal and intramuscular administration. Eur J Clin Pharmacol 1979; 15:51–56.

58. Graham AN, Johnson ES, Persaud NP, Turner P, Wilkinson M. Ergotamine toxicity and serum concentrations of ergotamine in migraine patients. Hum Toxicol 1984; 3:193–199.

59. Crooks J, Stephen SA, Brass W. Clinical trial of inhaled ergotamine tartrate in migraine. Br Med J 1964; 1:221–224.

60. Sutherland JM, Hooper WD, Eadie MJ, Tyrer JH. Buccal absorption of ergotamine. J Neurol Neurosurg Psychiatry 1974; 37:1116–1120.

61. Winsor T. Plethysmographic comparison of sublingual and intramuscular ergotamine. Clin Pharmacol Ther 1981; 29:94–99.

62. Tfelt-Hansen P, Paalzow L, Ibraheem JJ. Bioavailability of sublingual ergotamine. Br J Clin Pharmacol 1982; 13:239–240.

63. Lamb D, Persaud NP, Volans GN. Acute ergotamine poisoning. Hum Toxicol 1983; 2:424–426.

64. Friedman AP, Von Storch TJC, Araki S. Ergotamine tartrate: its history, action, and proper use in the treatment of migraine. NY State J Med 1959; 59:2359–2366.

65. von Storch TJC. Complication following the use of ergotamine tartrate. JAMA 1938; 111:293–300.

66. Goldfischer JD. Acute myocardial infarction secondary to ergot therapy: report of a case and review of the literature. N Engl J Med 1960; 262:860–863.

67. Pajewski M, Modai D, Wisgarten J, et al. Iatrogenic arterial aneurysm associated with ergotamine therapy. Lancet 1981; 2:934–985.

68. Fincham RW, Perdue Z, Dunn VD. Bilateal focal cortical atrophy and chronic ergotamine abuse. Neurology 1985; 35:720–722.

69. Henry PY, Larre P, Aupy M, et al. Reversible cerebral arteriopathy associated with the administration of ergot derivatives. Cephalalgia 1984; 4:171–178.

70. Harrison TE. Ergotaminism. JACEP 1978; 7:162–169.

71. Griffity RW, Grauwiler J, Hodel C, Leist KH, Mater B.Toxicologic considerations. In: Berde B, Schild HO, eds. Ergot alkaloids and related compounds vol 49, handbook of experimental pharmacology. New York: Springer-Verlag, 1978:805–851.

72. Lagier G, Castot A, Riboulet G, Boesh C. un Cas d'ergotisme mineur sembland en rapport avec une potentialisation de l'ergotamine par l'ethylsuccinate d'erythromycine. Therapie 1979; 34:515–521.
73. Carliner NH, Denune DP, Finch CS Jr, Goldberg LI. Sodium nitroprusside treatment of ergotamine-induced peripheral ischemia. JAMA 1974; 227:308–309.
74. Bagby RJ, Cooper RD. Angiography in ergotism: report of two cases and review of the literature. Am J Roentgenol 1972; 116:179–186.
75. Corrocher R, Brugnara C, Maso R, et al. Multiple arterial stenoses in chronic ergot toxicity. N Engl J Med 1984:310–261.
76. Fenely MP, Morgan JJ, McGrath MA, Eagan JD. Transient aortic arch syndrome with dysplasia due to ergotism. Stroke 1983; 14:811–814.
77. Carter ER. Bilateral thrombophlebitis after a single dose of ergotamine tartrate for migraine. Br Med J 1958; 2:1452–1453.
78. Merhof GC, Porter Jm. Ergot intoxication: historical review and description of unusual clinical manifestations. Ann Surg 1974; 180:773–779.
79. Perkin GD. Ischaemic lateral popliteal nerve palsy due to ergot intoxication. J Neurol Neurosurg Psychiatry 1974; 37:1389–1391.
80. Robert M, Derbaudrenghien JP, Blampain JP, et al. Fibrotic processes associated with long-term ergotamine therapy. N Engl J Med 1984; 311:601–602.
81. Taal BG, Spierings ELH, Hilvering C. Pleurpulmonary fibrosis associated with chronic and excessive intake of ergotamine. Thorax 1983; 38:396–398.
82. Stecker JF Jr, Rawls HP, Devine CJ Jr, et al. Retroperitoneal fibrosis and ergot derivatives. J Urol 1974; 112:30–32.
83. Eigler FW, Schaarschmidt K, Gross E, Richter HJ. Anorectal ulcers as a complication of migraine therapy. JR Soc Med 19xx; 79:424–426.
84. Horton BT, Peters GA, Blumentahl LS. A new product in the treatment of migraine: a preliminary report. Mayo Clin Proc 1945; 20:241–248.
85. Friedman MD, Wilson EJ. Migraine: its treatment with dihydroergotamine. Ohio State Med J 1947; 43:934–938.
86. Tillgren N. Treatment of headache with dihydroergotamine tartrate. Acta Med Scand 1947; 196(suppl):222–226.
87. Hoeldtke RD, Cavanaugh ST, Hughes JD, Polansky M. Treatment of orthostatic hypotension with dihydroergotamine and caffeine. Ann Intern Med 1968; 105:168–173.
88. deMetz JE, van Zwieten PA. Differential effects of dihydroergotamine on the circulatory actions of arterial and venous dilators in the rat. J Cardiovasc Pharmacol 1981; 3:217–227.
89. Anderson AR, Tflet-Hansen P, Lassen NA. The effect of ergotamine and dihydroergotamine on cerebral blood flow in man. Stroke 1987; 18:120–123.
90. Callaham M, Raskin NA. Controlled study of dihydroergotamine in the treatment of acute migraine headache. Headache 1986; 26:168–171.
91. Raskin NH. Repetitive intravenous dihydroergotamine as therapy for intractable migraine. Neurology 1986; 36:995–997.
92. van der Berg E, Walterbusch G, Gotzen L, et al. Ergotism leading to threatened limb amputation or to death in two patients given heparin–dihydroergotamine prophylaxis. Lancet 1982; 1:955–956.

93. Scherf D, Schlachman M. Electrocardiographic and clinical studies on the action of ergotamine tartrate and dihydroergotamine 45. Am J Med Sci 1948; 216:673, 679.

94. Belgrade MJ, Ling LJ, Schleevogt MB, Ettinger MG, Ruiz E. Comparison of single dose meperidine, butorphanol and dihydroergotamine in the treatment of vascular headache. Neurology 1989; 39:590-592.

95. Schran HF, Tse FL. Pharmacokinetics of dihydroergotamine following subcutaneous administration in humans. Int J Clin Pharmacol 1985; 23:1-4.

96. Hilke H, Kanto J, Kleimola T. Intramuscular absorption of dihydroergotamine in man. Int J Clin Pharmacol 1978; 16:277-278.

97. Kanto J. Clinical pharmacokinetics of ergotamine, dihydroergotamine, ergotixine, bromocriptine, methysergide and lergotrile. Int J Clin Pharmacol 1983; 21:135-142.

98. Raskin NH. Headache, 2nd ed. New York: Churchill Livingstone, 1988:151.

99. Iserson KV. Parenteral chlorpromazine treatment of migraine. Ann Emeg Med 1983; 12:756-758.

100. Lane PL, Ross R. Intravenous chlorpromazine—preliminary results in acute migraine. Headache 1985; 25:302-304.

101. Edmeads J. Emergency management of headache. Headache 1988; 28:675-679.

102. Basbaum AL, Fields HL. Endogenous pain control mechanisms: review and hypothesis. Ann Neurol 1978; 4:451-462.

103. Ramaswamy S, Bapna JS. Antagonism of morphine tolerance and dependence by metoclopramide. Life Sci 1987; 40:807-810.

104. Carrol JD. Migraine—general management. Br Med J 1971; 2:756-757.

105. Edmeads J. Management of acute attack of migraine. Headache 1973; 13:91-95.

106. Gallagher RM. Emergency treatment of intractable migraine. Headache 1986; 26:74-75.

9

Treatment of the Mixed Headache Syndrome

Seymour Diamond
Diamond Headache Clinic
Chicago, Illinois, and
Chicago Medical School
North Chicago, Illinois

CLINICAL RECOGNITION

In the patient with the mixed headache syndrome, the history, including the frequency and severity of the headaches, previous treatments, and the outcome of prior treatment, is the primary guide in selecting the appropriate treatment modalities. The patient presenting with mixed headaches will usually report a history of migraine headache superimposed upon a pattern of lower grade, but daily, headaches that may be described as muscle contraction headaches. Frequently, the patient may identify this pattern as the occurrence of periodic "hard" or "sick" headaches and a constant headache.

Several variations of the mixed headache syndrome have been described [1]. The first type is the presentation of headaches occurring on a periodic basis. The clinical symptoms are typical of migraine headache, and over the course of years, the migrainous symptoms subside. Eventually, the headaches become less distinctly migraine and progressively demonstrate features of muscle contraction headache. The second variation consists of headaches that predominantly present as muscle contraction types that intermittently occur, with features typical of migraine.

The third pattern presents as episodic migraine headaches. Over several years, another type of headache occurs during the interval betwen migraine attacks. These interval headaches have features that are common to muscle contraction headache. A less common, fourth pattern features a daily headache of constant duration over the course of many years. The headache may wax and wane in intensity, and the patient intermittently experiences symptoms that are related to migraine. However, the patient is unable to distinguish these symptoms because of the intensity of the headache and the occurrence of these symptoms on a daily, or nearly daily, basis.

Several factors have been implicated in the evolution of episodic migraine headaches into the mixed headache syndrome. Depression has been cited as a factor in the development of the mixed headache syndrome [2]. For example, patients with migraine headache may develop daily muscle contraction headaches that can be identified as symptoms of depression.

Other psychological factors, medical problems, and iatrogenic factors also have been implicated in leading to this transformation [3]. Mathew and his colleagues evaluated 80 subjects [3]. Of the 61 patients with daily headache, 70.5% had abnormal Minnesota Multiphasic Personality Inventory (MMPI) scores, as compared with 12.5% of the 19 patients with pure migraine. Over one-half of the patients with a daily headache had evaluations of 1.2 and 3 on the following scales: hypochondrias, depression, and hysteria. Most of these patients demonstrated a pattern that is designated, the neurotic triad. At least one abnormally high MMPI scale was present on the tests of 88.4% of the daily headache patients. On the Zung Self-Rating Depression Scale, 46% of the daily headache patients had clinical depression, compared with 5% of the pure migraine patients. Various life stresses, including family, marriage, work, social, and environmental problems, were observed in over two-thirds of the daily headache patients, as opposed to fewer than one-third of the migraineurs. The contribution of traumatic life events to their situations was noted by 13% of the patients.

Hypertension was also implicated; it occurred in 16% of the daily headache patients versus 2% of those with migraine. Supplemental estrogens were not identified as factors in the development of the daily headache. However, excessive amounts of medications used to treat the acute headache attacks, such as ergotamine preparations, narcotics, and caffeine-containing analgesics, were reported by over one-half of the patients with the daily headache pattern, compared with 6% of the pure migraine patients.

TREATMENT CONSIDERATIONS

A comprehensive approach to the treatment of the mixed headache syndrome is of paramount importance in achieving a successful outcome. This approach includes the use of medication for both prophylactic and abortive therapy. Nondrug modalities should also be considered in most patients with mixed headaches. The nondrug therapies include biofeedback, stress management, dietary considerations, counseling for stress factors and psychological problems, and physical modalities, such as exercise, physical therapy, and transcutaneous electrical nerve stimulation (TENS).

Adherence to a diet that limits foods containing vasoactive substances is especially important in those patients being treated prophylactically with the monoamine oxidase inhibitors (MAOIs). The diet restricts foods containing amines, such as tyramine, dopamine, and phenylethylamine. In addition, the patients should avoid alcoholic beverages, cured meats, and food additives, such as monosodium glutamate (MSG). Vasoactive amines are found in fermented foods, including dairy products, such as yogurt and sour cream, and in many cheeses, such as Emmentaler. Tyramine is also found in pickled herring, chicken livers, and overripe bananas. Consumption of citrus fruits should be limited, because tyramine is found in small quantities in these fruits. Dopamine is found in Italian broad green beans, also known as fava beans. Phenylethylamine is believed to occur in chocolate. Alcoholic beverages may also contain vasoactive amines. The nitrites and MSG do not interact with the MAOIs, but have been reported to cause headache in some patients (Table 1).

Abortive Therapy

Intermittently, patients with the mixed headache syndrome will experience acute headaches that require appropriate abortive therapy. The daily use of many of these abortive agents may also contribute to the development of a rebound, daily headache [4]. Special caution must be exercised to prevent iatrogenic complications of treatment. Strict limits on the use of potentially habituating medications must be established with these patients. In addition to obtaining a headache history, the physician should instruct the patient of differentiating the "hard" migraine headache from the lower-grade, daily muscle contraction headache. This patient education may be as important as selecting an appropriate abortive treatment. Patients experiencing classic migraine headaches that are preceded by the typical auras of migraine, or those patients with nonclassic migraine attacks that begin during the daytime, may be good candidates for the use of an ergotamine-containing preparation for the acute treatment of their migraine headaches. The ergotamine preparations exert vasoconstrictive effects on dilated extracranial arteries and have both agonist and antagonist activity on serotonin. These drugs remain the gold standard of the acute treatment of migraine headache.

If these agents are not taken as early as possible in an attack, the drug may not be as beneficial. Effective use of the ergots is difficult in those patients awakened from sleep because of the headache. Many patients with nonclassic migraine will benefit if the ergot preparation is taken at the first signs of an

Table 1 Tyramine Restricted Diet

Food	Foods allowed	Foods to avoid
Beverages	Decaffeinated coffee and soft drinks. Caffeine sources to be limited to 2 cups/day, including coffee, tea, and colas	Alcoholic beverages, for example, wine, ale, and beer Chocolate milk Buttermilk
Meat, fish, poultry	Fresh or frozen: beef, lamb, veal, pork, fish, turkey, chicken Eggs Tuna or salmon salad Shellfish	Aged, canned, cured, or processed meats, canned or aged ham, pickled herring, salted and dried chicken livers, aged game Hot dogs and fermented sausage (contains either nitrates or nitrites, such as bologna, salami, pepperoni, summer sausage) Any meat prepared with meat tenderizer or soy sauce
Dairy products	Cheese: American, cottage, farmer, ricotta, cream, Velveeta Homogenized, skim, and low fat milk Yogurt limited to ½ cup/day	Cheese: bleu, Boursault, brick, Brie, Camembert, cheddar, Swiss, Gouda, Rouquefort, Stilton, mozzarella, parmesan, romano, Emmentaler
Bread, bread substitutes	Commercial breads: white, whole wheat, rye, French, Italian English muffins, melba toast, Rye Krisp, bagels Crackers All hot and dry cereals Spaghetti, macaroni, other pasta	Hot, fresh, homemade yeast breads Fresh yeast coffee cakes, yeast doughnuts Sourdough breads Any breads, crackers, or cakes containing cheese, nuts, or chocolate
Vegetables	White or sweet potato, rice, asparagus, carrots, spinach, pumpkin, tomatoes, squash, corn, zucchini, broccoli, lettuce, cabbage, beets, cucumbers, etc.	Pole, bread, lima, fava, navy, pinto, garbonzo beans, lentils, snow peas, or pea pods Onions, except for flavoring Sauerkraut, olives, pickles
Fruits	Apples, cherries, apricots, peaches, pears, etc. Bananas limited to ½/day	Avocados, figs, raisins, papaya, passion fruit, red plums

Table 1 Continued

Food	Foods allowed	Foods to avoid
	Citrus fruits limited to ½ cup/ day, including orange, grape-fruit, lime, lemon, tangerine, pineapple	
Soups	Cream soups composed of foods allowed Homemade broths	Canned soups, including soup cubes, bouillon cubes, soup bases with autolyzed yeast or MSG *(read labels)*
Desserts	All cakes, pies, cookies, candy, except for those containing chocolate and nuts Gelatin products	Chocolate cakes, cookies, ice cream, pudding, and pies Mincemeat pies Chocolate syrup Carob products
Miscellaneous	Limited amounts of: salt, lemon juice, butter or margarine, cooking oils, whipped cream, white vinegar, commercial salad dressings	Soy sauce Foods that contain monosodium glutamate (MSG), such as meat tenderizers, Accent, seasoned salt Yeast, yeast extracts, and Brewer's yeast Mixed dishes: macaroni and cheese, pizza, lasagna, beef stroganoff, cheese blintzes Nuts and peanut butter Seeds, such as pumpkin, sesame, or sunflower Frozen TV dinners Pickled, preserved, or marinated foods *Read all labels on snack items*

imminent migraine attack. Patients with classic migraine may achieve resolution of the attack without entering the painful phase, if the ergot preparation is taken at the onset of the aura.

For the mixed headache patient, difficulties with the ergot preparation may result from several situations. Failure to recognize the onset of a migraine attack from the daily muscle contraction headache may lead to daily use of these agents, thereby triggering a rebound phenomenon. If the mixed headache patient usually experiences a daily headache, an acute migraine attack may not be detected early in the scenario, and the patient may be delayed in taking the ergot preparation, and thus fail in obtaining benefit from its use. Other patients may be extremely fearful of developing a migraine evolving from a muscle contraction headache, and they will use the ergots before the attack becomes migrainous. This situation increases the use of the agents, and the patient may require detoxification from the ergot preparation.

To prevent the development of ergotamine rebound headache, we instruct our patients on the strict limits placed on the total daily and weekly dosage of ergot. The limits are outlined in the literature supplied by the pharmaceutical manufacturers. In addition, we advise our patients that, regardless of the amount

Table 2 Ergotamine Therapy

Medication	Dosage
Ergotamine tartrate[a]	
Oral	
With caffeine (Cafergot, Wigraine)	2 tablets at onset, may repeat 1 tablet every ½ hr, up to 6/day, 10/wk
Sublingual (Ergomar, Ergostat)	1 tablet at onset, may repeat 1 tablet every ½ hr, up to 2/day, 5/wk
Rectal	
With caffeine (Cafergot, Wigraine suppositories)	Insert one suppository at onset, may repeat in 1 hr, up to 2/day, 5/wk
Inhalation (Medihaler-Ergotamine)	One inhalation every 5 min, up to 6/day, 10/wk
Dihydroergotamine[a]	
Intramuscular (DHE-45)	1 ml at onset, may repeat in 1 hr, up to 3 ml/day, 5 ml/wk
Isometheptene mucate	
Oral (Midrin)	2 capsules at onset, may repeat 1 capsule every 1 hr, up to 5/day, 15/wk

[a]A 4-day hiatus between uses is mandatory for any ergotamine preparation or dihydroergotamine

of doses of ergot used on the first day of an attack, they must observe a 4-day hiatus between uses (Table 2). Naproxen (Naprosyn) may be beneficial in ameliorating ergotamine rebound headache [5]. It has been our experience that patients undergoing ergotamine rebound will experience significant exacerbation of their headache during the initial 48 hr following withdrawal. A decrease in symptoms will occur after 2 days, which will be succeeded by another exacerbation of the headache during the fifth to seventh day after the offending agent has been discontinued.

A variety of ergotamine preparations are currently available in the United States. Ergotaine preparations may be administered in a variety of forms, including oral and sublingual tablets, rectal suppositories, and by inhalation. The inhaled and sublingual ergotamine preparations do not contain any additive. The injectable form of ergotamine is no longer available in the United States. However, an ergotamine derivative, dihydroergotamine (DHE-45), may be used for parenteral administration.

Selection of the form of ergot to utilize, involves consideration of the patient's previous response to ergots. Because gastric stasis may accompany migraine, and nausea is often associated with the acute migraine attack, some patients may not tolerate or may fail to obtain successful resolution of their headache with an oral preparation. An alternative method of administration may provide a more successful outcome. Other patients may not tolerate the caffeine additive in the oral and rectal forms, and may benefit from another administrative route. Oral preparations are familiar to most patients and may be better accepted and more convenient to utilize. Rectal suppositories are indicated for those patients in whom bed rest is possible after administration of the drug. The sublingual and inhaled forms of ergot are more rapid in their onset of action, when compared with the other forms. However, patients may find them distasteful or difficult to successfully self-administer. The injectable preparation of dihydroergotamine may be useful in those patients who can self-inject the agent, and in whom the other dosage forms have been unreliable or unsuccessful.

Many patients with the mixed headache syndrome do not benefit from the use of ergot or would not be good candidates for these drugs. The ergots are contraindicated in patients with ischemic cardiac disease, peripheral vascular disorders, and kidney and liver disease. For these patients, another agent containing isometheptene mucate, dichloralphenazone, and acetaminophen (Midrin), may be useful because it has vasoconstrictive effects without the risk of rebound headache. Midrin also contains a mild sedative agent that may be useful for the tension component of the headache. This action may be especially useful in those patients in whom the daily muscle contraction headache cannot be clearly distinguished from the migraine. It is also useful for those patients in whom the muscle contraction headache evolves into the migrainous headache.

The nonsteroidal anti-inflammatory agents (NSAIDs) are another alternative treatment option. The NSAIDs provide beneficial analgesic effects for acute muscle contraction headaches [6] and have also demonstrated good results in the relief of an acute migraine attack [7] (Table 3).

Simple over-the-counter (OTC) analgesics will often suffice for patients with episodic muscle contraction headaches. However, the patient with the mixed headache syndrome rarely finds these agents to be effective, in spite of the excessive quantities of the OTC drugs consumed by these patients. The overutilization of the OTC pain relievers may cause headache [8] whether or not the drugs contain caffeine.

Table 3 Nonsteroidal Anti-Inflammatory Agents in the Treatment of Vascular Headache

Agent	Abortive therapies (migraine)	Prophylactic therapies (migraine)	Menstrual migraine	Cluster headache variant and chronic paroxysmal hemicrania
Aspirin	900 mg/onset	650 mg bid	650 mg qid prn	
Flufenamic acid	400 mg/onset		250 mg/onset repeat every hour up to 750 mg/day	
Meclofenamate	100 mg/onset			
Mefenamic acid	500 mg/onset		250 mg/onset repeat every hour up to 750 mg/day	
Naproxen sodium	825 mg/onset repeat 275–550 mg every 30–60 min, up to 1375 mg/day	275–550 mg bid	250 mg tid	
Tolfenamic acid	200 mg/onset	100 mg tid		
Fenoprofen calcium		600 mg bid to qid	600 mg tid	
Ketoprofen		50 to 75 mg tid to qid	50–75 mg tid	
Indomethacin				12.5–75 mg tid
Naproxen		250–750 mg daily	250 mg tid	

Prescription analgesics and muscle relaxants may prove beneficial for the treatment of the muscle contraction component of their headaches. Narcotic analgesics should be avoided for abortive therapy of acute muscle contraction headache to prevent dependency problems. Several combination preparations that contain either aspirin or acetaminophen with a short-acting barbiturate agent, butalbital, may be used for an occasional acute headache. Because butalbital can be habituating, limits on the use of these agents should be established to prevent iatrogenic complications.

A variety of muscle relaxants are beneficial for the patient with muscle contraction headache. These agents include single-entity preparations that contain only the muscle relaxant, and combination preparations that also contain simple analgesics, such as aspirin or acetaminophen (Table 4). In general, these agents are well tolerated by most patients with muscle contraction headache. On occasion, sedation may occur with these agents, and patients should be cautioned about their use.

Prophylactive Therapy

Because of the frequent occurrence of attacks in the mixed headache syndrome, prophylactic therapy is the cornerstone of treatment and is essential for all patients with these headaches. Most of these patients experience two different types

Table 4 Muscle Relaxants

Drug	Dosage
Carisoprodol 350 mg	1 tablet, bid to qid
Carisoprodol 200 mg and aspirin 325 mg	1 or 2 tablets, bid to qid
Carisoprodol 200 mg, aspirin 325 mg, and codeine phosphate 16 mg	1 or 2 tablets, up to qid, not to be used on a daily basis
Chlorzoxazone 500 mg	½ to 1 tablet, bid to qid
Cyclobenzaprine 10 mg	1 or 2 tablets tid
Methocarbamol 500 mg	3 tablets tid maintenance dose: 2 tablets, bid to qid
Methocarbamol 400 mg and aspirin 325 mg	2 tablets, bid to qid
Metaxalone 400 mg	1 or 2 tablets, tid to qid
Orphenadrine citrate, 25 mg, aspirin 385 mg, and caffeine 30 mg	1 or 2 tablets, bid to qid
Orphenadrine citrate 50 mg, aspirin 770 mg, and caffeine 60 mg	1 tablet, bid to quid

of headaches. Therefore, prophylactic therapy of the mixed headache syndrome often includes agents that are prescribed to prevent both migraine and muscle contraction components of this syndrome. The use of several different agents, each directed at a specific aspect of the problem, is termed copharmacy.

Before discussing the copharmaceutic approach to the treatment of the mixed headache syndrome, it is necessary to review the limited number of studies that have utilized single agents in treating this syndrome. Studies have evaluated the use of the β-adrenergic blocking agents, including propranolol; the tricyclic anti-depressants (TCAs), such as amitripytline and doxepin; the MAOIs, such as phenelzine and isocarboxazid; and the ergot derivative, dihydroergotamine.

Mathew [9], in a randomized controlled study, administered propranolol, 20 mg, three times a day, increasing the dose within the first month to 40 mg, either three or four times a day, dependent on the patient's ability to tolerate the medication. Patients were continued on active treatment for a period of 6 months, following a 1 month pretreatment evaluation period. Thirty-eight patients completed the evaluation period. The weekly headache index was measured and compared with the index during both the pretreatment phase and the last 3 months of therapy. The index decreased from an average of 6.7 to 3.2, an improvement of 52%.

In the same study, Mathew [9] also assessed the efficacy of amitriptyline in the treatment of the mixed headache syndrome. Amitriptyline was administered at 25 mg every evening, gradually increasing to 50-75 mg nightly, based on patient tolerance. A decrease in the weekly headache index was observed in 31 evaluable patients from 7.8 to 3.1, a 60% improvement over baseline.

Bonoso and his colleagues evaluated the effects of amitriptyline in mixed headache [10]. In this study, 15 patients were treated with 75 mg of amitriptyline, every evening, for 2 months. The mean headache intensity decreased from 17, during the pretreatment phase, to 5.4 during the second month of therapy. In examining the number of hours that patients spent with headaches of different intensities, decreases were noted for each of the severity grades of headache, most notably in headaches of mild or moderate severity.

The use of a daily ergot derivative, dihydroergotamine, was also evaluated. The drug was given orally in a time-released preparation. The results indicated that the headache intensity decreased from an average monthly figure of 18.7 to 10.7 in the second month of treatment. However, when evaluating the number of hours with headache of a given intensity, significant decreases occurred in those headaches of severe or extreme ratings. Negligible decreases were noted in the mild and moderate headaches. These results coincided with a study by Fontanari and his associates [11] that used the time-released form of dihydro-ergotamine. In this study, only 40% of patients with mixed headaches benefited from this agent. Sixty percent of ten cases had less than a 10% decrease in the measured headache parameters of frequency, intensity, and duration.

Another tricyclic agent, doxepin was evaluated in a double-blind placebo-controlled crossover study [12]. Doxepin given in doses of 100 mg every evening, was compared with placebo during a 9-week treatment period; 14 patients completed the study. Although doxepin minimally decreased the number of days with headache, it demonstrated significant reductions in the headache indices and the amount of analgesic and ergotamine doses required by these patients.

In the treatment of the mixed headache syndrome, MAOIs may be used after other therapies have failed. In a recent study [13], the MAOIs, phenelzine and isocarboxazid, reduced the headache parameters of frequency and severity by over 50% in 12 of 16 patients. Almost complete amelioration of the headaches was achieved in 25% of the cases.

Only two studies of this syndrome have examined the use of combination therapy with two distinct agents used concurrently. Mathew (9) examined the results of using propranolol and amitriptyline concomitantly at the doses described previously. In 36 patients who completed the study, the weekly headache index increased from 7.4 in the pretreatment phase to 2.5 in the last 3 months of therapy, a 69% decrease from baseline. At the Diamond Headache Clinic, an MAOI (phenelzine or isocarboxazid) was used in combination with one of the following tricyclic antidepressants: amitriptyline, doxepin, trazadone, or trimipramine [14]. The choice of the MAOI and tricyclic antidepressants was based on the patient's ability to tolerate each of the given agents. The dosage was adjusted accordingly as the patient began to tolerate the medication. The patients were selected for the recidivist nature of their headaches and their failure to respond to all prior treatment with traditional headache prophylactic therapies. Six of the eight patients reported at least a 50% reduction in their headache parameters. Also, 25% of these patients experienced a complete remission of their headaches on this combination regimen.

Only limited studies have been undertaken to evaluate pharmacologic treatment of the mixed headache syndrome. Research has been minimal because of the complicated nature of this syndrome, the various factors which may impact on the frequency and severity of the headaches, and the outcome of the treatment. However, in clinical practice, we have found that numerous pharmacologic agents may be utilized in combination therapy to help reduce the occurrence of the mixed headache syndrome.

Assessment of the effects on the migraine headaches, independent of the effects on the muscle contraction headaches, may be helpful in selecting appropriate agents. For the migraine headache component, the β-adrenergic blocking agents, calcium channel blockers, NSAIDs, and MAOIs have demonstrated usefulness in the reduction of these headaches. The first avenue of therapy for muscle contraction headaches consists of the various tricyclic antidepressants. These agents should be tried before initiating MAOI therapy.

The β-blockers remain the agents of choice in migraine prophylaxis. A variety of these agents have been demonstrated as beneficial and have been discussed elsewhere in this text. If these drugs cannot be used because of complicating medical diseases, an inability to tolerate, or prove ineffective, then alternative agents should be considered. A calcium antagonist or NSAID may be the next choice of therapy. In female patients with menstrual migraine, or for those who experience migraine attacks at both menses and throughout the cycle, the NSAIDs may be the choice of therapy. Menstrual migraine may be refractory to therapy with other agents. The MAOIs may be indicated for those patients in whom more traditionally accepted agents have failed to achieve satisfactory results.

Selection of the tricyclic agent in the treatment of headache is based on the presence of a sleep disturbance. Patients who experience insomnia, in addition to headaches, will usually benefit from a tricyclic agent with sedative properties, such as amitriptyline, doxepin, or trazodone. The nonsedating antidepressants, such as protriptyline or nortriptyline, are more appropriate for the patients who complain of persistent fatigue or require prolonged sleep.

In selecting therapeutic agents, one must also consider side effects associated with these agents. Inevitably, patients treated with tricyclic antidepressants will experience some type of side effect. These reactions are usually mild and transient. The side effects may be beneficial, such as the sedating action of some agents. However, the side effects frequently prompt patients to dicontinue therapy. Slow titration of the doses, by small increments, may help decrease the severity of the side effects and result in a satisfactory outcome. In addition, the patient may require changing to a different tricyclic antidepressant if the side effects are severe and persistent. The physician should be cognizant of the side effects and the relationship of the specific antidepressant to the various neurotransmitters (Table 5).

If the patient fails to respond to the tricyclic agents, the MAOIs should be considered. The MAOIs may be used safely in combination with β-blockers and calcium antagonists. However, careful monitoring is essential to avoid a hypotensive reaction. The MAOIs may be used in combination with many of the tricyclic antidepressants [15]. However, the use of the tricyclic imipramine is verboten with MAOI therapy.

Inpatient Therapy

In treating the mixed headache syndrome, the physician must be aware that this patient is more likely to be refractory to most of the standard therapies. Also, these patients are more prone to dependency problems with a variety of analgesics or the ergotamine preparations. Failure with outpatient therapy may result in spite of aggressive use of pharmacologic agents and nondrug modalities.

In this group of recidivist patients, the appropriate use of an inpatient treatment may produce notable improvement. A retrospective study was undertaken

Table 5 Effects of Tricyclic Antidepressants

Drug	Serotonin inhibition	Norepinephrine inhibition	Dopamine inhibition	Sedative effects	Anticholinergic effects
Amitriptyline	Moderate	Weak	Inactive	Strong	Strong
Desipramine	Weak	Potent	Inactive	Mild	Moderate
Doxepin	Moderate	Moderate	Inactive	Strong	Strong
Imipramine	Fairly potent	Moderate	Inactive	Moderate	Strong
Nortriptyline	Weak	Fairly potent	Inactive	Mild	Moderate
Protriptyline	Weak	Fairly potent	Inactive	None	Strong

that evaluated 372 consecutive patients hospitalized at the Diamond Inpatient Headache Program at Louis A. Weiss Memorial Hospital, Chicago [16]. Ten percent of the respondents reported improvement during hospitalization, and they remained headache-free following discharge from the program. An additional 54% of the patients achieved a greater than 50% reduction in their headache index for all types of headache diagnoses. For the patients with the mixed headache syndrome who were not habituated, the headache index decreased from 0.9 to 0.48 at 1 month postdischarge, and a further decrease to 0.43, 6 or more months after discharge. In patients dependent upon caffeine-containing analgesics, the headache index improved from 0.95 to 0.41. However, they reported a slight increase at the final follow-up to 0.5. The mixed headache patients who were narcotic-dependent, demonstrated a decrease in the headache index from 0.99 to 0.55 at 1 month postdischarge, with minimal deterioration to an index of 0.58 at least 6 months after discharge. These results were comparable with the patients who were barbiturate-dependent, and whose index dropped from 0.98 to 0.64 at the time of the survey. Ergot-dependent patients experienced similar responses with the index decreasing from 0.95 to 0.58, at the time of the survey.

In another evaluation, a significant reduction in the utilization of health care facilities was noted in a long-term follow-up survey [Diamond Headache Clinic, unpublished data]. Evaluation consisted of 39 patients with the mixed headache syndrome, previously admitted to the inpatient unit, who may or may not have been habituated to analgesics or ergots. In the year before admission to the inpatient headache unit, these patients required 26 hospitalizations. Only three patients required subsequent readmission in the year following discharge from the inpatient headache unit. Emergency room visits for acute treatment of headaches also decreased substantially, from an average per patient of one visit every-other-month to one visit every 10 months.

Although significant benefits result from inpatient programs, some patients with the mixed headache syndrome are not suitable candidates for admission. Strict criteria for admission have been established. In addition, the program must be based upon a multidisciplinary approach, utilizing a variety of treatment strategies of pharmacologic management and nondrug modalities. The program should also be evaluated periodically to ensure long-term successful outcomes.

CONCLUSION

The patient with the mixed headache syndrome experiences two distinct headache problems, consising of periodic migraine headaches and daily headaches of the muscle contraction type. Successful management of these patients requires recognition of these separate entities and management strategies for each problem. Nonpharmacologic therapies are very important to these patients. However, the use of a carefully developed medical regimen is mandatory.

The pharmacologic management is divided into two categories, abortive and prophylactic therapies. For each of these categories, the use of agents specific for the two headache types is usually required. This form of therapy, with specific drugs aimed at a distinct aspect of the patient's headache problem, is termed copharmacy.

An essential part of the management of the mixed headache syndrome is avoidance of habituating medications. Dependence on analgesics or ergot preparations requires detoxification from these agents before initiating therapy. The use of an inpatient headache program provides for an excellent environment for detoxification and monitoring the patient during initiation of therapy. Of primary importance, the patient with the mixed headache syndrome deserves a continuity of care from the physician, who must be cognizant of the complex issues produced by this syndrome.

REFERENCES

1. Saper JH. The mixed headache syndrome: a new perspective. Headache 1982; 22:284–286.
2. Diamond S. Depression and headache. Headache 1983; 23:122–126.
3. Mathew NT, Stubits E, Nigam MP. Transformation of episodic migraine into daily headache: analysis of factors. Headache 1982; 22:66–68.
4. Wainscott G, Volans G, Wilkinson M. Ergotamine-induced headaches. Br Med J 1974; 2:274.
5. Mathew NT. Amelioration of ergotamine withdrawal symptoms with naproxen. Headache 1987; 27:130–133.
6. Diamond S. Ibuprofen versus aspirin and placebo in the treatment of muscle contraction headache. Headache 1983; 23:206–207.
7. Pradalier A, Rancurel G, Dordain G, Verdure L, Rascol A, Dry J. Acute migraine attack therapy: comparison of naproxen sodium and an ergotamine tartrate compound. Cephalalgia 1985; 5:107–113.

8. Kudrow L. Paradoxical effects of frequent analgesic use. In: Critchely M, et al., eds. Advances in neurology, vol. 33. New York: Raven Press, 1982: 335–341.

9. Mathew NT. Prophylaxis of migraine and mixed headache. A randomized controlled study. Headache 1981; 21:105–109.

10. Bonuso S, Di Stasio E, Barone P, Steardo L. Timed-release dihydroergotamine in the prophylaxis of mixed headache. A study versus amitriptyline. Cephalalgia 1983; 3(suppl 1):175–178.

11. Fontanari D, Perulli L, Conte F, Tambato E, Toso V, Zanetti R. Planned release dihydroergotamine in common migraine and "tension-vascular headache," multicentre clinical trial. Cephalalgia 1983; 3(suppl 1):189–191.

12. Morland TJ, Storli OV, Mogstad TE. Doxepin in the prophylactic treatment of mixed "vascular" and tension headache. Headache 1979; 19:382–383.

13. Freitag FG, Diamond S. The long-term use of monoamine oxidase inhibitors in the management of headache. In: Rose FC, ed. New advances in headache research. London: Smith-Gordon, 1989:301–304.

14. Freitag FG, Diamond S, Solomon GD. Antidepressant in the treatment of mixed headache: MAO inhibitors and combined use of MAO inhibitors and tricyclic antidepressants in the recidivist headache patient. In: Rose, FC, ed. Advances in headache research. London: John Libbey & Co, 1987:271–275.

15. Schuckit M, Robins E, Feighner J. Tricyclic antidepressants and monoamine oxidase inhibitors, combination therapy in the treatment of depression. Arch Gen Psychiatry 1971; 24:509–514.

16. Diamond S, Freitag FG, Maliszewski M. Inpatient treatment of headache: long-term results. Headache 1986; 26:189–197.

10

Pharmacologic Treatment of Cluster Headache

R. Michael Gallagher
University Headache Center
Moorestown, New Jersey, and
University of Medicine & Dentistry of New Jersey—
School of Osteopathic Medicine
Stratford, New Jersey

John Stirling Meyer, Makoto Ichijo
and Masahiro Kobari
Veterans Administration Medical Center
and Baylor College of Medicine
Houston, Texas

Jamshid Lofti
Baylor College of Medicine,
and St. Luke's Episcopal Hospital
Houston, Texas

INTRODUCTION

Although clinical descriptions of cluster headache first appeared in the late 1800s, the condition was fully described by Harris [1] in 1936 under the term "ciliary (migrainous) neuralgia." Horton [2] popularized the name "histaminic cephalgia" (Horton's syndrome), based on his suggestion that histamine played a primary role in the pathogenesis of this disorder, a view that is no longer tenable. A number of other syndromes, including erythromelalgia of the head [3], sphenopalatine neuralgia [4], vidian neuralgia [5], and greater superficial petrosal neuralgia [6], have been proposed by different authors to describe similar types of head pain. The fact that the headaches occur in clusters was noted by Kunkle et al. [7], and the term *cluster headache* was formally endorsed by the Ad Hoc Committee on Classification of Headache [8]. The term *cluster headache syndrome* is used in

131

the proposed Classification and Diagnostic Criteria for Headache Disorders, Cranial Neuralgias, and Facial Pain of the Internal Headache Society [9].

Cluster headache [10–13] is characterized by periodic, paroxysmal pain occurring almost exclusively on one side of the head. The excruciating, burning, and boring pain is located primarily behind and around one eye, although radiation of the pain to frontotemporal and facial areas is common. The head pain lasts from an average of 30–60 min and occurs one to many times a day. Headaches often occur late at night or early in the morning, causing the patient a miserable awakening. Accompanying autonomic nervous symptoms [11–14] are common. They include ipsilateral lacrimation, conjunctival injection, nasal obstruction, rhinorrhea, facial flushing, and unilateral or bilateral sweating of the face. Partial Horner's syndrome, including ptosis and miosis involving the affected eye, is occasionally observed during the headache [14,15]. In the episodic form, headache clusters, accompanied by autonomic nervous symptoms, occur daily for several weeks to several months and, then, are followed by complete remission for months or years. In the chronic form, the prolonged remissions are absent.

Cluster headache occurs preponderantly in males, with a male/female ratio of about 5:1 [12]. The onset of cluster headache can be at any age, but mostly it first appears in persons between 20 and 40 years of age. Conservatively, it is estimated that approximately 400,000 men and 80,000 women suffer from cluster headache in the United States, with the prevalence rate of about 0.4% for men and 0.08% for women [13].

The precise pathogensis of cluster headache is still unknown, although involvement of the cephalic vascular system is widely accepted [11,14,16]. The effectiveness of earlier treatments were often unpredictable and accompanied by considerable side effects, which have sometimes led to suicidal attempts. Over the last several years, newer therapies have been developd that show considerable promise and hope for the afflicted cluster sufferer.

PATHOGENESIS AND CEREBRAL HEMODYNAMICS OF CLUSTER HEADACHE

Pathogenesis

Histamine is a well-established vasoactive substance [17], with primarily vasodilator properties that precipitate headache in normal volunteers [18]. Since Horton et al. [3] presented cases in whom attacks of headache were induced by the subcutaneous injection of histamine, vascular components have been thought to be involved in the mechanisms of cluster headache. In the classification of headache proposed by the Ad Hoc Committee in 1962 [8], cluster headache was classified under "vascular headache of migraine type." Although cluster headache appears to be a distinct clinical entity from migraine, and its etiology is still unproved, many investigators believe that vascular changes play an important role in its development [11,14,17]. Several lines of evidence supporting the vascular etiology have been reported. The clinical observation that attacks of cluster headaches are ameliorated in some patients by digital compression of the superficial temporal or carotid artery on the involved side suggests involvement of extracranial or intracranial circulation, or both, during the attack of head pain [19]. Occasionally, engorgement of the superficial temporal arteries on the affected side can be observed during the attack. The attacks of cluster headache are regularly induced by the consumption of alcohol [3,10] or administration of nitroglycerine [20], both of which are well known to be cerebral vasodilators. Changes in the cerebral vascular caliber, although not frequent, have been directly observed by carotid angiography during attacks of cluster headache [21]. Changes of intracerebral and extracerebral blood flow that have been measured during attacks of cluster headache will be discussed later and they, likewise, support a vascular etiology [16]. Although cephalic vascular changes certainly occur during cluster headaches, whether this is the primary cause of symptoms or a secondary phenomenon remains to be clarified.

Some of the autonomic nervous symptoms accompanying the headache, such as unilateral lacrimation, conjunctival injection, nasal obstruction, rhinorrhea, and facial flushing, are usually attributed to the hyperactivity of the parasympathetic or to dysfunction of the sympathetic nervous system, by either peripheral or central mechanisms [11-14,22]. Ptosis and miosis, which are symptoms of a partial Horner's syndrome, are attributed to temporary impairment, vascular or otherwise, of the sympathetic nerves during the headache [14,15].

There is a pathway of peptidergic neurons originating from the nerve cells of the trigeminal ganglion, that accompanies the first and second divisions of the trigeminal nerve. This innervates the ipsilateral cerebral vessels and is called the *trigeminovascular pathway* [23]. Hardebo [24] contends that almost all the symptoms of the cluster headache could be caused by activation of this pathway. Substance P [23], and probably calcitonin gene-related peptide (CGRP) [25], seem to be neurotransmitters for this system. Changes in cerebral spinal fluid (CSF) and plasma levels of histamine [26,27], serotonin [26], acetylcholine [28], and opioid peptides (e.g., β-endorphin) [29,30], all have been reported during cluster headache. These substances are not only vasoactive [17,31], but some of them are neurotransmitters, suggesting participation of both vascular and neurogenic factors.

Although the precise pathogenic mechanisms for cluster headache remain unknown, there are vascular changes during the characteristic headache that seem to play an important role in its genesis [11,14,16]. Whether the vascular involvement is primary or secondary, and whether intra- or extracerebral vessels mainly participate in the pathogenesis of cluster headache, remain a subject for further investigation. However, alterations in the neurogenic regulation of the cerebral vessels seem to be an important factor related to the pathogenesis of cluster headache [24].

Cerebral Hemodynamics

Broche et al. [32], in 1970, were among the first to investigate cerebral hemodynamics in patients with cluster headache. They applied implantable electromagnetic flowmeters to both internal carotid arteries in a 51-year-old woman who had suffered from cluster headaches for about 15 years. However, they were unable to record any changes in mean or pulsatile blood flow in either carotid artery during attacks of headache. Norris at al. [33], utilizing the ^{133}Xe intracarotid injection method, fortuitiously measured cerebral blood flow (CBF) during the course of a cluster headache in a 32-year-old man. The first study, performed about 10 min after the onset of headache, showed CBF values to be at the upper limits of normal. Later, after partial relief of pain by the administration of ergotamine tartrate, the CBF showed abnormally high values. They attributed the CBF increases either to reactive hyperemia or as a response to the head pain.

Sakai and Meyer [34], in 1978, were the first to systematically investigate regional CBF changes during cluster headache with the ^{133}Xe inhalation technique. Mean gray matter flow values measured in seven patients during typical cluster headaches were significantly higher than the values during headache-free intervals measured in five patients. The average increase of gray matter flow during headaches was 44.5% among three patients who were measured repeatedly. Unlike those of migraine, the CBF values tended to return to normal values rapidly after cessation of the headache. They also calculated the extracerebral flow index (EFI) to estimate the percentage of contribution by the extracerebral circulation [34]. This index showed significant increases during cluster headaches, indicating increases in extracerebral blood volume or flow. They also found that, whereas CO_2 responsiveness of the cerebral vessels was impaired during cluster headaches, the vasoconstrictive response to O_2 inhalation was excessive [35]. This finding was in clear contrast with migraineurs, whose O_2 responsiveness was not increased during headaches.

Nelson et al. [36] measured CBF in four patients during spontaneous cluster headaches and in an additional group of patients during cluster headache provoked by nitroglycerin, alcohol, and histamine; however, CBF changes, were not uniform during headache attacks. They concluded that CBF changes do occur during cluster headache, and the vascular involvement is not confined to the extracerebral circulation. However, they were not of the opinion that CBF changes were primarily involved in the mechanism of cluster headache. Krabbe et al. [37], more recently, attempted to apply single-photon emission tomography, using ^{133}Xe inhalation, to obtain tomographic CBF images in 18 patients with cluster headache. Mean CBF values determined after successful induction of headache by alcohol or nitroglycerin, or both, did not show significant changes compared with resting CBF values. However, there were increases of regional CBF in the central and basal regions of the brain, as well as in a small portion of the right parietotemporal region. These regional CBF increases were thought, possibly, to be due to activation by pain.

There have been some inconsistencies in reported results of CBF measurements during cluster headache [32–37]. This may be attributable to differences in the methodology applied and, certainly, to differences that exist between spontaneously occurring attacks versus drug-induced attacks. There are also problems with the brief duration and fluctuating nature of cluster headaches themselves. However, there is a good deal of evidence that both the intracerebral and extracerebral circulation are involved in the pathophysiology of cluster headache, as reviewed by Meyer et al. [16] in 1987.

PHARMACOLOGIC TREATMENT OF CLUSTER HEADACHE

Calcium Channel Blockers

Calcium channel blockers or antagonists are a relatively new class of drugs, which have been shown to be useful in the treatment of cluster headache (Table 1). Compared with many other drugs, they are preferred because of their high patient tolerance and low incidence of side effects.

Calcium antagonists are a group of drugs that dilate vessels and inhibit myocardial contraction by blocking the entry of calcium ions through the calcium channels (slow channels) of the vascular smooth muscle and myocardium [38–41].

Table 1 Cluster Headache Treatment

Medication	Episodic	Chronic
Nifedipine	x	xx
Nimodipine	x	xx
Verapamil	x	xx
Prednisone	xxx	a
Triamcinolone	xxx	a
Ergotamine	xx	x
Methysergide	xx	xx
Lithium	x	xx
Cyproheptadine	x	x
H_1 and H_2 antagonists	x	xx
Histamine	xx	xx
Pizotyline	x	x
Indomethacin	x	x

x---------------xx---------------xxx
Least effective   Most effective

aNot suited for this form.

They exert strong vasodilator effects on the coronary arteries and, because of their inhibitory effects on the myocardium, they were first successfully applied to the treatment of ischemic heart disease [38–40]. Later, their vasodilator effects on cerebral vessels gained attention [40,41]. There are now several calcium antagonists available. Some of them, such as nimodipine, nicardipine, and diltiazem, are useful for their relatively selective vasodilator effects on the cerebral vessels [40,41]. Some of the other calcium antagonists, such as flunarizine, exert more protective effects on nerve cells [40]. Basic aspects of the calcium antagonists, including their pharmacologic properties and their effects on cerebral vessels and nervous tissue, have been described in detail elsewhere in this book when discussing their prophylactic use in the treatment of migraine (see Chap. 7). Calcium antagonists are now undergoing clinical investigation in several neurological disorders, including migraine [20–23,42–44], vasospasm following subarachnoid hemorrhage, cerebral ischemia, cerebral anoxia, hypoglycemia, epilepsy, dementia, vertigo, and tremor [40]. Recently, cluster headache has been added to the list of disorders that benefit from prophylactic treatment with calcium antagonists [40,45].

In 1983, Meyer et al. [42] reported the effectiveness of a calcium antagonist, nimodipine (Nimotop), among patients with chronic cluster headache. In a study that used a double-blind, crossover, randomized protocol, nimodipine (60 or 120 mg/day) significantly reduced the frequency of headache within 2 months after starting the treatment. The frequency of headache was further reduced during the following 2 months. Later, nimodipine (30–240 mg/day) was shown to reduce not only the frequency, but also the severity, of headaches [44]. The incidence and severity of side effects have been minimal with nimodipine, and the development of tolerance was extremely rare. Through various open studies, nifedipine (Procardia) (30–120 mg/day) and verapamil (Calan, Isoptin) (160–720 mg/day) were shown to decrease the frequency and severity of cluster headache [43]. Side effects were less common with verapamil than with nifedipine and included postural hypotension, constipation, and skin rash.

Later, Jonsdottir et al. [45] reported that the percentage of cluster headache patients who improved with nifedipine was 60%, with verapamil 79%, and with nimodipine 53%. However, there appeared to be no significant differences in the effectiveness among these three calcium antagonists for control of cluster headache. Because the incidence of side effects and tolerance is higher for verapamil and nifedipine than for nimodipine, the suggested preference for the prophylactic treatment of cluster headache would be nimodipine, verapamil, and nifedipine, in that order [21].

The effectiveness of calcium antagonists in the treatment of cluster headache has been supported by several other investigators. Mullally et al. [46] reported that nifedipine, 40 mg/day, was effective in six of seven patients with chronic cluster headache who had not benefited from treatment with methysergide,

ergotamine, lithium, or indomethacin. The side effects were minimal and confined to postural light-headedness. By applying probability analysis, de Carolis
et al. [47] reported that nimodipine, 120 mg/day, stopped clusters in 7 out of
13 patients with episodic cluster headaches within 10 days of treatment. Reports
were made by Diamond et al. [48] in the treatment of intractable cluster headache
among patients refractory to agents such as lithium, methysergide, corticosteroids,
or calcium antagonists. When these patients with intractable cluster headache were
treated in combination with histamine desensitization (intravenous administration
of histamine phosphate over a 10-day course with H_1 and H_2 antagonists), the
calcium antagonist verapamil (240 mg/day) was effective in 13 of 14 patients.
The only negative report of calcium antagonists in the prophylactic treatment of
cluster headache was that of Watson et al. [49]. They reported that various calcium
antagonists, such as nifedipine, diltiazem, verapamil, and nimodipine, were ineffective in 11 of 12 patients with chronic cluster headache. The reason for this
sharp difference from other authors reporting beneficial effects is unknown. There
are no reports, to date, concerning flunarizine in the treatment of cluster headaches.
This is a potent calcium antagonist for the treatment of migraine.

The mechanisms by which calcium antagonists reduce the frequency and improve the severity of headache attacks are unproved at present. The assumed
similarity in the etiology between migraine and cluster headache was the initial
rationale for the use of calcium antagonists in the treatment of cluster headache.
Although vascular factors are certainly involved in the pathogenesis of cluster
headache [11,14,16], migraine and cluster headache are usually thought to be
separate clinical entities. It is also noteworthy that, although most of the
vasodilators (e.g., alcohol [3,10] and nitroglycerin [20]), provoke attacks of cluster
headache, calcium antagonists, which are also cerebral vasodilators, ameliorate
the attacks of headache. It is presumed that reduction of vasomotor tone of the
intra- or extracerebral vessels by calcium antagonists render them less vulnerable
to the hemodynamic changes occurring during cluster headaches.

As yet, there are no completely satisfactory agents for the prophylactic treatment of cluster headache. Calcium antagonists appear to exert a high rate of effectiveness in decreasing the frequency and severity of cluster headaches, especially in the chronic form of the disease. Calcium antagonists have little in the
way of major side effects, and development of tolerance is infrequent. If one takes
efficacy, side effects, and tolerance into account, calcium antagonists are considered by some clinicians to be the treatment of choice in cluster headache.

Corticosteroids

Corticosteroids can be remarkably effective in the treatment of cluster headache
and were first suggested by Horton [50]. Their exact mechanism of action is as
yet unknown, although it is assumed that a precipitating humoral mechanism is

suppressed. Corticosteroid therapy is reserved for those patients, episodic and chronic, who are or become refractory to other forms of therapy.

The potential for long-term adverse effects with corticosteroids is significant. However, the unrelenting repeated attacks and the excruciating pain experienced by sufferers often justify the risks. Therapy is initiated at higher doses and tapered over a period of 1 month, in most cases. Some episodic cluster patients will experience a termination [51] of attacks, whereas, the headaches return as the dose is decreased in others. The headaches usually return in chronic cluster patients, but the period of relief may benefit the patient psychologically and "buy time" while other therapies are instituted.

Prednisome (Deltasone) [52] is the most commonly used oral corticosteroid. The dosage must be titrated to the individual. An average starting daily dosage is 60–80 mg, which is decreased each five to seven days to complete the steroid course in 30 days. Although most patients will benefit, some will experience recurrence of attacks as the dosage is lowered. In those patients whose attacks are to recur, the daily dosage will usually be below 20 mg [53] (Table 2).

Triamcinolone (Aristocort) is effective [54] and, by some clinicians, is considered to be the preferred corticosteroid in cluster therapy. There are reports of it being effective in patients who were unresponsive to full-dose prednisone [51]. The usual starting daily dosage is 16 mg, which is decreased every five days to complete its course in 30 days. Particularly difficult patients can be started at 32 mg/day and weaned in the same fashion over 35 days (see Table 2).

The long-lasting injectable corticosteroids triamcinolone acetanide (Kenolog), methylprednisolone (Depo-Medrol), or dexamethasone (Decadron-LA) also can be utilized [55]. By administering the long-acting forms intramuscularly, a gradual

Table 2 Sample Steroid Schedule

	a.m.	Noon	p.m.	Late p.m.
Prednisone				
Day 1–5	20 mg	20 mg	20 mg	20 mg
6–10		20 mg	20 mg	20 mg
11–15		20 mg		20 mg
16–20		10 mg		10 mg
21–25				10 mg
26–30				5 mg
Triamcinolone				
Day 1–7	4 mg	4 mg	4 mg	4 mg
8–14		4 mg	4 mg	4 mg
15–21		4 mg		4 mg
22–30				4 mg

tapering corticosteroid level can be achieved. This process can be repeated several times, but, thereafter, should be discontinued because of potential adverse reactions.

It should be kept in mind that corticosteroid therapy can be remarkably effective in the treatment of severe cluster sufferers. However, serious adverse effects can occur and strict adherence to usual steroid precautions is imperative. Side effects include fluid retention, weight gain, Cushing's syndrome, gastrointestinal disturbances (including ulcer), and lethargy. Corticosteroids are contraindicated in severe hypertension, diabetes, peptic ulcer disease, infection, active immunizations, or pregnancy.

Ergotamine

Until recently, ergotamine tartrate [56] preparations were the most widely accepted treatment of choice for the prevention of cluster headache. They can be extremely useful in both the prophylactic and abortive treatment of this headache. It has significant vasoconstrictive effects as well as central activity, which is discussed in Chapter 8. Generally, ergotamine is well tolerated by most, but individual sensitivity varies greatly from patient to patient. Careful monitoring of patients for untoward reactions or vascular complications is a necessity. The total daily dosage should be restricted to 1–2 mg/day, and the total weekly dosage should not exceed 14 mg.

Ergotamine, or its derivatives, can be found in various products, which include Cafergot, Wigraine, Medihaler-Ergotamine, Ergomar, Ergostat, Bellergal-S, and DHE-45 (Table 3).

Ergotamine, 1 mg (Cafergot, Wigraine), or 0.6 mg (Bellergal-S) can be given once or twice daily to prevent cluster attacks. In many patients this will not suffice, and the addition of another medication, such as indomethacin (Indocin), steroids, lithium (Eskalith, Lithobid), cyproheptidine (Periactin), antidepressants, or phenothiazines will be necessary. Patients who experience only nocturnal attacks may benefit by administering the ergot, 1–2 mg in tablet or suppository form, at bedtime.

Because of the brief duration of cluster attacks and the strict limitations of ergotamine use, the abortive treatment with ergotamine is of limited value. In such patients who experience infrequent or breakthrough attacks while taking other preventive medications, it can be tried. The suppository (Cafergot, Cafergot PB, Wigraine), inhalation (Medihaler-Ergotamine), or sublingual (Ergomar, Ergostat) forms are best suited because of rapid absorption. Again it must be emphasized that careful monitoring of amounts taken is imperative.

Ergonovine, 0.2 mg (Ergotrate), can be useful in the preventative treatment of cluster headaches. Some clinicians feel that it is as effective as methysergide, with better tolerance and fewer restrictions. It is given three to four times daily

Table 3 Ergot Preparations

Route of administration and brand name	Composition			
Preparation	Ergot alkaloid (mg)	Caffeine (mg)	Belladonna (mg)	Barbiturate (mg)
Oral				
Caffergot	Ergotamine, 1	100		
Wigraine	Ergotamine, 1	100		
Ergotrate	Ergonovine, 0.2			
Bellergal-S	Ergotamine, 0.6		0.2	Phenobarbital 40
Rectal				
Caffergot suppository	Ergotamine, 2	100		
Wigraine suppository	Ergotamine, 2	100		
Inhalation				
Medihaler	Ergotamine, 0.36			
Sublingual				
Ergomar	Ergotamine, 2			
Ergostat	Ergotamine, 2			
Injectable				
DHE 45	Dihydroergotamine 1			

as a single entity or in combination with other medications. Patients should be monitored closely for untoward effects.

Dihydroergotamine (DHE-45) can be self-administered intramuscularly to abort attacks. It is injected at the onset of the attack and is limited to a maximum of two injections in 1 day or six injections in 1 week. Although effective in some patients, the relief may be temporary and the completion of the headache merely delayed. Investigational studies on a nasal inhalatory form of dihydroergotamine suggest effectiveness [57].

Methysergide

Methysergide (Sansert, Deseril) is considered to be the prophylactic medication of choice in the treatment of episodic cluster by many clinicians (see Chap. 7). It is an ergotamine derivative and a potent serotonin inhibitor that is effective in approximately 60% of patients. In the early course of the disease, it appears to be effective. However, as patients become older, effectiveness often decreases [58].

Methysergide is administered in divided doses throughout the day for a total of 4–8 mg/day. Many patients experience an initial transient nausea, vomiting, muscle aches, and insomnia during the first 3 day of treatment. Consequently, some physicians administer methysergide in increasing doses over the first several days. If the foregoing initial side effects persist longer than 3 days the drug should be discontinued. All patients receiving this therapy should be monitored closely, with special attention to the renal, peripheral vascular, and cardiovascular systems. Methysergide should not be used in the presence of peripheral vascular or cardiovascular insufficiency, hypertension, active peptic ulcer disease, cardiac valvular disease, hepatic or renal insufficiency, or pregnancy.

Continuous treatment with methysergide is not recommended for more than 4–6 months. There should be an interruption of therapy or "drug holiday" for 1 month between use periods; otherwise a fibrosis in the retroperitoneal region, lungs, and heart valves may develop. This condition is usually reversible on cessation of the drug; thus making the drug holiday mandatory. In episodic cluster the headache period is usually fewer than 4 months and continuous use should not be a problem.

In patients who experience only partial relief or who do not respond, concomitant therapy with other drugs can be considered. Other concomitant drugs frequently utilized are corticosteroids, nonsteroidal anti-inflammatory drugs, and antidepressants.

In chronic cluster patients who do not respond to the usual medicaments, methysergide could be utilized. In such patients who do respond to methysergide, careful monitoring of the amounts of medication prescribed is necessary. Desperate patients are sometimes tempted to hoard tablets and continue its use during the mandatory drug holidays, without the knowledge of the physician.

Lithium

Lithium carbonate (Eskalith, Lithobid), which is often used in the treatment of manic–depressive disorders, has been effective in chronic cluster headache patients [59–61]. The mechanism of action is not completely understood, but is thought to be related to its effect on cyclic changes in serotonin and histamine [62]. It also affects sodium, calcium, and magnesium metabolism, inhibits the action of antidiuretic hormone, and reduces the rapid eye movement (REM) stage of sleep [12]. Lithium appears to be less effective in episodic cluster headaches.

The therapeutic dosage of lithium varies from patient to patient and must be titrated. In general 300–1200 mg/day is administered. A good beginning dose is 300 mg every 12 hr, which can be adjusted as necessary. Most patients who do respond will do so within 2 weeks of therapy. In some unresponsive patients the judicious addition of ergotamine can be extremely effective and well tolerated [63].

Lithium toxicity can occur; therefore, serum lithium levels must be monitored and maintained below 1.2 mEq/l. Nonsteroidal anti-inflammatory drugs [64], diuretics, salt-restricted diets, and salt loss through increased perspiration, as seen in the summer, increase the risk of toxicity [65]. Patients should be advised to avoid diuretics and follow normal salt diets.

The side effects of lithium therapy include fatigue, tremor, sleepiness, diarrhea, decreased thyroid function, goiter, fluid retention, blurred vision, and exacerbation of dermatological conditions. It should not be given to patients with significant renal, cardiovascular, or thyroid disease, in combination with nonsteroidal anti-inflammatory drugs or thiazide diuretics. The addition of low-dose propranolol (40–80 mg) will often ameliorate any lithium-induced tremors.

Histamine Desensitization

There is some evidence to suggest that histamine plays a role in cluster headache. It can be used as a provocative agent in susceptible individuals. Administered subcutaneously, a characteristic cluster attack can be precipitated [50] in 5–30 min. Headaches also can be provoked in normal individuals, but the headache is more generalized and is associated with pressure and flushing of the face. Increased levels of histamine have been demonstrated in the serum [66] as well as in the urine [67] in sufferers shortly after attacks. Some clinicians believe that the cluster attacks are the result of the sudden release of histamine from body stores [68]. Whether histamine is involved as a primary precipitating mechanism or is a secondary resultant event is not yet clear.

Histamine desensitization became popular following the initial suggestion by Horton that histamine was closely involved in the cluster mechanism. Various subcutaneous and intravenous methods and protocols were utilized, with mixed results, leading many physicians to abandon its use. However, there has been a renewed interest in histamine desensitization, and it is often an integral part of inpatient treatment programs.

Histamine desensitization usually is reserved for those patients who do not respond to other treatment. Usually, it is utilized in conjunction with prophylactic medications. These medications include H_1 and H_2 antagonists, lithium, nonsteroidal anti-inflammatory drugs, antidepressants, ergotamine, or phenothiazines.

At the Diamond Headache Clinic a solution of 5.5 mg of histamine and 250 ml of 5% dextrose and 0.5 N saline solution (D5/1/2NSS) is utilized. The solution is given by slow intravenous infusion every 12 hr for a total of 21 treatments. The patient controls the infusion rate starting with 10 drops/min. The rate is increased 10 drops for each 15 min as tolerated. Most patients will reach a rate that will precipitate flushing or mild headache, at which time the rate is decreased. Occasionally, a full-blown headache can be precipitated by a too rapid rate.

Histamine desensitization by the subcutaneous route has been reported to be successful by some clinicians [68,69]. However, it is rarely as effective as the intravenous method. Histamine acid phosphate 0.275 mg/ml is utilized: 0.1 ml is injected the first day and increased by 0.05 ml each successive day to a maximum of 1.0 ml. If a headache should occur within 1 hr of treatment, the dose is reduced by 0.05 ml, and this remains the maintenance dose. Injections are continued once daily until the headaches cease or until it is evident that the treatment will not be successful.

Combination H_1 and H_2 Antagonists

It appears that there are H_1 and H_2 receptors in the carotid vascular bed [70]. The concomitant use of H_1 and H_2 antagonists seems reasonable because H_1 antagonists only partly reverse histamine-induced vasodilatation [71]. Anthony et al. [72] and Russell [73] reported poor results, whereas Cuypers et al. [74] reported some success. Although more investigative study is needed, it does appear that some patients may benefit from this combination therapy.

Cimetidine (Tagamet), 300 mg four times daily, or rantidine (Zantac), 150 mg twice daily, are most often utilized as the H_1 antagonist. Cyprohepadine (Periactin), 4 mg four times daily; hydroxyzine (Atarax, Vistaril), 10–25 mg four times daily; clemastine fumarate (Tavist), 1.3–2.6 mg four times daily; or chlorpheniramine maleate (Chlor-Trimeton), 4 mg four times daily, can be used as the H_2 antagonist. Side effects are minimal, with tiredness and weight gain being most often reported.

Antihistamines

Nasal congestion, rhinorrhea, stuffiness, and lacrimation are common symptoms experienced with cluster attacks. This has led many sufferers to try antihistamines in the hope of preventing attacks. Anecdotally there are many reports of success, to some degree. However, most of these patients experience the relief only in the early stages of cluster.

Our experience has been poor with antihistamines used as a single-entity therapy. However, some patients will respond to antihistamines, such as cyproheptadine, hydroxyzine, clemastine fumarate, or chlorpheniramine, in combination therapy. Drugs commonly used in combination are methysergide, ergotamine, nonsteroidal anti-inflammatory drugs, H_2 antagonists, and calcium channel blockers.

Pizotyline

Pizotyline (Sandomigran), which is not available in the United States, is an antiamine that is sometimes used in the preventative treatment of migraine (see Chap 7). Several clinicians [75,76] have reported effectiveness in cluster prophylaxis. It is administered 1.5 mg three times daily and is well tolerated by most patients. Side effects include weight gain, drowsiness, or dizziness.

Indomethacin

Indomethacin (Indocin) is a nonsteroidal anti-inflammatory drug with significant analgesic effects. It is particularly effective in the treatment of a cluster variant, chronic paroxysmal hemicrania [79], and is helpful to some cluster patients [55]. It is administered orally, 25–50 mg four times daily. Side effects usually are related to the gastrointestinal tract and include nausea, cramps, epigastric burning, ulceration, constipation, and diarrhea. Some patients may benefit from the suppository form, when the oral form cannot be tolerated. Other side effects include dizziness, headache, fatigue, tinnitis, and, in rare instances, hematological or renal disorders.

Oyxgen

Oxygen inhalation can be quite dramatic in relieving symptoms of a cluster headache attack (Table 4). Seventy-five percent of patients can abort symptoms

Table 4 Cluster Abortive Treatment

Treatment	Effectiveness
Oxygen inhalation	xxx
Cocaine drops	xx
Lidocaine drops	xx
Ergotamine	
DHE-45	xx
Tablet[a]	x
Inhalation	xx
Suppository	xx
Analgesics	x
NSAIDs	x
Antihistamines	Noneffective

x---------------xx---------------xxx
Least effective   Most effective

[a]Longer attacks.

within 12 min [78]. It is presumed that oxygen creates a reactive vasoconstriction. Oxygen is administered at a rate of 7–8 L, by facial mask, at the onset of an attack. There appears to be no preventative benefit from oxygen. Although usually effective, the apparatus is heavy and cumbersome, making it impractical for some patients. Oxygen is well tolerated and side effects are almost nonexistent.

Cocaine and Lidocaine

The application of cocaine to the sphenopalatine foramen has been shown to abort cluster attack [79]. It is presumed to produce local anesthesia and vasoconstriction. A 5–10% cocaine solution is mixed in a saline solution and applied intranasally.

Proper body position and application of the solution is extremely important. The patient lies on the back with the neck extended 30–45° toward the floor. The head is turned toward the side of pain and ½ dropperful is dripped into the nostril. This position should be maintained for 60 sec and the procedure repeated, if necessary, but not to exceed two applications over 4 hr. In some cases, when nasal congestion is significant, a decongestant spray can be used before the cocaine solution.

Kitrelle reported that a 4% solution of lidocaine can be effective [80]. This enables treatment in many, without resorting to cocaine, which carries with it an addiction risk. The procedure is identical with that for cocaine, and pretreatment with a nasal decongestant may be necessary.

Other Medications

Other medications, either singly or in combination with those already mentioned, may be helpful in the prevention of cluster headache in some patients. These include phenothiazines, such as chlorpromazine (Thorazine) or promethazine (Phenergan), 100–200 mg/day; benzodiazepines, such as diazepam (Valium), 20–40 mg/day; or chlordiazepoxide (Librium), 30–100 mg/day; antidepressants, such as amitriptyline (Elavil, Endep), nortriptyline (Pamelor, Aventyl), doxepin (Adapin, Sinequan), 50–200 mg/day; fluoxetine (Prozac), 20–60 mg/day; phenelzine (Nardil), 30–75 mg/day; β-blockers, such as propranolol (Inderal), 120–320 mg/day, or nadolol (Corgard), 80–120 mg/day; timolol (Blocadren), 10–30 mg/day, metoprolol (Lopressor), 50–200 mg/day; and nonsteroidal antiinflammatory drugs, such as ketoprofen (Orudis), 200–300 mg/day, naproxen (Naprosyn), 1000 mg/day, ibuprofen (Motrin, Rufen), 2400 mg/day. Tiospirone, an investigational serotonin antagonist, have been shown to be effective [81] in a preliminary study.

Analgesics and Sedatives

The effectiveness of analgesics in the symptomatic treatment of cluster is variable. The short duration of attacks and possible poor absorption of medication during acute pain [52] often make oral analgesics impractical. However, a trial of various narcotic or nonnarcotic analgesics can be attempted. Although usually of limited help, these medications may aid the patient psychologically during difficult periods and reduce associated anxiety. Unmonitored use of such medications, however, should be avoided because potential habituation or toxicity can develop.

COMBINATION THERAPY

The treatment of the unresponsive cluster headache patient often can be a formidable task. Simple single-drug therapy is ideal, but many sufferers simply do not respond. Corticosteroids are considered by many to be the most effective drugs in use today. However, a considerable percentage of patients still require more to achieve a control of symptoms. The combining of two or more therapeutic agents may afford relief, when each by itself is ineffective.

Ergotamine or methysergide are often combined with corticosteroids, lithium, nonsteroidal anti-inflammatory drugs, antihistamines, or antidepressants. Antihistamines are often combined with nonsteroidal anti-inflammatory drugs, H_2 antagonists, or calcium channel blockers. The various combinations are many, and the possibilities are left to the experience and imagination of the clinician. A medication program should be tailored to suit the particular sufferers, always keeping in mind drug interactions and possible additive adverse effects.

Some cluster sufferers experience residual scalp, face, or neck pain following attacks. Persistent tension headaches between, or overlaying the clusters, as a result of anxiety and frustration are common. In these situations the addition of an antidepressant, muscle relaxant, or nonsteroidal anti-inflammatory drug can be helpful.

REFERENCES

1. Harris W. Ciliary (migrainous) neuralgia and its treatment. Br Med J 1936; 1:457–460.
2. Horton BT. Histamic cephalgia (Horton's headache or syndrome). M State Med J 1961; 10:178–203.
3. Horton BT, MacLean AR, Craig WMck. A new syndrome of vascular headache, results of treatment with histamine: preliminary report. Proc Staff Meet Mayo Clin 1939; 14:257–260.
4. Sluder G. The syndrome of sphenopalatine-ganglion neurosis. Am J Med Sci 1910; 140:868–878.
5. Vail HH. Vidian neuralgia. Ann Otol Rhinol Laryngol 1932; 41:837–856.

6. Gardner WJ, Stowell A, Dutlinger R. Resection of the greater superficial petrosal nerve in the treatment of unilateral headache. J Neurosurg 1947; 4:105–114.

7. Kunkle EC, Pfeiffer JB Jr, Vilhoit WM, Hamric LW Jr. Recurrent brief headache in "cluster" pattern. Trans Am Neurol Assoc 1952; 77:240–243.

8. Ad Hoc Committee on Classification of Headache. Classification of headache. JAMA 1962; 179:127–128.

9. Ad Hoc Committee of the International Headache Society. Proposed classification and diagnostic criteria for headache disorders; cranial neuralgias and facial pain. Copenhagen: B Stougaard Jensen, 1988.

10. Friedman AP, Mikropoulos HE. Cluster headaches. Neurology 1958; 8:653–663.

11. Kudrow L. Cluster headache, mechanisms and management. Oxford: Oxford University Press, 1980.

12. Diamond S, Dalessio DJ. Cluster headache. In: Diamond S, Dalessio DJ, eds. The practicing physician's approach to headache, 4th ed. Baltimore: Williams & Wilkins, 1986:66–75.

13. Kudrow L. Cluster headaches. In: Blau JN ed. Migraine: clinical, therapeutic, conceptual and research aspects. London: Chapman & Hall, 1987:113–133.

14. Ekbom K. Pathogenesis of cluster headache. In: Blau JN, ed. Migraine: clinical, therapeutic, conceptual and research aspects. London: Chapman & Hall, 1987:433–448.

15. Nieman EA, Hurwitz LJ. Ocular sympathetic palsy in periodic migrainous neuralgia. J Neurol Neurosurg Psychiatry 1961; 24:369–373.

16. Meyer JS, Hata T, Imai A. Evidence supporting a vascular pathogenesis of migraine and cluster headache. In: Blau JN, ed. Migraine: clinical, therapeutic, conceptual and research aspects. London: Chapman & Hall, 1987:265–302.

17. Gross PM. Cerebral histamine: indications for neuronal and vascular regulation. J Cereb Blood Flow Metab 1982; 2:3–23.

18. Meyer JS, Dalessio DJ. Toxic vascular headache. In: Dalessio DJ, ed. Wolff's headache and other head pain, 5th ed. New York: Oxford University Press, 1987:136–171.

19. Ekbon K. Some observations on pain in cluster headache. Headache 1975; 14:219–225.

20. Ekbom K. Nitroglycerin as a provocative agent in cluster headache. Arch Neurol 1968; 19:487–493.

21. Ekbom K, Greitz T. Carotid angiography in cluster headache. Acta Radiol Daign 1970; 10:177–186.

22. Spierings ELH. The involvement of the automomic nervous system in cluster headache. Headache 1980; 20:218–219.

23. Moskowitz MA. The neurobiology of vascular head pain. Ann Neurol 1984; 16:157–158.

24. Hardebo JE. The involvement of trigeminal substance P neurons in cluster headache: a hypothesis. Headache 1984; 24:294–304.

25. Edvinsson L, McCulloch J, Kingman TA, Uddman R. On the functional role of the trigemino-cerebrovascular system in the regulation of cerebral circulation. In: Owman C, Hardebo JE, eds. Neural regulation of brain circulation. Amsterdam: Elsevier Science Publishers, 1986:407–418.

26. Anthony M, Lance JW. Histamine and serotonin in cluster headache. Arch Neurol 1971; 25:225-231.
27. Medina JL, Diamond S, Fareed J. The nature of cluster headache. Headache 1979; 19:309-322.
28. Kunkle EC. Acetylcholine in the mechanism of headaches of migraine type. Arch Neurol Psychiatry 1959; 81:135-141.
29. Mosnaim AD, Diamond S, Freitag F, Chevesich J, Volf ME, Solomon G. Plasma and platelet methionine-enkephalin levels in chronic cluster patients during an acute headache episode. Headache 1987; 27:325-328.
30. Hardebo JE, Ekman R. CSF neuropeptides in cluster headache. Headache 1986; 26:316-317.
31. Kobari M, Gotoh F, Fukkuuchi Y, Amano T, Suzuke N, Uematsu D, Obara K, Gogolak I, Sando P. Effects of (D-Met^2,Pro^5)-enkephalinamide and naloxone on pial vessels in cats. J Cereb Blood Flow Metab 1985; 5:34-39.
32. Broch A, Horven I, Nornes H, Sjaastad O, Tonjum A. Studies on cerebral and ocular circulation in a patient with cluster headache. Headache 1970; 10:1-8.
33. Norris JW, Hachinski VC, Cooper PW. Cerebral blood flow changes in cluster headache. Acta Neurol Scand 1976; 54:371-374.
34. Sakai F, Meyer JS, Regional cerebral hemodynamics during migraine and cluster headaches measured by the ^{133}Xe inhalation method. Headache 1978; 18:122-132.
35. Sakai F, Meyer JS. Abnormal cerebrovascular reactivity in patients with migraine and cluster headache. Headache 1979; 19:257-266.
36. Nelson RF, du Boulay GH, Marshall J, Russell RWR, Symon L, Zilkha E. Cerebral blood flow studies in patients with cluster headache. Headache 1980; 20:184-189.
37. Krabbe AE, Henriksen L, Oleson J. Tomographic determination of cerebral blood flow during attacks of cluster headache. Cephalalagia 1984; 4:17-23.
38. Fleckenstein A. Specific pharmacology of calcium in myocardium cardiac pacemakers, and vascular smooth muscle. Annu Rev Pharmacol Toxicol 1977; 17:149-166.
39. Braunwald E. Mechanism of action of calcium-channel-blocking against. N Engl J Med 1982; 307:1618-1627.
40. Kobari M, Gotoh F, Tomita M. Calcium antagonists and cerebral circulation. Jpn J Stroke 1984; 6:371-387.
41. Greenberg DA. Calcium channels and calcium channel antagonists. Ann Neurol 1987; 21:317-330.
42. Meyer JS, Hardenberg J. Clinical effectiveness of calcium entry blockers in prophylactic treatment of migraine and cluster headaches. Headache 1983; 23:266-277.
43. Meyer JS, Dowell R, Mathew N, Hardenberg J. Clinical and hemodynamic effects during treatment of vascular headaches with verapamil. Headache 1984; 24:313-321.
44. Meyer JS, Nance M, Walker M, Zetusky WJ, Dowell RE Jr. Migraine and cluster headache treatment with calcium antagonists supports a vascular pathogenesis. Headache 1985; 25:358-367.
45. Jonsdottir M, Meyer JS, Rogers RL. Efficacy, side effects and tolerance compared during headache treatment with three different calcium blockers. Headache 1987; 27:364-369.

46. Mullally WJ, Livingstone IR. The treatment of chronic cluster headache with nifedipine. Headache 1984; 24:264-165.
47. de Carolis P, Baldrati A, Agati R, de Capoa D, D'Alessandro R, Sacquegna T. Nimodipine in episodic cluster headache: results and methodological considerations. Headache 1987; 27:397-399.
48. Diamond S, Freitag FG, Prager J, Gandhi S. Treatment of intractable cluster. Headache 1986; 26:42-46.
49. Watson CPN, Evans RJ. Chronic cluster headache: a review of 60 patients. Headache 1987; 27:158-165.
50. Horton B. Histamine cephalgia. Lancet 1952; 2:92-98.
51. Raskin NH. Cluster headache. In: Headache. New York: Churchill Livingstone, 1988: 243-244.
52. Couch JR. Cluster headache: characteristics and treatment. Semin Neurol 1982; 2:30-49.
53. Couch JR, Ziegler D. Prednisone therapy for cluster headache. Headache 1977; 17:15-18.
54. MacNeal PS. Useful therapeutic approaches to the patient with "problem headache." Headache 1975; 15:186-189.
55. Campbell JK. Cluster headache, In: Rose FC, ed. Management of headache. New York: Raven Press, 1988:115-126.
56. Ekbom K. Ergotamine tartrate orally in Horton's "histamine cephalgia:" a new method of treatment. Acta Psychiatry Neurol Suppl 1947; 46:105-113.
57. Anderson P, Jespersen, L. Dihydroergotamine nasal spray in the treatment of attacks of cluster headache. Cephalalgia 1986; 6:51-54.
58. Kudrow L. Cluster headache. Clin J Pain 1989; 5:29-38.
59. Kudrow L. Lithium prophylaxis for chronic cluster headache. Headache 1977; 17:15-18.
60. Mathew N. Clinical subtypes of cluster headache and response to lithium therapy. Headache 1978; 18:26-80.
61. Ekbom K. Lithium for cluster headache: review of the literature and preliminary results of long-term treatments. Headache 1981; 21:132-139.
62. Diamond S, Medina J. Newer drug therapies for headache. Postgrad Med 1980; 68:134.
63. Stagliano R, Gallagher RM. Combination ergotamine and lithium therapy in the chronic cluster headache patient. Headache 1983; 23:147.
64. Gallagher RM, Frietag F. Cluster headache: diagnosis and treatment. J Osteopath Med 1987; 1(5):10-18.
65. Saper J. Cluster headache. In: Headache disorders. Boston: John Wright, 1983:108-109.
66. Anthony M, Lance JW. Histamine and serotonin in cluster headaches. Arch Neurol 1971; 25:225-231.
67. Sjaastad O, Sjaastad OV. The histaminuria in vascular headaches. Acta Neurol Scand 1977; 46:331-342.
68. Ryan R, Ryan R. Other types of vascular headaches. In: Headache and head pain. St. Louis: CV Mosby, 1978:186-207.

69. Stern FH. Histamine cephalgia—an often overlooked cause of headache. Psychosomatics 1969; 10:53.

70. Saxena PR. The significance of histamine$_1$ and H$_2$ receptors on the carotid vascular bed in the dog. Neurology 1975; 25:681-687.

71. Hardebo JE, Krabbe AA, Gjerris F. Enhanced dilatory response to histamine in large extracranial vessels in chronic cluster headache. Headache 1980; 20:316-320.

72. Anthony M, Lord GDA, Lance JW. Controlled trails of cimetidine in migraine and cluster headache. Headache 1978; 18:261-264.

73. Russell D. Cluster headache: trial of a combined histamine H$_1$ and H$_2$ antagonist treatment. J Neurol Neurosurg Psychiatry 1979; 42:668-669.

74. Cuypers J, Altenkirch H, Bunge S. Therapy of cluster headache with histamine H$_1$ and H$_2$ receptor antagonists. J Eur Neurol 1979; 18:345-347.

75. Ekbom E. Prophylaxis treatment of cluster headache with a new serotonin antagonist BC 105. Acta Neurol Scand 1969; 45:601-610.

76. Nelson RF. Cluster migraine can be relieved but is seldom recognized. Mod Med 1971; 39:115.

77. Matthew N. Indomethacin responsive headache syndrome. Headache 1981; 21:147-150.

78. Kudrow L. Response of cluster headache to O^2 inhalation. Headache 1981; 21:1-4.

79. Barre F. Cocaine as an abortive agent in cluster headache. Headache 1982; 22:69-73.

80. Kitrelle J, Grouse D, Seybold M. Cluster headache, local anesthetic abortive agents. Arch Neurol 1985; 41:496-498.

81. Diamond S, Freitag F, Gallagher R. Tiospirone in the treatment of cluster headache. Headache 1989; 29:312.

11

Treatment of Muscle Contraction (Tension) Headache

William G. Speed III
The Johns Hopkins University
School of Medicine
Baltimore, Maryland

INTRODUCTION

Before discussing the treatment of muscle contraction, or tension headaches it is necessary to understand what is meant by the use of these terms. All headaches that result from tension are not necessarily caused by muscle contraction, and not all headaches that fit the criterion of muscle contraction headache have demonstrable excessive muscle contraction. For the sake of one's sanity and the avoidance of confusion, only the term *muscle contraction headache* will be used, whether or not there is a demonstrable tension etiology [1–3].

For many, many years excessive contraction of muscles of the neck and head have been thought to be the explanation for the headache of this disorder. Indeed, there are complex neurological mechanisms involved in the maintenance of muscle tone, the degree of which is determined by the state of activity of a special population of the anterior horn cells, called fusimotor cells, or γ-efferent neurons. These act on the α-motor neurons, supplying the extrafusal muscles, which, in turn, are further influenced by inhibitory cells such as the Renshaw cell and many others [4,5]. Although the role of supraspinal control on the γ-efferent system has not been established, it is quite probable that there are cortical, subcortical, and limbic afferent and efferent pathways connected to this sytem. It is the interaction among these systems that maintains the state of muscle control. It is highly likely, therefore, that various spinal, cortical, or limbic factors, which may have an adverse influence on this maintenance system, cause it to malfunction and permit the persistence of abnormal muscle contraction. This concept may eventually prove to be correct, but as yet, there is no hard evidence to support it.

There is a growing belief, at least among clinicians, that there may also be a central disturbance of neurotransmitter–receptor function or dysfunction of pain-modulating systems, resulting in the production of chronic head pain with a clinical appearance identical with that called muscle contraction headache. This thought is particularly enticing in relation to Raskin's article *Headache May Arise from Perturbation of the Brain* [6]. He described 15 patients, previously headache-free, who underwent electrode implantation in the periaquaductal gray and/or the somatosensory region of the thalamus, who immediately at the time of implantation, or within a few days thereafter, reported severe continuous head pain. In most of these patients, the headaches recurred or persisted for months to years. Although most of these headaches were interpreted by Raskin as resembling migraine, the important point to be gained from this article is the strong implication that the brain itself may contain headache-generating mechanisms.

It is probable, therefore, that muscle contraction headache, from the standpoint of etiology, does not occur as the result of a single malfunction. It may occur from sustained muscle contraction, from primary neuronal abnormalities, from neurotransmitter disturbances, from dysfunction of pain-modulating systems, or from any combination of these. These concepts are important in the considerations one must give to the various modalities that are used in the management of this disorder.

Acute and Muscle Contraction Headache

Muscle contraction headaches may be classified as acute or chronic. The acute type is common and, at some time, is experienced by almost everyone. It is mild to moderate in intensity. The pain involves the bilateral temporofrontal, vertex, or occipitocervical areas, either individually or in any combination. It is described as tight, pressing, squeezing, or aching sensations, and may be triggered by such things as fatigue, acute family crises, peaking of stressful workloads, or any other temporary stressful situation. It usually subsides following the cessation of the offending stimulus, or it may be relieved by various over-the-counter analgesics. Most patients with this variety of headache do not seek the services of a physician.

Chronic muscle contraction headache, on the other hand, presents with quite a different picture. Although the same areas may be involved as in the acute type, the pain itself is usually constant and unremitting, and may be present for weeks, months, years, or decades. The description of the pain characteristics are similar to those of the acute variety, but in addition, there may be feelings of soreness, weightlike sensation, tight bands, crawling sensations, and, occasionally, superimposed intermittent jabbing, stabbing, piercing components.

Such headaches may be seen in association with nasal or paranasal inflammation; temporomandibular joint dysfunction (perhaps better called myofascial pain dysfunction syndrome); disorders of the neck (e.g., degenerative arthritis, ankylosing spondylitis, and discogenic disease); local cranial inflammation secondary to systemic disorders (e.g., viral infection and lupus); after head trauma; and with high cervical or posterior fossa tumors. Most of these disorders can be diagnosed without difficulty. The large majority of muscle contraction headaches, however, are due to none of these disorders. They may be associated with anxiety, depression, repressed hostility, and so forth. However, it is by no means always clear, even in the obvious presence of these emotional symptoms, that they are the sole explanation for these headaches. Many chronic headache disorders are due to either the chronic use of analgesics or of ergot compounds. Most headaches that result from the chronic use of ergot compounds are migraine because, as a rule, ergot is used to treat intermittent migraine, which may then become chronic as the use of ergot approaches a daily or near daily occurrence. Nevertheless, some physicians [7] consider that this variety of chronic headache is best categorized as muscle contraction or mixed-type headaches, rather than migraine. The frequent or chronic use of analgesics can lead to a state of chronicity for the migraineur, but also can lead to the chronic variety of muscle contraction headache [8].

These various reasons will still leave a large group that will remain unexplained. It is this unexplained group that may ultimately be resolved by a further understanding of the central nervous system abnormalities that must certainly underlie in at least some who have this disorder. It is important to keep all of these concepts in mind when considering the management of chronic muscle contraction headache because pharmacotherapeutic agents that have no recognized muscle-relaxing effect are known to have therapeutic benefit in the treatment of this disorder.

MANAGEMENT

Withdrawal of Chronic Analgesic Use

If the patient is taking analgesics, it is first of the utmost importance to discontinue these before proceeding to the use of other medications. All analgesics are capable of perpetuating these headaches, whether they are bought over-the-counter or require a prescription from a physician. This includes aspirin, as well as acetaminophen [9–13]. It has not yet been determined whether or not the various nonsteroidal anti-inflammatory drugs (NSAIDs) are capable of contributing to this pain process, but there is some suspicion that they might.

When these patients are abruptly withdrawn from the constant use of analgesics, their headaches may temporarily exacerbate, normally for a period of 3–5 days, and then a diminution of the pain intensity usually begins; frequently, much to the surprise of the patient. During the initial withdrawal phase, no pain medication of any sort should be given, but ice compresses may be applied to the head or towels may be pulled tightly about the head. If nausea or vomiting occurs the use of suppositories of promethazine, prochlorperazine, hydroxyzine, or chlorpromazine may be useful. About the only analgesic that should not be withdrawn abruptly is one containing a short-acting barbiturate such as butalbitol (Phrenilin, Esgic, Fiorinal, Axotal Repan) and related compounds. Such abrupt withdrawal can precipitate a seizure. However, abrupt withdrawal can be accomplished; the physician should add, beginning at the time of withdrawal, 3 tablets of phenobarbital, 30 mg, at bedtime and decrease the dose by 1 tablet each week. Also, if birth control pills are being used, these should be discontinued, even though there does not appear to be any vascular component to muscle contraction. When birth control pills are continued, they may interfere with the therapeutic response of appropriate medication, and if there is no improvement, the physician will not know whether this is because of the birth control pills or a basic failure to respond to the chosen medication. Prophylactic medication may be started as soon as the patient agrees to stop the use of analgesics or birth control pills. To do so before this commitment on the part of the patient is to invite failure and frustration.

Pharmacotherapy

Antidepressants

There are many pharmacotherapeutic agents that are beneficial to the patient with chronic muscle contraction headache. Tricyclic antidepressants (Table 1) are the most effective of all pharmacotherapeutic agents used in the treatment of this disorder [1,15]. The effectiveness of these agents is not contingent upon the presence of concurrent depressive symptomatology [14]; hence, their mode of action, although not understood for the control of chronic muscle contraction headache, is not necessarily dependent on their antidepressant properties. Those tricyclic agents that have the most impact on the neuronal reuptake of serotonin and have a high degree of anticholinergic activity appear to be the most effective, but unfortunately, they also exhibit the most side effects. Amitriptyline or doxepin may be tried as a first-line choice, and the dose is usually given at bedtime to avoid the sedative effect, which normally will lessen by morning. The usual starting dose is 25 mg, which may be increased by 25 mg every third or fourth night. If needed, the dose can be increased as tolerated, to as much as

Table 1 Antidepressants

Generic name	Trade name	Dosage
Tricyclic agent,		
Amitriptyline	Elavil, Endep	50–150 mg in divided doses or at bedtime
Doxepin	Sinequan, Adapin	50–150 mg at bedtime
Fluoxetine	Prozac	20–60 mg in divided doses
Imipramine	Tofranil	50–150 mg in divided doses or at bedtime
Nortriptyline	Pamelor, Aventyl	50–150 mg in divided doses or at bedtime
Amoxapine	Asendin	150–300 mg at bedtime
Protriptyline	Vivactil	15–40 mg in divided doses
Desipramine	Norpramin, Pertofrane	75–150 mg in divided doses or at bedtime
Maprotiline	Ludiomil	75–200 mg in divided doses or at bedtime
Trimipramine	Surmontil	50–150 mg in divided doses or at bedtime
Trazodone	Desyrel	100–300 mg in divided doses or at bedtime
MAOI		
Phenelzine	Nardil	45–90 mg in divided doses
Tranylcypromine	Parnate	30–60 mg in divided doses

150 mg, although some patients may require more. Although a response may
be seen within the first week, it is not unusual for the maximum response to take
2–3 weeks.

Sedation, dryness of the mouth, constipation, cardiac irritability, and weight
gain are the most common unwanted side effects of many of the tricyclic compounds. However, patients should be monitored on a regular basis, because other
side effects can occur. The anxiety and frustration induced by excessive weight
gain could induce another trigger for maintaining the headache. Therefore, patients who have difficulty keeping their weight under control must be carefully
watched for excessive weight gain.

There are many tricyclic, or closely related, compounds that may be used,
and some, in certain patients, may be more effective and have fewer side effects
than others. These are imipramine, nortriptyline, maprotiline, trimipramine, amoxapine, protriptyline, desipramine, and trazodone.

Monoamine oxidase (MAO) inhibitors are useful for a small subset of individuals who prove to be completely resistant to the various combinations of tricyclic compounds and β-blockers. Phenelzine sulfate is the MAO inhibitor most often used. Physicians who prescribe this medication must be certain that they are very familiar with its properties because it has potentially serious side effects. In addition, it should never be given to a poorly compliant patient nor to one of less-than-average intelligence. When this medication is used with these comments in mind, and with appropriate restrictions, it is a generally safe medication.

Phenelzine sulfate was originally used for the treatment of severe migraine by Anthony and Lance [17] and later by others [18,19]. However, it is also effective in the treatment of chronic muscle contraction headache, and it may be safely employed with amitriptyline [20,21]. The combination of one of the β-adrenergic blockers, amitriptyline, and phenelzine sulfate may be used. The dosage of phenelzine is 15 mg three times daily. Occasionally, if there are no side effects, this dosage may be slowly increased to a maximum of 30 mg three times daily. If there has been no improvement in the headache after 3 weeks of this combination, then it should be discontinued because a longer trial is unlikely to prove beneficial. It must be remembered that the restrictions applied to phenelzine must be continued for a period of 2 weeks after the medication has been discontinued because of the risk of a reaction with inappropriate foods or medication is likely to persist for that period.

A hypertensive crises may occur if significant amounts of tyramine are ingested [22,23] while the patient is taking phenelzine. Therefore, the following foods must be avoided: chocolate, wine, beer, pickled herring, liver, dry sausage (including salami, pepperoni, and bolgna), fava bean pods, cheese, yogurt, yeast extract, spoiled, or improperly refrigerated protein-rich foods such as meats, fish, or dairy products. It is also essential to avoid any sympathomimetic drugs [24] that may be contained in nose drops, eye drops, or pills, whether bought over-the-counter or prescribed. This included sympathomimetics that may be used by dentists. Some analgesics, such as meperidine (Demerol) are also contraindicated. To be safe, patients taking phenelzine should be advised not to take any medication that is not cleared first with the physician who is prescribing phenelzine.

The most common side effects are orthostatic hypotension, insomnia, fluid retention and constipation; a few patients feel jittery and charged up and some may gain weight. In general, however, most patients tolerate this medication quite well, and the above mentioned combination may prove very beneficial to certain resistant chronic muscle contraction headache patients.

Beta Adrenergic Blockers

Beta adrenergic blockers are effective in the treatment of this disorder and the combination of these medications with the tricyclic compounds are more effective

Table 2 β-Adrenergic Blockers

Generic name	Trade name	Dosage
Propranolol	Inderal, Inderal LA	80–160 mg in divided doses or once daily
Nadolol	Corgard	20–160 mg in 2 divided doses or once daily
Timolol	Blocadren	20–40 mg in 2 divided doses
Atenolol	Tenormin	50–100 mg in 2 divided doses or once daily
Metoprolol	Lopressor	100–400 mg in 2 divided doses

than either drug used alone [16]. Propranolol was the first of these drugs to become available. The dose may vary from 20–40 mg given four times a day, or 60–160 mg given in long-acting form once daily. One should begin with the lower dose and increase as needed. There are contraindications to its use such as: asthma, heart failure, and Raynaud's phenomenon. Side effects include lethargy, dizziness, brachycardia, blurred vision, and decreased physical stamina. Sometimes short-term memory loss can be signficiant and may require that the medication be discontinued, but recovery is always prompt.

There are other β-adrenergic blockers that are beneficial, and, like the tricyclic compound discussed previously, some patients may respond better and have less side effects with some than with others. These are: nadolol, timolol, atenolol, and metoprolol. Several weeks use of these medications, are needed before determining that they are ineffective. The β-blockers can be combined with tricyclic antidepressants for more difficult headache patients.

Dihydroergotamine

In 1986, Raskin [25] reported on the successful use of repetitive doses of dihydroergotamine (DHE-45) in the treatment of migraine. This treatment has been almost as effective in the treatment of chronic muscle contraction headaches.

Table 3 Muscle Relaxants

Generic	Trade name	Dosage
Carisoprodol	Soma	350 mg 3–4 times per day
Chlorzoxazone	Parafon DSC	1 tablet 3–4 times per day
Metaxalone	Skelaxin	2 tablets 3–4 times per day
Cyclobenzaprine	Flexeril	1 tablet 2–3 times per day
Orphenadrine	Norflex	100 mg 2 times per day
Methocarbamol	Robaxin	750–1500 mg 2–3 times per day

For this therapy, patients need to be hospitalized for 3–5 days to receive intravenous DHE-45 every 8 hr, provided there are no contraindications to its use. The initial dose is 0.5 mg and, if this is satisfactorily tolerated, then the remaining doses are each 1 mg.

Calcium Channel Blockers

Although there are no published reports on the use of calcium channel blockers in muscle contraction headache, I have noted response in some patients when using these medications. This must mean, therefore, that either there are vascular components in this disorder that are not otherwise recognized, or these medications have actions that have not yet been defined. Nevertheless, when more conventional measures fail, a trial of verapamil or diltiazem may be warranted [26]. The control of headaches with the use of calcium channel blockers may be slow; therefore, one must not assume that a trial is ineffective until a period of 6–8 weeks has elapsed.

Muscle Relaxants

Muscle relaxants are sometimes effective, but are not as dramatic as their name might imply. Carisoprodol, cyclobenzaprine, chlorozoxazone, metaxalone, orphenadrine, and methocarbamol may be tried in some cases (Table 3). The muscle relaxants are given in divided doses and are tolerated by most patients. Fatigue is the most common adverse side effect.

Tranquilizers

Tranquilizers, such as diazepam, chlordiazoproxide, and meprobamate (Table 4), are of limited value in these headaches, but they have been shown to have a response better than that of a placebo [27]. There is a potential danger of habituation, as well as increasing the degree of underlying depression, and they should be used with appropriate caution. Fatigue is the most common side effect.

Table 4 Tranquilizers

Generic name	Trade name	Dosage
Alprazolam	Xanax	0.25–0.5 mg 3–4 times per day
Chlordiazopoxide	Librium	5–10 mg 3–4 times per day
Clorazepate	Tranxene	3.75–7.5 mg 2–3 times per day
Diazepam	Valium	5–10 mg 3–4 times per day
Lorazepam	Ativan	0.5–1 mg 3–4 times per day
Meprobamate	Equanil	5–10 mg 3–4 times per day
Oxazepam	Serax	10–15 mg 3–4 times per day
Prazepam	Centrax	5–10 mg 2–4 times per day

Table 5 Nonsteroidal Anti-Inflammatory Drugs

Generic name	Trade name	Dosage
Indomethacin	Indocin	75–150 mg in 3–4 divided doses
Ibuprofen	Motrin, Rufen	800–2400 mg in 3–4 divided doses
Tolmetin	Tolectin	600–1200 mg in 3–4 divided doses
Meclofenamate	Meclomen	200–400 mg in 3–4 divided doses
Naproxen	Naprosyn, Anaprox	250–375 mg in 2–3 divided doses
Piroxicam	Feldene	10–20 mg once daily
Fenoprofen	Nalfon	800–1800 mg in 3–4 divided doses
Sulindac	Clinoril	300–400 mg in 2 divided doses

Nonsteroidal Anti-Inflammatory Drugs

The nonsteroidal anti-inflammatory drugs have been shown to be effective in the treatment of acute muscle contraction headache (Table 5). However, some patients who suffer with chronic muscle contraction headache will benefit from continuous therapy. Indomethacin, ibuprofen, napoxen, fenoprofen, meclofenamate, tolmetin, piroxicam, or sulindac can be tried. Gastric irritation and ulceration are the most common side effects.

Biofeedback

Biofeedback training is a useful modality to employ in many patients with chronic muscle contraction headache [29–32]. Eletromyographic (EMG) feedback, general body relaxation, and finger-warming (thermal) techniques are utilized. A high level of motivation, an ability to concentrate, and a signficiant level of self-discipline to ensure daily practice of what is learned in the training program are prerequisites for a successful outcome. The purpose of biofeedback is to train patients to use their thought processes to overcome the physiological abnormalities that produce muscle contraction headache. Those who obtain good results may still require the use of prophylactic medication to maintain good headache control, but some can indeed reduce the use of such medications, and a fortunate few may need only the employment of their biofeedback training.

CONCLUSION

In the overall management of chronic muscle contraction headache, it is important that a strong effort be made to provide patients with an understanding of their headaches and to help them recognize that a concerted effort on the part of both the physician and the patient is essential to the ultimate resolution of their problem. A few patients may need counseling in addition to biofeedback and pharmacotherapy. It is generally agreed that emotional components may be a precipitant for these headaches, perhaps by the translation of anxiety into a physical symptom or a symbolic representation of psychiatric distress, and such patients may require a psychiatric referral. There are no published results, however, that establish the efficacy of this modality in the treatment of this disorder [33].

REFERENCES

1. Simons D, Day E, Wolff G. Experimental studies on headache: muscles of the scalp and neck as sources of pain. Assoc Res Nerv Dis 1943; 23:228–244.
2. Philips C. Tension headaches: theoretical problems. Behav Res Ther 1978; 16:249–261.
3. Pozniak-Patewicz E. "Cephalic" spasm of head and neck muscles. Headache 1976; 15:261–266.
4. Chusid JG. The neurologic basis of muscle tone. In: Correlative neural anatomy and functional neurology, 17th ed. Lange Medical Publications, 19xx:167–169.
5. Clark RG. Essential of clinical neuro-anatomy and neurophysiology, 5th ed. Philadelphia: FA Davis, 19xx:13–16.
6. Raskin NH, Hosobuchi Y, Lamb S. Headache may arise from perturbation of the brain. Headache 1987; 27:416–420.
7. Mathew NT Reuveni U, Perez F. Transformed or evolutive migraine. Headache 1987; 27:102–106.
8. Rapaport A, Weeks R, Sheftell F. Analgesic rebound headache: theoretical and practical implications. Cephalalgia 1985; 5(suppl 3):448–449.
9. Kudrow L. Paradoxical effects of frequent analgesic use. Adv Neurol 1982; 33:335–341.
10. Rapaport A, Weeks RE, Sheftel FD. The analgesic wash-out period, a critical variable in the evaluation of headache treatment efficacy [Abstract]. Neurology 1986; 36(suppl):100–101.
11. Henry P, Dartigues JF, Benetier MP. Ergotamine and analgesic induced headaches. In: Rose FC, ed. Migraine: proceedings 5th international migraine symposium, London. 1984:197–205.
12. Saper JR. Changing perspectives on chronic headache. Clin J Pain 1986; 2:19–28.
13. Saper JR. Drug treatment of headache: changing concepts and treatment strategies. Semin Neurol 1987; 7:178–191.
14. Lance JW, Curan DA. Treatment of chronic tension headache. Lancet 1964; 1:1236–1239.
15. Diamond S, Baltes BJ. Chronic tension headache treated with amitriptyline—a double blind study. Headache 1971; 11:110–116.
16. Mathew NT. Prophylaxis of migraine and mixed headache. A random controlled study. Headache 1981; 21:105–109.
17. Anthony M, Lance JW. Monamine oxidase inhibition in the treatment of migraine. Arch Neurol 1969; 21:263–268.

18. Raskin NH, Schwartz RK. Interval theory of migraine: long-term results. Headache 1980; 20:336–340.
19. Lance JW. The pharmacotherapy of migraine. Med J Aust 1986; 144:85–88.
20. Lader M. Combined use of tricyclic antidepressants and monoamine oxidase inhibitors. J Clin Psychiatry 1983; 44:20–24.
21. White K, Simpson G. The combined use of MAOIs and tricyclics. J Clin Psychiatry 1984; 45:67–69.
22. Blackwell B, Price J, Taylor D. Hypertensive interaction between monoamine oxidase inhibitors and foodstuffs. Br J Psychiatry 1967; 113:349–365.
23. Blackwell B, Mabbitt LA. Tyramine in cheese related to hypertensive crises after monoamine oxidase inhibition. Lancet 1965; 1:938–940.
24. Marley E. Monoamine oxidase inhibitors and drug interactions. In: Grahame-Smith DG, ed. Drug interactions. Baltimore: University Park Press, 1977:171–194.
25. Raskin NH. Repetitive intravenous dihydroergotamine as treatment for intractable migraine. Neurology 1986; 36:995–997.
26. Raskin NH. Tension headache. In: Headache, 2nd ed. New York: Churchill Livingstone, 1988:223.
27. Friedman AP. The treatment of chronic headache with meprobamate. Ann NY Acad Sci 1957; 67:822–827.
28. Friedman AP. Treatment of chronic headache. Int J Neurol 1962; 3:388–397.
29. Diamond S, Medina J, Diamond-Falk J. The value of biofeedback in the treatment of chronic headache. A 5 year retrospective study. Headache 1979; 19:90–96.
30. Beaty ET, Haynes SN. Behavioral intervention with muscle contraction headache. A review. Psychosom Med 1979; 41:165–180.
31. Bruhn P. Controlled trial of EMG feedback in muscle contraction headache. Ann neurol 1979; 6:34–36.
32. Budzynski T, Stoyva J, Adler C. Feed-back induced muscle relaxation: application to tension headache. Behav Ther Exp Psychol 1970; 1:205.
33. Dalessio DJ. Wolff's headache and other head pain, 4th ed. New York: Oxford University Press, 1980:377.

12

Treatment of Psychogenic Headache

Brian E. Mondell
Baltimore Headache Institute and
The Johns Hopkins University
School of Medicine
Baltimore, Maryland

> Listen to the patient. He is trying to tell you what is wrong.
>
> Sir William Osler

INTRODUCTION

Every physician recognizes that headache has both physical and/or psychological determinants [1-4]. An objective differentiation of these determinants is practically impossible because they are so closely interrelated. Therefore, when evaluating the patient presenting with headache, one must take into account not only the symptom of headache, but also the patient's psychodynamics. Many times the patient has a problem that he has tried to solve with an illness—headache. The symptom of headache permits him to complain; whereas, he was unable to complain about his true problem. In other instances, emotional factors play some part in perception and reaction to physiological pain. Therefore, psychogenic headaches are headaches resulting from delusional or conversion reactions in which peripheral pain mechanisms are nonexistent, or hypochondriacal or depressive states in which peripheral disturbances responsible for headache are minimally operational.

TERMINOLOGY AND DIAGNOSIS

Delusional Headache

Delusional headache represents the expression of psychiatric illness of psychotic proportion. In the psychotically depressed, the patient may be convinced—through a somatic delusional system—that headache is the result of a tumor or "decaying brains." In others, headache is perceived to be pain inflicted by demons, designed to punish them. Still others feel that headache is caused by incurable illnesses. Headache may also be a complaint in patients with schizophrenia. These patients believe that their head pains result from external influences, such as someone having control over their thoughts or poisoning them with external toxins. In schizophrenic patients, the mechanism is easily tied back to their underlying thought disorder. Whether the result of major depression or of defective thinking, such headache is well localized and bizarre in characterization. Typically, the patient localizes the pain with a single pointing finger. The pain is often accompanied by unusual sounds, such as banging, rattling, sputtering, and grinding. Psychotic thinking may thereby manifest itself in a delusional manner as this form of headache.

Conversion Headache

Conversion headache expresses a psychiatric stress or conflict. This physical complaint, lacking any organic cause, is the major symptom of an underlying psychiatric disorder. The expression of a psychological conflict or need, this disturbance, is not under voluntary control; the entire process occurs outside of awareness. The hallmark of a conversion reaction is the patient's apparent lack of concern for a symptom that, in others, would and should cause concern. Janet described this as "la belle indifference" [5].

An internal conflict or need may be kept out of awareness by onset or exacerbation of headache. Headache can also enable an individual to avoid potentially stressful or otherwise undesired activity. This physical pain represents the conversion or transfer from emotional disturbance to headache.

This type of psychogenic headache is often described in a very dramatic manner by a patient who typically is a young woman. Apparently, quite common several decades ago, conversion headache is not now as frequently encountered, and many cases are seen in men in military settings, particularly during times of warfare. Expansive gesticulations and mannerisms accompany the description of headache. The quality and location of headache vary, but consistently vivid, descriptive terms abound. The headache may be unrelenting and poorly responsive to any medical intervention. Characteristically, this patient denies emotional disturbance and downplays past psychological trauma. Moreover, the patient's affect does not coincide with the description of pain. In summary, despite bitter complaining, there is a satisfied indifference on the patient's part to conversion headache, thereby delaying proper diagnosis and effective treatment. Mental conflict, instead of being consciously experienced, is converted into the functional symptom of headache. The headache serves to allay a deeper anxiety, thereby giving way to a calmness in the patient's expression of his pain. It is when such an affective indifference exists toward a pain that is disabling—preventing employment and social integration—that the diagnosis of conversion headache can be made.

Hypochondriacal Headache

Hypochondriacal headache, sometimes referred to as anxiety headache, is induced by either worry or concern in patients with certain preexisting personality characteristics. Characteristically, they have a poor sense of self-worth and feelings of incompleteness, in which a sense of identity depends upon the presence of another. These inadequate, insecure, and passive self-perceived individuals complaining of headache turn to physicians. These patients are preoccupied with a fear or belief of having a serious disease, which persists despite medical reassurance. Such twisted thinking causes dysfunction in social activities and occupational performance. The nature, location, and duration of the pain vary from individual to individual. Associated symptoms of anxiety are universally present and include tachycardia, palpitations, hyperventilation, light-headedness, paresthesias, gastrointestinal distress, tension, and muscle aches, as well as fatigability.

Even though hypochondriacal headache is most often a psychoneurotic phenomena, it may reach delusional proportions. Moreover, hypochondriacal headache in adolescents or young adults may indicate an underlying thought disorder. Therefore, hypochondriacal headache can clearly be more than an obsessive preoccupation with physical disease.

Depression Headache

Depression headache, now ranking first among the psychogenic types of headache, is a psychobiological disorder, most probably related to diminished brain serotonin. This form of headache varies in all parameters, except for its persistent and intractable nature. Notwithstanding, patients often describe such headache as a general pressure that substantially interferes with all manner of physical and mental activity. Headache is worse in the morning and less pronounced later in the day. Accompanying phenomena, by definition, must include some combination of the following: poor appetite with significant weight loss or increased appetite with significant weight gain; alterations in bowel habits; insomnia or hypersomnia; psychomotor agitation or retardation; loss of interest or pleasure in usual activities in the social and work environment; decreased or increased libido; loss of energy; feelings of worthlessness; impaired attention and concentration; and suicidal thoughts. Clearly, headache and these vegetative symptoms represent a very common and painful disorder—depression headache.

TREATMENT

To successfully manage psychogenic headache, one must understand the relationship between mind, body, and environment. In patients with severe, recurrent headaches, psychological factors may be identified as primary etiologic factors that are treatable. Psychological aspects may, however, be difficult to discern because of biological variables; such as heredity, neurobiochemistry, and physical surroundings. It is essential to heed psychological aspects, as character may predispose to headache, crisis may precipitate headache, and conflict may aggravate headache. Psychological distresses of the mind, biochemical disturbances of the brain, and environmental stressors together, clearly cause head pain.

To treat this headache patient, one must perform a comprehensive psychological evaluation, as well as a detailed medical examination. An understanding of the patient's past experiences is needed to make sense of the presenting complaint of headache. A profile of the type of person suffering from head pain emerges from psychological developmental history in which one pays close attention to the patient's prior successes and failures at overcoming obstacles. This profile uncovers stressors that may be acting as precipitants of headache, as well as predisposition to headache.

Upon completion of a thorough history and physical examination, one can diagnose and initiate treatment. In the psychogenic headache patient, the diagnosis is benign, and this fact must be related to the patient in an assuring fashion to alleviate the patient's fear of serious disease. For those patients whose minds cannot be put easily at rest, one must establish an empathic, long-term relationship. Availability and genuine concern will permit one to learn more about the patient's ongoing headache status and psychodynamics.

An obstacle to successful treatment may be increased preoccupation with headache as a symptom and resentment to caregivers who must have missed "the correct diagnosis." Increasingly, some patients become morbidly absorbed in headache and related bodily disturbances. Beyond the subjective responses to headache, some objective behavioral manifestations occur and interfere with management. Patients overuse a variety of medications and withdraw from life. Additionally, marital or family strain results, accompanied by anger, guilt, and frustration, causing significant intrapsychic conflicts. Emotional and behavioral dysfunction coexist in psychogenic headache and must be addressed with psychotherapeutic interventions.

Also important in the treatment of major personality disturbances expressed as headache are a variety of psychotropic medications. These agents may be may be classified into neuroleptics, antidepressants, and anxiolytic sedatives (Table 1).

Table 1 Psychogenic Headache Medications

Generic name	Brand name	Daily dosage[a]
Neuroleptics (major tranquilizers)		
Phenothiazines		
Aliphatic		
Chlorpromazine	Thorazine	30–600
Promazine	Sparine	40–600
Piperidine		
Mesoridazine	Serentil	25–200
Thioridazine	Mellaril	50–400
Piperazine		
Fluphenazine	Prolixin	1–10
Perphenazine	Trilafon	4–20
Trifluoperazine	Stelazine	2–30
Miscellaneous allied compounds		
Thioxanthene		
Thiothixene	Navane	6–30
Butyrophenone		
Haloperidol	Haldol	1–10
Dihydroindoline		
Molindone	Moban	25–100
Dibenzoxazepine		
Loxapine	Loxitane	10–100
Antidepressants		
Tricyclic derivatives		
Amitriptyline	Elavil	20–300
Desipramine	Norpramin	25–200
Doxepin	Sinequan	25–300
Imipramine	Tofranil	30–300
Nortriptyline	Pamelor	30–100
Protriptyline	Vivactil	15–60
Tetracyclic derivatives		
Maprotiline	Ludiomil	50–200
Monoamine oxidase inhibitors		
Hydrazines		
Isocarboxazid	Marplan	10–30
Phenelzine sulfate	Nardil	15–75
Nonhydrazines		
Tranylcypromine sulfate	Parnate	10–30
Lithium salts		
Lithium carbonate	Eskalith	600–1500

(continued)

Table 1 *(continued)*

Generic name	Brand name	Daily dosage[a]
	Cerebral stimulants	
Methamphetamine	Desoxyn	2.5–10
Methylphenidate	Ritalin	10–30
	Novel antidepressants	
Amoxapine	Asendin	50–250
Fluoxetine	Prozac	20–80
Trazodone	Desyrel	50–300
	Anxiolytic agents (minor tranquilizers)	
	Carbamate derivative	
Meprobamate	Equanil	600–1600
	Diphenylmethane antihistamine derivative	
Hydroxyzine	Atarax, Vistaril	50–200
	Benzodiazepine derivatives	
Alprazolam	Xanax	1–4
Chlordiazepoxide	Librium	10–100
Clorazepate	Tranxene	15–60
Diazepam	Valium	2–40
Lorazepam	Ativan	2–8
Oxazepam	Serax	30–90
	Antianxiety with antidepressants	
Perphenazine/ amitriptyline	Triavil 2/10, 4/10 2/25, 4/25, 4/50	3–4 tablets
Benactyzine/ meprobamate	Deprol	3–4 tablets
Chlordiazepoxide/ amitriptyline	Limbitrol 5/12.5, DS	3–4 tablets

[a]All dosages are in milligrams (mg) unless otherwise stated.

Neuroleptics

Neuroleptics modify psychotic behavior and are major therapeutic agents that have the capacity to modify affective states without significantly impairing cognitive functioning. Not only do they modify behavior through their reaction upon the central nervous system, but they also affect the functioning of the extrapyramidal tracts and the autonomic nervous system. They principally act as dopamine-blocking agents. Representative members of the neuroleptics include phenothiazines, butyrophenones, thioxanthenes, dihydroindolines, and dibenzoxazepines.

Phenothiazines

Of all neuroleptics, phenothiazines have the largest role in the treatment of psychogenic headache. The fact that the aliphatic and piperidine series are more sedating than the piperazine series may or may not be desirable. The piperazine group contains the more potent compounds which, however, are more likely to cause parkinsonism or other basal ganglia dysfunction.

With the use of phenothiazines, there is a disruption in activities regulated by the hypothalmus. Thermoregulation is impaired; adrenocorticotropic hormone (ACTH) secretion is diminished; and growth is reduced. Another endocrine effect is the lowering of urinary gonadotropins. In women, libido and ovulation may be decreased. Infertility often occurs, and there may even be untimely lactation. In men, plasma testosterone may be lowered.

Other disturbances arise from the use of phenothiazines. Orthostatic hypotension may occur; therefore, caution should be exercised in using these medications in patients with atherosclerotic heart disease or any condition in which a sudden drop in blood pressure would be dangerous. In addition to postural hypotension, the cholinergic effects and dopaminergic-blocking effects may provoke electrocardiographic changes and even ventricular tachyarrhythmias. Skin reactions occurring in patients treated with phenothiazines include photosensitivity, abnormal skin pigmentation, and occasionally jaundice. Although infrequent, blood dyscrasias may occur. Other important toxicological reactions include the extrapyramidal syndromes—parkinsonian akathisia, and tardive dyskinesia. Finally, sudden death could occur as a result of neuroleptic malignant syndrome.

Antidepressants

Tricyclic Antidepressant Agents

Chemically related to phenothiazines are tricyclic antidepressants. They act by diminishing cellular permeability, thereby reducing the reuptake of norepinephrine and serotonin at the synaptic cleft, thus increasing the action of these neurotransmitters. Limbic structures may be stimulated. Resultant change in mood and behavior becomes noticeable, usually after 2 or 3 weeks of therapy.

Tricyclic antidepressants should be continued at a maintenance level after clinical improvement has occurred because symptoms may recur with premature withdrawal.

Tricyclic antidepressants have, for the most part, minor side effects. Dry mouth and difficulties in accommodation are frequently encountered. In the elderly and otherwise sensitive individuals, dizziness, tachycardia, and postural hypotension may occur. Caution should be exercised in prescribing these agents if there is a history of glaucoma or urinary retention. Rarely, have incoordination, tremor, and convulsion been noted. Overusage, however, may bring about excessive anticholinergic blockade, leading to agitation, delirium, choreoathetosis, myoclonus, hyperpyrexia, and coma.

Monoamine Oxidase Inhibitors

In addition to tricyclic compounds, monoamine oxidase inhibitors are important antidepressants. Both the hydrazine and nonhydrazine derivatives increase the amount of intraneuronal serotonin and catecholamine neurotransmitters, such as epinephrine, norepinephrine, and dopamine, by inhibiting the activity of the enzyme monoamine oxidase. Obviously, then, in employing these medications, a diet low in vasoactive substances must be followed, and similarly sympathomimetic medications must be restricted to avoid a hypertensive reaction. A therapeutic response may be accompanied by the common side effects of hypotension expressed as dizziness or fainting. Additionally, constipation and peripheral edema are common. Anticholinergic effects, such as dry mouth and blurred vision, may be seen. Otherwise, clinically desired central nervous activation may be accompanied by hyperreflexia, tremors, insomnia, restlessness, and even hypomania.

Lithium

Besides tricyclic compounds and monoamine oxidase inhibitors, lithium salts represent another antidepressant medication. Modifications of brain amine metabolism by lithium are responsible for its therapeutic response. Lithium inhibits the release of norepinephrine and serotonin, increases the reuptake of norepinephrine, and increases synthesis and the turnover rate of serotonin. There is little effect on dopaminergic systems. Additionally, lithium alters the concentrations of α-aminobutyric acid and glutamate. Lithium also increases cortisol excretion, modifies aldosterone excretion, and lowers protein-bound iodine. Toxic symptoms of lithium include nausea, abdominal cramps, vomiting, diarrhea, polydypsia, polyuria, coarse tremors and muscle twitching, ataxia, slurred speech, and lethargy. Convulsions, coma, and even death may ensue from significant disturbances of electrolyte balance with resultant cardiac and pulmonary dysfunction.

Antidepressants are, indeed, complex and diverse pharmacologic drugs. In addition to tricyclic compounds, monoamine oxidase inhibitors, and lithium salts, some other drugs that affect biogenic amines, with resultant antidepressant effects, include cerebral stimulants—for example, amphetamine derivatives and methlyphenidate—as well as the newer, more novel agents such as fluoxetine.

Anxiolytics

The final group of psychotropic medications used to treat psychogenic headache are those therapeutic agents classified as anxiolytics. Representative members of anxiolytic sedatives include carbamates, antihistamines, and benzodiazepines. Unlike neuroleptics, they do not pharmacologically affect the extrapyramidal or the autonomic nervous systems. As a group, anxiolytics are indicated for the treatment of psychogenic headache in which anxiety and neuromuscular tension are evident. Although carbamates and diphenylmethane antihistamines have been more prominent, benzodiazepines are now more frequently used. They act by reducing the turnover of norepinephrine and serotonin and elevate brain choline and acetylcholine. Even though these medications generally are particularly safe to prescribe, tolerance and significant withdrawal reactions may occur. Drowsiness or hyperactivity, mood alterations, impaired concentration, ataxia, and dysarthria may occur. Prescribed normally, respiratory depression, hypotension, hypothermia, or coma rarely occur.

β-Blocking agents may also alleviate anxiety states operational in psychogenic headache. Both central and peripheral mechanisms of action have been suggested to explain such a beneficial effect. Peripheral blockade, however, of symptoms of anxiety seems to be the more important mechanism.

Treatment Guidelines

The selection of appropriate psychogenic headache medication(s) depends upon the nature of the psychopathology of the individual patient. The dosage and type of drug(s) will be varied depending upon the individual patient's tolerance. Treatment of psychogenic headache must be individualized, but the following guidelines do apply.

In treating delusional headache, one employs phenothiazines or allied compounds and the selective use of antidepressants, while exploring through psychotherapy the disordered thinking in this psychotic state. In treating conversion headache, antianxiety and antidepressant medications serve as a useful adjunct to facilitate supportive and dynamic psychotherapy for the primary psychiatric condition. In treating hypochondriacal headache, one must avoid the trap of symptomatically treating individual headaches. Instead, one must carefully design and rigidly follow a program of insight-oriented treatment and cotherapy with some combination of major or minor tranquilizers, α-adrenergic blockers, and antidepressants. In treating depression headache medical management with tricyclic compounds, tetracyclic agents, monoamine oxidase inhibitors, some of the newer, more novel antidepressants, direct cerebral stimulants, and perhaps lithium carbonate combines well with psychotherapy to attack the underlying problem—depression.

For optimal therapeutic response, one should utilize all modalities—one or more psychoactive drugs and a good physician–patient relationship permitting effective psychological intervention directed specifically at the underlying cause of psychogenic headache.

REFERENCES

1. Adler CS, Adler SM, Packard RC. Psychiatric aspects of headache. Baltimore: Williams & Wilkins, 1987.

2. Ad Hoc Committee on Classification of Headaches. Special report. JAMA 1962; 179:717–718.
3. American Psychiatric Association. Diagnostic and statistical manual of mental disorders, 3rd ed, rev. Washington, DC: American Psychiatric Association, 1987.
4. Headache Classification Committee of the International Headache Society. Classification and diagnostic criteria for headache disorders, cranial neuralgias and facial pain. Cephalalgia 8(suppl 7).
5. Janet P. The major symptoms of hysteria. New York: Macmillan, 1920.

13

Pharmacologic Therapy for Headaches in Children

Gerald S. Golden
Boling Center for Developmental Disabilities
University of Tennessee
Memphis, Tennessee

INTRODUCTION

Headache is one of the three most common neurological complaints in children seen in an ambulatory setting, being surpassed in frequency only by seizure disorders and problems of behavior and learning. The onset of recurrent or chronic cephalgia in a child is an unsettling experience for the family because they are certain that the child has either a severe, life-threatening illness or that he or she is using imaginary symptoms to control those about him or her. The first step in treatment, after establishment of an appropriate diagnosis, is achieving a level of understanding on the part of the family that will ensure their cooperation in the therapy program.

DIFFERENCES IN THE TREATMENT OF PEDIATRIC HEADACHES

Several issues complicate the treatment of headaches in the pediatric-aged group [1,2]. First, a specific diagnosis may be more difficult to achieve than in an adult. Migraine in preadolescent children, and especially in the preschool-aged group rarely has a classic pattern. The headaches are typically bilateral, unaccompanied by prominent gastrointestinal symptoms, and unassociated with an aura. As the child becomes older, classic symptoms of migraine begin to evolve. The diagnosis can be aided by a search for associated features, such as a family history of migraine, nocturnal awakening with cephalgia, headaches that are present in the morning, and a tendency for attacks to cluster in time. Complicated migraine may present with major neurological signs and little or no headache, although the diagnosis usually is clearer as the child becomes older. Migraine equivalents are more common in children than in adults, and always present a difficult diagnostic problem. Further increasing the clinical complexity of headaches in children is that the pattern typically changes over time. This often necessitates revision of the initial diagnosis, but will generally clarify the diagnostic problems.

A second difference between children and adults is the smaller role that psychological factors play in the origin and maintenance of headaches in the pediatric-aged group. Psychological symptoms usually develop because of the chronic pain, rather than being the causal agent [3,4]. Depression presenting as chonic headaches does occur in children, but is much less common than in adults.

A third issue relates to the use of pharmacologic agents in treatment (Table 1). Many useful drugs have not been approved for children under 12 years of age; even fewer are approved for patients under 6 years of age. This generally means that the manufacturer has not carried out the studies needed to obtain approval, not that the drug represents any specific hazard for children. There are no legal constraints on the use of these medications in patients in a specific aged group. Any approved medication can be used for an unlabeled indication, if necessary [5]. The practitioner should make a full explanation of the drug's status to the family, and document this thoroughly in the patient's chart.

An additional problem with the use of unapproved drugs is that there often is inadequate information concerning pharmacodynamics in children. This makes it difficult to calculate an appropriate dose and timing schedule. In addition, there may be side effects that are peculiar to the pediatric-aged group and have not been previously reported. In general, children 12 years or older can take standard adult doses of most medications.

There is a reluctance to use certain groups of drugs in children. Strong analgesics, such as narcotics, are rarely prescribed because of their high addiction potential. Drugs such as methysergide maleate, which have been associated with serious long-term side effects, are also prescribed infrequently.

TREATMENT

Strategies Prior to the Use of Medication

There is a popular belief that many headaches in children are caused by eyestrain. This situation is actually quite rare, although the child with severe hyperopia may fatigue after reading for a prolonged period. The myope does not have this

Table 1 Drugs for Headaches in Children

Drug	Dose	Daily maximum	Approved	Pediatric form
Symptomatic treatment				
Aspirin	7–10 mg/kg	30–65 mg/kg	Yes	Chewable
Acetaminophen	5–7 mg/kg	30–40 mg/kg	Yes	Liquid
Ibuprofen	200–400 mg	1200–3200 mg	No	None
Codeine	0.75–1 mg/kg	4 mg/kg	Yes	None
Propoxyphene	0.5–0.75 mg/kg	2–3 mg/kg	Yes	None
Abortive treatment				
Isometheptane mucate	65–130 mg	260–520 mg	No	None
Ergotamine tartrate	1–6 mg	10 mg/wk	No	None
Prophylactic treatment				
Propranolol	10–80 mg	160–240 mg	Yes	None
Cyproheptadine	2–4 mg	4–16 mg	Yes	Syrup
Amitriptyline	10–25 mg	40–100 mg	No	None
Ergonovine maleate	0.2 mg	0.4–0.6 mg	No	None
Antinauseants				
Trimethobenzamide	100–200 mg	400–800 mg	Yes	Suppository
Prochlorperazine	2.5–5 mg	7.5–15 mg	>2	Suppository
Metoclopramide	2–10 mg	10–15 mg	Yes	Syrup

problem. Other conditions of the eyes, ears, nose, throat, and sinuses rarely, if ever, cause chronic headaches in children. More specific symptoms of the underlying condition should be present, and the child and family can be spared a costly and time-consuming laboratory evaluation if there is no other clinical evidence of disease.

The issue of dietary precipitation of migraine in children is even more controversial than it is in adults. It is important to avoid restricting the child's diet unnecessarily and, rather than empirically restricting certain foods or classes of foods, the family should keep a headache and food diary. This will allow the determination of any correlation with diet. The lay public, and many physicians, are convinced that hypoglycemia is a common cause of headaches. Reactive hypoglycemia is rare in children, if it exists at all. If hypoglycemia is documented, the child requires a detailed evaluation for several serious metabolic and endocrine disorders.

Other headache triggers are also unusual in childhood. The most common is exercise. If this a major problem, it is better to treat the child prophylactically with medication than to restrict sports and other forms of strenuous exercise.

Symptomatic Therapy

Analgesics, such as salicylates and acetaminophen, are often effective for relieving the pain of both muscle contraction headaches and mild or moderate migraine
headaches in children, and they are the first-line drugs to be used for symptomatic
therapy [6,7]. Aspirin can be given in a dose of 7–10 mg/kg every 3–4 hr for
two to three doses. Children are less likely to have gastric irritation than are adults,
and it is not usually necessary to use buffered or enteric-coated preparations, unless
there is a personal or family history of peptic ulcer disease or the child complains
of abdominal discomfort. A chewable 80-mg pediatric tablet is available. Treatment with aspirin should not continue for more than 1 or 2 days, to prevent the
development of toxicity. There is some controversy concerning the role of aspirin
in the development of Reye's syndrome, and therefore, its use should be avoided
if the headache is an accompaniment of influenza or varicella [8].

Acetaminophen is used in doses of 5–7 mg/kg every 3–4 hr for two to three
doses. It is safe to give the second dose within 2 hr of the first, as long as a daily
dose of 30–40 mg/kg per day is not exceeded. Acetaminophen is available in a
liquid preparation, 160 mg/5 ml, making it useful for younger children. This drug
has virtually no side effects in therapeutic doses.

Ibuprofen, 200 mg every 4–6 hr is also an effective analgesic, although the
tablets are not scored, and it is difficult to use in patients under the age of 12
years. The drug has not been approved for use in children. Ibuprofen cross-reacts
with salicylates, and should not be used in a patient who is sensitive to aspirin.
It can also produce gastric irritation.

There are several proprietary drugs that are mixtures of caffeine, a short-
to intermediate-acting barbiturate, and either aspirin or acetaminophen. These
are useful if simple analgesics do not provide sufficient relief of pain, although
caution should be used when prescribing barbiturates to children. It is advisable
to set a limit on the number of pills that can be taken for a single headache or
during a week. If the pain continues, or is very severe, codeine 0.75–1 mg/kg
every 4–6 hr or propoxyphene hydrochloride 0.5–0.75 mg/kg every 6 hr may
be used. These drugs are often combined with aspirin or acetaminophen. Most
pediatricians avoid the use of strong natural or synthetic opioids in all but the
most unusual situations.

Vomiting may be a severe accompaniment to migraine. If it is a problem
that is serious enough to require more than symptomatic treatment, suppositories
of trimethobenzamide or prochlorperazine can be used. One or two trimethobenzamide suppositores can be given to children who weigh more than 15 kg, and
repeated in 6 hr if needed. The dose of prochlorperazine for children weighing
more than 20 kg is 2.5–5 mg by suppository. Metoclopramide is also a potent
antiemetic, but must be given parenterally if nausea and vomiting are present.
Children over 6 years of age can be given 2–10 mg intramuscularly. Unfortu-

nately, the incidence of acute extrapyramidal reactions with these drugs is higher in children than in adults; consequently, they should be used only if necessary to prevent dehydration. These side effects can be treated with the intravenous administration of 25-50 mg of diphenhydramine hydrochloride.

Abortive Therapy

The use of abortive therapy in children presents a number of special problems. Classic migraine is unusual before adolescence, and in the absence of an aura, there is no opportunity to take medication before the pain begins. The child may not be able to differentiate which headache will be severe and require abortive therapy, and which will respond to less potent analgesics. Young children cannot take independent responsibility for carrying medicine with them and taking it in an unsupervised setting; therefore, it may not be available when it is needed. Some schools cooperate with the physician, and a treatment plan can be developed; in other cases, the school may be unwilling to take responsibility for administration of any drug but aspirin.

Isometheptene mucate, a sympathomimetic agent, is useful for older children with migraine. Proprietary preparations include a mild sedative and acetaminophen or caffeine and acetaminophen. The patient can take the adult dose of two capsules initially followed by one capsule every hour to a total of five capsules. It is difficult to treat children under 8-10 years of age, as only the adult form is available. Some children may have feelings of anxiety after taking several doses.

If the patient does not have an adequate response to isometheptane mucate, but the headaches are severe and clearly vascular, ergotamine compounds are the drugs of choice. These are available in any one of a number of formulations, some of which also contain barbiturates, caffeine, and belladonna alkaloids in various combinations. The preparations containing belladonna alkaloids are useful for children because they help reduce the vomiting that may be part of the headache or induced by the ergot compound. The physician should become comfortable with an oral preparation and one which can be given by suppository. An inhaler that administers a dose of 0.36 mg with each inhalation is now available. The adult dose is up to six inhalations per attack and up to 15 a week, but a recommended dose for children has not been determined. Cardiovascular side effects of ergot compounds are rare in children. The major problem is sedation caused by the barbiturate.

Most of these compounds are not available in pediatric formulations; therefore, the dose must be reduced appropriately. The usual limit for adults of 4-6 mg of ergotamine for a single headache, and 10 mg/week should be converted to the equivalent dose for the child. These medications are not commonly used for children under 6 years of age.

Prophylactic Therapy

There is a natural reluctance to treat children with any medication for long periods; consequently, prophylactic therapy is used less frequently than when treating adults. The first indication is the presence of repeated severe headaches, especially if they interfere with the child's function at home, in school, or with peers. A second indication is the presence of complicated migraine that is accompanied by major neurological abnormalities before or during the headache.

It is difficult to document the effectiveness of prophylactic therapy, because migraine tends to be a cyclic disorder, with periods of spontaneous remission. Prensky and Sommer reported that one-half of children with migraine had a 50% reduction in headache within 6 months, irrespective of the treatment used [9].

Propranolol is widely used as a prophylactic agent in adults, and it is now being used commonly in younger children [7,10]. This drug may be particularly useful for patients with complicated migraine. The usual plan is to start with doses as low as 10 mg twice a day and to gradually increase the dose until a therapeutic response is obtained. This may require as much as 160-240 mg daily and take 4-6 weeks. A long-acting preparation may be effective given daily. Side effects, such as lethargy, significant bradycardia, and postural hypotension, are rarely troublesome. The drug should be avoided or used with caution in children with asthma because it may precipitate respiratory problems. If high doses are being administered, propranolol should always be discontinued gradually in step-wise fashion. There has been one report that this drug is no more effective than placebo, and that it might lengthen the duration of headaches, but this needs to be documented more completely [11].

Cyproheptadine has both antihistamine and antiserotonin effects. This has become a popular medication in the armamentarium of pediatricians, despite little or no published data documenting its effectiveness and the fact that treatment of headache is not an approved indication. A dose of 4 mg two to four times daily is used. The most common side effects are sedation and increased appetite with excessive weight gain.

Tricyclic antidepressants, particularly amitriptyline, are useful in treating chronic headaches in adults [12]. Although there is not a significant association between depression and headache in preadolescent children, amitriptyline appear to have some usefulness. It is useful for children who are clinically depressed, especially if there is a family history of bipolar depressive disorder. The drugs have also been recommended for those children in whom headaches are present on awakening or are associated with sleep disturbance [2]. An initial dose of 10 mg at bedtime can be increased until a therapeutic result is obtained, side effects supervene, or a maximum dose of 40-100 mg/day is reached. Other psychotropic drugs and anxiolytic agents, rarely used in children.

There also has been little published experience concerning the use of calcium channel blockers in children. In adolescents, the same drugs and doses can be used as are prescribed for adults. Because new compounds are being introduced regularly, no specific recommendation would remain current.

Long-term prophylactic administration of ergot derivatives is not used commonly in children, having been replaced by propranolol and cyproheptadine. If other drugs are not effective, a trial of ergonovine maleate, in a dose of 0.2 mg two or three times daily must be useful.

Abnormalities on the electroencephalogram (EEG) are commonly found in children with migraine, especially those patients who are refractory to the usual therapeutic modalities and are referred to a pediatric neurologist. In this selected subgroup, nearly 25% of children have paroxysmal abnormalities, although many of these patients have never had a seizure [9,13]. It has become common practice by some clinicians, for this reason, to prescribe anticonvulsants for children with refractory headaches. In many cases, this is done even if there are no abnormalities on the EEG. There is little or no documentation that this approach is any more effective than the administration of placebo. There does, however, appear to be a specific entity of headache as a seizure manifestation. These headaches are diffuse or bifrontal, start abruptly, and are typically associated with nausea and vomiting [14]. Treatment with anticonvulsants appears to be effective in these patients.

The most commonly used anticonvulsants are phenytoin and carbamazepine. Phenytoin therapy is begun at a dose of 4–5 mg/kg per day. The desired blood concentration is 10–20 μg/mg. Dose related side effects include ataxia and, rarely, sedation. An occasional child will have a hypersensitivity reaction with a rash; this requires discontinuing the drug. Carbamazepine is begun at a dose of 100–200 mg daily and increased to a level of 20–30 mg/kg per day, attempting to achieve a blood concentration of 6–12 μg/ml. Barbiturates should be avoided, because of the high incidence of adverse effects on cognition and behavior.

Methysegide maleate, a potent antiserotonin agent, is an effective prophylactic agent for migraine in adults. Because of the potential for severe side effects, such as retroperitoneal fibrosis, it is rarely used in children and adolescents. Therefore, there is little information available concerning an appropriate dose schedule, duration of therapy, or protocol for monitoring for the development of side effects.

Cluster headaches rarely occur before late adolescence. Treatment is the same as in adults, with methysergide maleate, propranolol, prednisone, and lithium being effective in individual patients [2]. The dose and dosage schedule is the same as that recommended for adults.

Nonpharmacologic Therapy

Personality and behavior problems do not appear to be important precipitating causes of migraine in childhood. It appears that the recurrent pain and social disability from the headaches have an influence on these psychological factors, and those children with more severe headaches are more likely to be adversely affected [3]. Although children with migraine are not more stressed or anxious than their peers, children with headaches respond to normal levels of stress and anxiety with this symptom rather than other physical complaints [4].

Biofeedback and other relaxation techniques appear to be effective in some children and adolescents with either muscle contraction or migraine headaches. Olness et al. reported that self-hypnosis was more effective in treating migraine than either placebo or propranolol [15]. This work needs to be replicated before being incorporated into routine management.

CONCLUSION

Chronic or recurrent headaches in children raise a great deal of anxiety in the child and the family. It is important that this aspect of management not be neglected and that sole reliance not be put on pharmacologic management [1]. The first step is to assure the family, following a careful history and neurological examination and any special studies that are indicated, that the child does not have serious neurological disease. It is important to then help them accept that the child does, in fact, have headaches and that this is a common problem in childhood and adolescence. Many parents feel that if the child does not have a neurological disorder, the complaint of headache is not valid. A quick cure should not be promised. Although all children will have a remission of their symptoms, exacerbation in the future is to be expected. The parents and child should be prepared for this eventuality. Finally, the parents should be helped to feel comfortable in not providing excessive secondary gain to the child, and not allowing him or her to use the symptoms to manipulate the persons in his environment.

REFERENCES

1. Golden GS. The child with headaches. Dev Behav Pediatr 1982; 3:114–117.
2. Gascon GG. Chronic and recurrent headaches in children and adolescents. Pediatr Clin North Am 1984; 31:1027–1051.
3. Cunningham SJ, McGrath PJ, Ferguson HB, Humphreys P, D'Astrous J, Latter J, Goodman JT, Firestone P. Personality and behavioural characteristics in pediatric migraine. Headache 1987; 27:16–20.
4. Cooper PJ, Bawden HN, Camfield PR, Camfield CS. Anxiety and life events in childhood migraine. Pediatrics 1987; 79:999–1004.
5. FDA Drug Bulletin. Use of approved drugs for unlabeled indications. 1982; 12:4–5.
6. Golden GS. Management of headaches in children. Nurse Pract 1987; 12:38–44.
7. Drugs for migraine. Med Lett 1984; 26:95–96.
8. Arrowsmith JB, Kennedy DL, Kuritsky JN, Faich GA. National patterns of aspirin use and Reye syndrome reporting, United States, 1980 to 1985. Pediatrics 1987; 79:858–863.

9. Prensky AL, Sommer D. Diagnosis and treatment of migraine in children. Neurology 1979; 29:506–510.

10. Rosen JA. Observations on the efficacy of propranolol for the prophylaxis of migraine. Ann Neurol 1983; 13:92–93.

11. Forsythe WI, Gillies D, Sills MA. Propranolol (Inderal) in the treatment of childhood migraine. Dev Med Child Neurol 1984; 26:737–741.

12. Couch JR, Ziegler DK, Hassanein R. Amitriptyline in the prophylaxis of migraine. Neurology 1976; 26:121–127.

13. Guidetti V, Fornara R, Marchini R, et al. Headache and epilepsy in childhood: analysis of a series of 620 children. Funct Neurol. 1987; 2:323–341.

14. Swaiman KF, Frank Y, Seizure headaches in children. Dev Med Child Neurol 1978; 20:580–585.

15. Olness K, MacDonald JT, Uden DL. Comparison of self-hypnosis and propranolol in the treatment of juvenile classic migraine. Pediatrics 1987; 79:593–597.

14

Headaches in the Elderly

Frederick G. Freitag
Diamond Headache Clinic and
University of Chicago
School of Medicine
Chicago, Illinois

INTRODUCTION

In the elderly patient with headache, drug therapy represents a special and complex problem for the clinician. Although headache disorders, such as migraine and muscle contraction headache, usually occur in the prime of life, these headaches may continue to occur or even begin de novo within this age group. Standard therapies may be helpful for these patients. However, other therapies may be more appropriate for them. Also, adjustments in the dosage of pharmacologic agents may be indicated because of alterations in drug metabolism that are associated with aging. Finally, certain headache disorders are usually present only in older individuals and, therefore, need to be specifically addressed.

MIGRAINE, CLUSTER, AND MUSCLE CONTRACTION HEADACHES

Epidemiological Considerations

A detailed evaluation of the epidemiological considerations of headache disorders has been presented elsewhere in this text. However, headaches should be examined specifically relative to their occurrence and resolution in the later years of life. Other medical factors involved with their occurrence must also be considered.

Several epidemiologic surveys of headache and neurological disorders have been conducted. Waters [1], in a survey of British general practitioners, found an annual incidence of headache between 53 and 66%, in the aged group from 55 to 74 years. These findings were a sampling from the Welsh community of Pontypridd, which also demonstrated a 53% annual incidence of headache in this aged group. Further evaluation of these populations revealed that unilateral headaches occurred in between 37 and 49%. In vascular headache patients, especially migraineurs, there was a warning of an imminent headache occurrence in 19–26% of those surveyed. Associated symptoms of nausea or vomiting occurred in 25–30% of the population.

Ziegler and associates [2] surveyed a group of 1809 nonmedical volunteers. In their study, they found a lower prevalence for headache than had Waters. In the 55–64 aged group, the incidence of headache was only 15%, but increased to 21% in the aged group over 65. Within these aged groups, severe or disabling headaches occurred in fewer than 2% of this population.

In a New Zealand study, the prevalence of headache in older adults [3] declined progressively with age. In the ages from 50 to 59, slightly more than 30% of men, and a fraction under 50% of women, experienced headache. In the next 10-year bracket, the incidence in men was about 25%, and slightly under 40% of women continued with headaches. By the age of 70 and older, however, the prevalence had declined to approximately 20% in males and 30% in females. Interestingly, the rate at which these individuals experienced their headaches demonstrated a higher frequency of attacks with increasing age.

A recent study [4] of the incidence of headache was determined by reviewing the rates of diagnosis according to the diagnosis-related groups (DRG) classification for Medicare patients. Two classifications involve these types of headaches. The category of DRG 24 relates to seizure and headache occurring in the ages 70 and older, and DRG 25 for the same diagnosis for those under aged 70. Complications and comorbidity factors are included for DRG 24, but are not contained in DRG 25. The 4-year incidences for these two DRG groups were between 39 and 48%. These results were dependent on the community studied for DRG 24, and between 4 and 7% for DRG 25 for the two different communities.

Kaganov and co-workers [5] examined the occurrence of various symptoms of headache that they attributed to either a vascular or musculoskeletal etiology in different aged groups. In the 55- to 79-year-old group, the incidence of musculoskeletal symptoms with headache had remained fairly constant, occurring in approximately 14% of their population. Associated symptoms of vascular headache had declined to fewer than 12% of patients.

Goldstein and Chen [6] reported several studies that examined the incidence of migraine headache. The incidence of migraine between the ages of 55 and 64 ranged from 2 to 19.2% of men and 4.5 to 29.1% of women. After aged 65, the incidence dropped to 0.6-12.7% of men and 1.3-22.9% of women.

In the later years of life, the first occurrence of various headache types progressively diminishes with advancing age. Lance [7] found fewer than 5% first occurrence rate for migraine in those individuals aged 50-60. The rate decreased to a lower rate, with no new occurrence of migraine in the 70 year olds. However, he found that the initial onset of tension headache developed until the age of 80, although it diminished from a 10% frequency in the 50 year olds to fewer than 5% in those in their 70s. Similarly, initial onset of cluster headache decreased in frequency from approximately 6% in the 50s to about 1% in the 60s, and no initial onsets in the 70s.

Blau [8] conducted a survey to determine the age at which migraine ceased and the reasons for its resolution. In 52 patients who met the criteria for migraine headache, and had been free of their attacks for at least 3 years, 19 reported migraine remission in their 50s, 13 in their 60s, and the final 6 in their 70s. The average age of cessation was 55.5 years after an average migraine history of 33 years. A variety of factors were identified, by patients as significant in obtaining a remission of their migraine attacks. Eleven patients related psychological factors as the reason, nine dietary avoidance, and 13 the occurrence of menopause, either surgically induced or natural occurrence. Five patients treated for concomitant diabetes mellitus or hypertension, identified medical therapies as contributing to the cessation of their migraine attacks. Only ten patients did not identify a cause for their migraine remission. Various other measures were also identified. A vascular etiology for migraine headache was suggested by the occurrence of stroke in young patients, with no other risk factors other than a history of migraine, and the increased risk of complications of angiography in patients with migraine headache [9]. Because of these factors, Waters and colleagues [10], predicted a higher mortality among patients with migraine headache. In their study of 1310 women, between the ages of 45 and 64, however, they found that the mortality was lower in those with a history of headache. Analyses for the cause of death in headache patients compared with those without headache, and further comparison with those in whom the headaches had migrainous features, revealed a higher mortality from cancer, ischemic heart disease, and cerebrovascular accidents in nonheadache subjects. Cerebrovascular accident as a cause of death occurred in 3.3% of subjects without a history of headache, and in 2.2% of those whose headaches had at least two associated migrainous features.

Several studies have attempted to evaluate risk factors or changes in human physiology associated with aging that may provide clues to headache in the elderly. Hale and his colleagues [11] studied 1284 persons in a health-screening program in Florida. They found an 11% prevalence of headache in women and a 5% in men. No correlation was found between the occurrence of headache and age. Systolic or diastolic blood pressures, use of coffee, alcohol, or tobacco, time spent viewing television, and sleep were found to be factors. There was a 5.4% lower incidence of headache in subjects who obtained at least 7 hr of sleep a night than in those who slept less than 7 hr. In women, a correlation was noted between the likelihood of having headache and the total number of other diseases or bodily symptoms experienced by an individual. In this group the headaches were usually generalized or frontal in location, with 18% of women and 21.4% of men describing their headaches as occurring on only one side.

In contrast, Serratice and his group [12] observed that headache sufferers were less likely to consume tobacco, alcohol, or coffee. Subjects with headache were also more likely to live in poorer housing conditions and to exercise less regularly.

Previous work has demonstrated alterations in serum enkephalins in migraine and cluster headache [13,14]. Genazzani and his colleagues [15] have demonstrated that in midlife, serum β-endorphin levels continue to show a trend to peak levels, then subside with advancing age. However, cerebral spinal fluid endorphin levels show a progressive decline from the early years of life through old age. It has not been determined if these changes in endorphins cause the changes in the occurrence of vascular or other headaches with age.

Treatment

The nature of these headache disorders is usually of major consequence during the prime years of life. Therefore, well-controlled trials of various therapeutic agents for conditions have focused on the age group from 18 to 60 years. No specific studies have been undertaken to evaluate treatment within the older-aged groups who continue to experience headaches. Aging causes alterations in cardiac, renal, and central nervous system function. These changes may significantly affect the treatment of headaches. Evaluation and selection of therapeutic agents, abortive and prophylactic treatment of headaches may need to be modified. Various treatments for migraine, cluster, and muscle contraction headaches have been reviewed in entirety in other sections of this book. Concomitant medical conditions in the later years of life occur more frequently; consequently further considerations in the selection of drug therapies should include the use of agents that may be useful to treat several conditions simultaneously.

The development of atherosclerotic changes of the arterial system occurs with the normal aging process. The restriction of blood flow may lead to the development of cerebrovascular disease as it contributes to headache in the elderly. It may also trigger the onset of ischemic heart disease and hypertension and its accompanying complications, including alteration in renal function. Decreased exercise tolerance as a result of atherosclerotic disease may occur because of changes in heart function, with diminished cardiac output and angina pectoris associated with exertion. Intermittent claudication from atherosclerotic narrowing of the peripheral arterial circulation to the legs may also develop.

Diabetes mellitus, whether insulin-dependent or controlled with oral hypoglycemics, also may have a bearing on the selection of agents for headache treatment. Complications of diabetes mellitus on the vascular system may exacerbate atherosclerotic changes previously noted. Renal disease may result from the complications of diabetes mellitus or atherosclerotic disease involving the renal arteries. With increasing age, a general decrease in the function of the glomerular filtration system in the kidneys occurs, resulting in a general impact on the metabolism of many pharmaceutic agents.

Metabolic changes accompanying the aging process may lead to the development of osteoporosis. Although this condition of itself if not directly linked with headache, its treatment with estrogen may complicate and contribute to migraine headache. Occult thyroid disease may be seen in the elderly, and the typical myxedematous symptoms of thyroid disease, such as fatigue, weight gain, and hair loss, may not be seen. However, headache may occur as a symptom of the hypothyroidism, which may be detected only by abnormalities in results from laboratory studies of thyroid function.

Pulmonary function partially declines as a result of aging. The use of tobacco, however, may accelerate this process and lead to complications, such as chronic bronchitis, which may have therapeutic implications for the treatment of headache.

In the occurrence of cerebrovascular disease and the headache that may accompany it, other neurological ramifications of aging may be observed. Parkinson's disease often occurs within this aged group and may represent part of the involutive changes accompanying aging. Certain medications that may have an influence on this condition, may also cause headache [16]. Ophthalmologic disease, such as glaucoma, occurs more prevalently in this aged group. Many medications used in the treatment of headaches, such as the antidepressants, may have an effect on glaucoma.

Degenerative changes involving the cervical spine or temporomandibular joint, may produce headaches. Arthritis present in other joints should be considered in the selection of a therapeutic agent.

Abortive Therapy

The selection of an abortive agent for migraine headache may become more limited within the geriatric population. The ergotamine preparations (Cafergot, Wigraine), although extremely beneficial in the treatment of acute migraine headaches, may be contraindicated because of the development of atherosclerotic disease. The vasoconstrictive effects exerted by these agents may lead to vascular complications. These complications may be manifested as acute anginal episodes or resting claudication. More severe complications may also occur, eventually producing complete vascular occlusion and its ramifications. The use of ergot preparations in those patients with evidence of atherosclerotic disease should be avoided. In general, the use of ergot preparations in this aged group is to be avoided because atherosclerotic disease may be occult, and the risk of precipitating an acute complication from the ergotamine agent is greater.

For an alternative abortive agent, isometheptene mucate (Midrin) is used frequently for acute migraine episodes. This agent does not appear to carry the risks of the ergotamine preparations. However, isometheptene has sympathomimetic actions that hamper its use in patients undergoing treatment for hypertension.

In the treatment of muscle contraction headache, the use of muscle relaxants may be beneficial. These agents have sedating effects, which may be manifested greatly in the elderly patient. Additionally, the use of orphenadrine citrate (Norflex) is restricted in those patients with glaucoma, because of the drug's anticholinergic effects, which could further elevate intraocular pressure.

An effective modality for the abortive treatment of cluster headaches is the use of 100% oxygen, delivered by a face mask, for periods of 10–15 min. In most elderly patients, this therapy would be indicated. However, in patients with significant pulmonary disease, this particular use of oxygen could lead to suppression of the central nervous system driving mechanism on respiration. Appropriate assessment of pulmonary function and arterial blood gas levels should be obtained before initiation of this mode of treatment for patients with cluster headache and clinical evidence of pulmonary disease.

Prophylactic Therapy

In the elderly patient with headache, many of the traditionally recognized methods of treatment may be restricted. It is, therefore, appropriate to consider prophylactic therapy in patients who are disabled by their headaches or in whom the attacks frequently occur. A variety of agents have been useful in reducing the frequency and severity of migraine, cluster, and muscle contraction headaches. Selection of the pharmaceutic agent for treatment of these headaches is based on the same considerations for the elderly as for other headache patients.

In migraine prophylaxis, the β-adrenergic blocking agents remain the standard therapy for most patients. The mechanism by which these agents reduce the frequency and severity of migraine headaches is not understood. These agents are also beneficial in the treatment of hypertension and cardiac disease. Agents such as propranolol (Inderal) and metoprolol (Lopressor) may also improve the outcome of myocardial infarction and prevent the occurrence of repeat infarctions. The membrane-stabilizing effects of propranolol and other β-blockers may also be of clinical benefit for those patients with some forms of cardiac dysrythmias. However, it is well recognized that those β-blocking agents that have the additional pharmacologic action of a partial β-agonist are not useful in migraine prophylaxis.

Propranolol, nadolol (Corgard), metoprolol, atenolol (Tenormin), and timolol (Blocadren), have demonstrated positive clinical benefits in migraine. From clinical experience, these agents also appear beneficial for the elderly patient with migraine. In a study by Avorn and associates [17] concern was raised about the use of the β-adrenergic blocking agents in the elderly. These researchers noted an increased use of the antidepressant agents in patients receiving β-adrenergic blocking agents compared with patients receiving other unrelated medical therapeutic agents. However, their research was seriously criticized in subsequent reports [18].

The calcium channel antagonists may also be useful in the prophylactic treatment of migraine headache and, possibly, in chronic cluster headache. In some patients, these agents have been successfuly used in angina pectoris, hypertension, cardiac arrhythmias, and possibly the variant form of angina, Prinzmetal's angina. Of those agents currently available in the United States, only verapamil (Calan, Isoptin) has consistently proved beneficial for migraine. In those patients with cardiac migraine, a migraine equivalent syndrome, which may present with variant angina, verapamil may be the treatment of choice. Current research is ongoing with an experimental calcium channel antagonist, flunarizine. This drug appears to be devoid of cardiovascular effects, although it may be useful as a prophylactic agent for migraine. The use of this agent in the elderly must be undertaken with caution because high doses of a generic preparation of flunarizine resulted in the development of parkinsonian symptoms in several patients.

The antidepressant agents are useful for the treatment of both the depressive disorders and a variety of pain-related disorders, including migraine, muscle contraction headaches, and the mixed headache syndrome. The antidepressants may be divided into several classes. The tricyclic antidepressants are the oldest, most-recognized, and most-utilized agents. This group amitriptyline (Elavil), doxepin (Adapin, Sinequan), protriptyline (Vivactil), and imipramine (Tofranil). The second group of antidepressants are the monoamine oxidase inhibitors (MAOIs), including phenelzine (Nardil) and isocarboxazid (Marplan). The third group of agents is heterogeneous and includes chemically unique agents that are modifications of the basic tricyclic molecule, such as the bridged tricyclics and tetracyclics, but also includes drugs that are chemically unrelated to this basic moiety, such as trazodone (Desyrel) and fluoxetine (Prozac).

The tricyclic agents are generally effective in reducing the frequency and severity of migraine and muscle contraction headaches, occurring individually or combined. Their mode of action to relieve headache and other pain complaints is not understood. However, it may include direct analgesic effects, or it may relieve depression, which manifests itself as headache. These agents possess characteristics that are similar pharmacologically in their actions on the neurotransmitters. However, the action on these sites vary in degree. These differences account for the variations in adverse effects associated with tricyclic use. All of these agents possess anticholinergic effects, which contraindicate their use in patients with increased intraocular pressures.

In the elderly, these same anticholinergic effects may also contribute to constipation problems and difficulty initiating the urine stream; these difficult special problems exist for those patients who have concomitant prostatic hypertrophy. The anticholinergic effects may also contribute to central nervous system complications because the elderly appear to be more sensitive to these effects and may develop dementia secondary to their use. The cardiovascular toxicities associated with tricyclic use are in the form of increased risk of cardiac dysrythmias. Of the tricyclics, doxepin appears to have the widest safety margin for cardiac complications. However, doxepin also has significant sedative and antihistaminic effects that may contribute to increased appetite and weight gain, thereby seriously affecting patients with concomitant diabetes mellitus.

Initiation of tricylic agents in this aged group should be undertaken with caution. After carefully selecting a tricyclic agent for the treatment of headache, especially after consideration of any other complicating medical conditions, the patient should be started on therapy with the smallest dosage of the agent. An adequate trial time to allow the patient to adapt to the agent should be allowed before increasing the dose. Younger patients may only require several days to adapt to therapy; as long as several weeks, may be necessary for the older patient. In spite of these precautions, many older patients will poorly tolerate these agents and may rapidly discontinue therapy. A close patient–physician relationship should be developed and frequent contact with the patient is essential during initiation of the tricyclic antidepressant therapy if the patient is to continue on a pharmacologic regimen for reduction of their headaches.

For those patients who are unable to take tricyclic agents because of complicating medical conditions, a nontricyclic antidepressant may be useful. Trazodone appears to be well tolerated by many older patients with headache. It has less cardiotoxic risk than the tricyclics and minimal anticholinergic effects. Trazodone, and the recently developed agent fluoxitine, are highly specific for the serotonergic system and are often well tolerated, compared with the tricyclic antidepressants. However, fluoxitine is very stimulating and may produce insomnia in some patients. In contrast, trazodone is often extremely sedating, which some patients may find disturbing.

The MAOIs, such as phenelzine and isocarboxazid, may be well tolerated and effective in many elderly patients with headache. The use of the MAOIs should be reserved for those patients who have failed to respond to more standard therapies, or who are unable to tolerate the other antidepressants, either because of concomitant medical conditions or intolerable side effects. These patients must be capable of compliance with the dietary and medical restrictions associated with safe MAOI use. Diamond and colleagues [unpublished study] observed that the MAOIs were more effective in older patients than in younger patients with similar headache complaints. Because of the blood pressure-lowering effects of the MAOIs and other adverse reactions, initiation of treatment should be accomplished within an inpatient setting dedicated to headache patients.

Other medical therapies may also be useful in the treatment of headache in the elderly, including the nonsteroidal anti-inflammatory agents (NSAIDs). The NSAIDs have demonstrated useful effectiveness in the abortive and prophylactic therapy of migraine headaches and, possibly, in the prevention of cluster headache. In some cases of migraine, clonidine hydrochloride (Catapres) has also proved useful. It acts as an α-agonist agent and, through its central action on the adrenergic system, appears to exert an antihypertensive effect. Initiation of this agent must be undertaken cautiously in the elderly, as it may produce a profound orthostatic hypotension. If clonidine is stopped abruptly, significant reflex hypertension may ensue.

The drug therapy of migraine, muscle contraction, and cluster headache, may continue into the later decades of life. Because the occurrence of other concomitant medical conditions is more common in this aged group, the selection of prophylactic and abortive agents for headaches requires a more comprehensive medical evaluation before initiating therapy. Possible complications that may develop in these other medical conditions must be considered. Because the elderly are more likely to be under treatment for these conditions, the treatment plan must include methods to reduce the number of drugs required by these patients. Because drug metabolism is reduced during the normal aging process, lower doses of drugs may be indicated to avoid drug interactions that may occur during treatment of patients with multiple medical conditions.

OTHER CAUSES OF HEADACHE IN THE ELDERLY

A variety of medical conditions may cause or exacerbate headache in the elderly, including giant cell arteritis, cerebrovascular ischemic disease, heart disease, ophthalmologic disease, and degenerative joint disease. The progressive degenerative changes involving the joint spaces and ligaments associated with cervical spondylosis and temporomandibular joint arthritis, can lead to the development of muscle contraction headaches. The occurrence of these physiological changes may also contribute to chronic muscle contraction headache or to other causes, such as depression.

Cervical spondylosis is usually found on radiological studies. In the later years of life, this condition may be asymptomatic [20]. In 40% of cases of symptomatic spondylosis, headache may be a presenting symptom. Headache caused by spondylosis may arise from the involved apophyseal joints or from associated muscle spasm. Osteophytic pressure on vertebral arteries and nerve roots has also been cited as a possible contributing effect on this condition. Rheumatic conditions, such as rheumatoid arthritis and ankylosing spondylitis, may also involve the cervical spine and contribute to muscle contraction headache, similar to cervical spondylosis.

In the elderly, treatment of arthritic conditions, which may cause headache, requires evaluation and assessment of the etiologic components causing the headache. Determination of whether the headache results from reflex muscle spasm, depressive manifestations, or cervical spondylosis, must be clarified to select an appropriate treatment regimen for the patient. The use of antidepressants or muscle relaxants, or both, may be indicated. A variety of NSAIDs may be selected in the treatment of cervical or temporomandibular joint spondylosis. In selection of an NSAID for this condition, the following factors should be considered: previous response to NSAIDs, complicating medical conditions such as peptic ulcer disease, and patient compliance with the drug regimen. Because the NSAIDs at any given dosage, may require up to 3 weeks to exert notable benefit, the patient should be instructed to allow a sufficient trial to thoroughly assess a drug's clinical benefits.

The anti-inflammatory agents may be divided into three major classes. The carboxylic acids, oxicams, and pyrazole derivatives. The carboxylic acid derivatives may be further subdivided into the salicylates, acetic acid derivatives, propionic acids, and the fenamates [21]. All of these agents exert at least a portion of the anti-inflammatory effect through inhibition of cyclooxygenase. The dosage regimens of these agents vary considerably (Table 1).

The analgesic, phenacetin, was linked to development of interstitial nephritis. Subsequent studies have suggested that the salicylates and NSAIDs may also be linked to changes in renal function [22]. Studies with aspirin have produced variable results in assessing changes in renal function associated with long-term ingestion of aspirin [23,24]. Other diseases, such as rheumatoid arthritis and systemic lupus erythematosus, may affect the outcome of these renal function studies. The NSAIDs have been implicated in renal function including edema, increased serum potassium levels, acute renal failure, nephrotic syndrome, and papillary necrosis [25]. Several studies involving large patient groups failed to document a signficant contribution to renal disease from the NSAIDs [26]. In patients with mild renal disease, the use of sulindac (Clinoril) may be preferred to ibuprofen (Motrin, Rufin) [27].

Gastrointestinal complaints related to aspirin and the NSAIDs are common. These agents have been associated with blood loss, even with episodic use. Gastrointestinal bleeding and ulcer formation may also occur with NSAID therapy. However, the risk of developing gastrointestinal bleeding from aspirin has been evaluated in approximately 15 cases per 100,000 patients per year, who use aspirin at least 4 days a week. Similarly, the risk of developing gastric ulcer from aspirin use is approximately 10 cases per 100,000 per year. The author [28] indicates that the incidence of complication from aspirin use is four to eight times lower than the risk of developing thrombophlebitis from oral contraceptives. The incidence of this complication has been calculated to be an acceptable safe risk rate of 60 cases per 100,000 per year.

Table 1 Nonsteroidal Anti-inflammatory Drugs (NSAIDs)

Classification	Name	Route of administration	Dosage
Benzothiazine	Piroxicam	Oral	20 mg QD
Indoles	Indomethacin	Oral	25 mg BID to 50 mg QID
		Sustained release	75 mg QD to BID
		Rectal	50 mg QID
	Sulindac	Oral	150–200 mg BID
	Tolmetin	Oral	400 mg BID to QID
Propionic acids	Fenoprofen	Oral	600 mg BID to QID
	Ibuprofen	Oral	300 mg BID to 800 mg QID
	Naproxen	Oral	250 mg BID to 500 mg BID
	Ketoprofen	Oral	50 mg BID to 75 mg TID
	Flubiprofen	Oral	50 mg BID to 100 mg TID
Anthranilic acid	Meclofenamate	Oral	100 mg TID
Salicylates and related drugs	Acetylsalicylic acid	Oral	325–1300 mg BID to QID
	Choline magnesium salicylate	Oral	750 mg to 1500 mg BID
	Salsalate	Oral	500 mg to 750 mg TID
	Diflunisal	Oral	250 mg to 500 mg BID
	Diclofenac	Oral	50 mg BID to 75 mg TID

Compliance problems with medical regimens are well known in clinical practice for all aged groups. In the elderly, patient compliance with multiple drugs, used to treat multiple conditions, is especially important because the patients may require multiple doses per day.

Glaucoma may develop at any age, although it becomes more prevalent in the elderly. Visual problems may develop with a slow increase in the intraocular pressure headaches. However, symptoms are unlikely to occur until sustained intraocular pressure of 70–80 mmHg is attained. The headache or orbital pain may be minimal. However, if acute-angle closure glaucoma develops with a rapid rise in the intraocular pressure, severe eye pain and headache may ensue if the intraocular pressure attains 40–50 mmHg. Treatment of these conditions includes the use of topical preparations, such as the miotics and β-adrenergic blocking agents, to reduce the intraocular pressure. Oral carbonic anhydrase inhibitors may also begin to block the production of the aqueous humor. Surgical intervention may be necessary to effectively treat glaucoma.

Hypertension and its treatment may also cause headache in the elderly. Several medications used to treat hypertension are known to trigger headache. Vasodilators, such as hydralazine and the calcium channel antagonist nifedipine, are useful antihypertensives, but frequently precipitate headache. The old standards of hypertension therapy, reserpine and methyldopa, have fallen out of popular use. These agents have long been identified as headache precipitants, possibly through the development of depression and the headache associated with this disorder.

Hypertension is an uncommon cause of headache. Traub and Koreyn [29] found nocturnal and early-morning headaches more prevalent in those patients with hypertension for whom the blood pressure readings were in excess of 170 mmHg systolic, or 110 mmHg diastolic. However, these results were not statistically significant. Disappearance of the headache and the degree of decrease in blood pressure did correlate with treatment. Generally, the occurrence of headache was less common, regardless of the degree of elevation of blood pressure, in individuals beyond the age of 50. This phenomena has repeatedly been observed in elderly patients with headache.

With advancing age, the occurrence of ischemic heart disease and other cardiac diseases may occur. In the treatment of ischemic heart disease, the standard of therapy for acute attacks of angina has been nitroglycerin. Many patients treated with this agent report the occurrence of headache after its use. Nitroglycerin is also known to precipitate acute attacks of cluster headache. With the initiation of treatment, long-term use of nitroglycerin therapy to minimize the occurrence of angina related to ischemic heart disease is common. The headache associated with nitroglycerin use is often mild, transient, and tends to diminish with continued daily use of nitroglycerin. However, the headache condition may require alternative treatment for ischemic cardiac disease, such as the β-adrenergic blocking agents or calcium channel antagonists, to reduce the frequency of anginal attacks.

Headache as a manifestation of angina in ischemic heart disease has been reported by Fleetcroft and Maddocks [30]. The cited case reported episodes of headache that could occur independently or associated with chest pain. The headache attacks were often precipitated by activities, such as climbing stairs or moving from a warm to a cold room. In this patient, treatment with nifedipine and nitroglycerin resulted in amelioration of the headaches.

The implantation of pacemakers may be required in the treatment of certain cardiac diseases associated with arrhythmias. Several cases of headache have been reported by individuals after pacemaker implantation. Das [31] reports on a younger patient who developed headache following implantation of a VVI-type pacemaker. The headaches were severe, episodic, and frontal, lasting from minutes to hours and subsiding gradually. They were not associated with activity. Other symptoms were absent, and the physical and neurological examination were normal. Electrophysiological studies of the pacemaker function revealed the headaches occurred during pacemaker activity with venticular atrial pacing. Replacement of the pacemaker with an AV sequential pacemaker resulted in cessation of the headaches. A subsequent report of headache discussed a patient with an AV sequential pacemaker [32]. This patient developed a chronic full–headed–type headache after implantation of this category of pacemaker. The headache was unrelated to other symptoms or activities. The development of headache in the elderly after pacemaker implantation may require cardiac electrophysiological evaluations and possible changes in the pacemaker to resolve the headache.

CEREBROVASCULAR DISEASE AND HEADACHE

Several studies have examined the relationship between cerebrovascular disease and headache [33–35]. These studies found varying degrees of headache incidence related to transient ischemic attacks (TIA) and stroke. In TIA, the incidence ranges from 17% to as high as 64.7% of patients presenting with headache as one of the complaints. The occurrence of headache associated with TIA also varied with location. In carotid versus vertebrobasilar location, the headache complaint was more common with a carotid location of the ischemic event. In ischemic events culminating with stroke, considerable variation has been reported in the incidence of headache associated with the event, ranging from 17% for lacunar infarcts to as high as 57% with parenchymal hemorrhage, with 25–30% of patients complained of associated headache. Although generalization may be made about location and associated neurological characteristics associated with these headaches, there are more exceptions than rules.

The pathophysiology of headache associated with TIAs is not completely understood. Edmeads [36] has advanced a hypothesis for these headaches that is associated with platelet aggregations and the subsequent release reaction associated with platelet degranulation. This release reaction, leading to the production of prostaglandins and serotonin, has been previously associated with migraine headache.

Therapy for TIA may utilize one of several pharmacologic approaches, as well as surgical therapy. Anticoagulants have been evaluated in several studies and have been previously [37] reviewed. Few studies have exercised well-controlled study methodology to gauge the benefits of anticoagulants in the prevention of stroke in patients with TIA. In general, the use of anticoagulants tends to show a slightly improved risk of suffering from ischemic stroke. However, these benefits are more likely observed during the months immediately after the TIA. The use of anticoagulants, however, was found to greatly increase the risk of intracranial hemorrhage. The inappropriate use of anticoagulants with excessively prolonged prothrombin times was not demonstrated. However, correlation was found with the use of anticoagulants beyond 1 year and, in particular, in those elderly patients with hypertension.

Antiplatelet agents have also been examined in this same context [38]. Three different agents have been studied, including aspirin, sulfinpyrazone, and dipyridamole. The outcome evaluation parameters of ischemic stroke or death did not demonstrate any clinical benefit with dipyridamole, some positive benefits have been observed with sulfinpyrazone. A short-term study, over 12 weeks, demonstrated signficant reduction in the frequency of TIA events with sulfin-pyrazone, 80 mg/day, compared with placebo, and improved survival rates in patients with a history of previous stroke treated with 600 mg/day. A long-term study of sulfinpyrazone, however, failed to show any clinical benefit in reduced mortality. Several studies have examined the role of aspirin in treating TIA. These studies have suggested a possible small benefit to accrue from the use of aspirin in patients with TIA, in which stroke, occurrence of other TIA events, or death were used as end points. Positive results were found more likely to occur in male normotensives whose TIA symptoms were multiple in occurrence, and whose symptoms were specific for the involved artery.

In patients who experience stroke, depressive symptoms may occur during the recovery phase. The use of the antidepressant, trazodone, has been demonstrated as effective for increasing the level of activity in patients with ab-normal Zung Self-Rating Scores for depression or patients with a clinical diagnosis of depression. Patients who did not meet these criteria had similar levels whether taking trazodone or placebo [38].

In patients who experience headache as a manifestation of TIAs there is little evidence to suggest that anticoagulant therapy or the use of platelet-inhibiting agents, except aspirin, has any benefit in reducing the morbidity or mortality associated with these events. The hypothesis of Edmeads [36] may explain the occasional observation of those whose migraine headaches clinically improved with these agents. The low risk of significant adverse events related to the use of these medications may possibly make them beneficial for use in the elderly in reducing headache associated with cerebrovascular disease.

GIANT CELL ARTERITIS (TEMPORAL ARTERITIS)

In headache and other symptoms associated with a tender distended nodular artery, the diagnosis can be confirmed with laboratory evidence of inflammatory disease, such as an elevated sedimentation rate by Westergren method and temporal artery biopsy. However, atypical presentations in headache characteristics, such as loca-tion, absence of headache, occurrence of other presenting symptoms not involv-ing the head, and normal sedimentation rates, are frequently reported in the medical literature. Negative biopsy findings may occur because of skips in the lesion of the affected artery.

The use of corticosteroids remains the standard treatment for giant cell arteritis. Aggressive therapy with these agents should be initiated immediately after the clinical diagnosis is suspected and a sedimentation rate is obtained. Delaying therapy by awaiting biopsy results may lead to increased risk of complications, such as blindness, from this disease. A number of studies have been conducted that reviewed the results of treatment with corticosteroids in this disease and the occurrence of complications related to their use.

In a review article, Gerber [39] has recommended the use of 0.5 mg/kg per day of prednisone (Deltasone) or its equivalent such as prednisolone or methylprednisolone (Medrol). If the patient fails to respond, or if the sedmentation rate is not decreased by at least 50% within 2 weeks, the dosage should be increased. A decrease in the dosage of steroids can be accomplished in 5-mg decrements, based on the patient's clinical picture and sedimentation rate. The dosage can be maintained at 5–15 mg/day of prednisone.

Allen and Studenski [40], in their review, recommended prednisone 40–60 mg/day, in divided doses, for initiation of therapy. In patients acutely ill with disease, 60–80 mg/day of methylprednisolone succinate (Solu-Medrol), parenterally administered, is recommended. Doses of up to 500 mg of this agent should be administered intravenously over 1 hr if the patient presents with a sudden onset of blindness. However, no study has ever demonstrated the reversal of blindness by therapy. If a patient failed to respond to the initial dose of steroids, increased dosages of prednisone, up to 100 mg/day, may be administered. The initial dosage level of prednisone should be continued for at least 3–6 weeks, when resolution of the clinical symptoms and the sedimentation rate normalizes. A progressive tapering by 10-mg decrements every 2–4 weeks may be undertaken until the prednisone dosage is 40 mg/day. At dosages of 40 mg, decreasing to 20 mg of prednisone, the dosage should be similarly decreased but by 5-mg and 2.5-mg decrements, over similar periods, until a maintenance dosage of 5–7.5 mg/day is achieved. This dosage level should be continued for at least several months, at which time 1 mg every 1–3 months can be undertaken, with total treatment extending over periods of at least 6 months and up to 2 years.

A 25-year study of 42 patients with temporal arteritis [41] found that relapses of the disease occurred in 11 patients. Only one patient was taking at least 7.5 mg of prednisone per day and seven patients had discontinued corticosteroid therapy. Eventually, 33 patients discontinued therapy and were followed for periods up to 19 years. Twenty-three of the patients were treated for 1 year or less with steroids, and 14 underwent therapy no longer than 7 months. Dosages of prednisone in excess of 20 mg/day were used for an average of 2 months.

Similarly, Koorey [42] followed 27 cases during a 20-year period. Dosages of 40–80 mg/day of prednisone were given initially, and 2.5–10 mg/day was the maintenance dosage. Treatment was continued for an average of 22 months. In most patients, early withdrawal of corticosteroids resulted in relapse.

A long-term Swedish study of 90 patients revealed that longer treatment periods were used [43]. These patients were followed for periods up to 16 years from the time of diagnosis. The average length of treatment was 5.8 years. At 5 years after diagnosis, 43% were still receiving corticosteroid therapy, and 15% continued to receive treatment at 9 years after diagnosis. Maintenance doses of 1.25–10 mg of prednisolone were used in these patients. Relapse occurred in 50% of the cases when steroid therapy was withdrawn, regardless of the length of active treatment. Almost all relapses occurred within the first year after discontinuation of treatment, and nearly 50% experienced the relapse within the first month after treatment termination.

Complications of corticosteroid therapy are common and may depend on the dose and length of treatment. Up to 50% of patients will experience a complication [40]. The most common complication is compression fracture of the vertebrae. Other complications include myopathy, cataracts, and exacerbation of diabetes mellitus. More serious complications related to the use of corticosteroid therapy are rare. The use of calcium carbonate 1–1.5 g/day, along with 50,000 units of vitamin D twice a week, may help reduce the osteoporotic complications of steroid therapy.

Alternative treatments to the corticosteroids have been suggested, including cyclophosphamide (Cytoxin), azathioprine, chlorambucil (Leukeran), and methotrexate. Only one controlled trial has been undertaken in the treatment of patients with polymylagia rheumatica, giant cell arteritis, or both conditions [44]. The study involved 31 patients studied for 1-year. The patients received a titrated dose of prednisolone, based on clinical response, and were given either placebo or azathioprine 100–150 mg/day. No statistically significant difference in the dosage of prednisolone required by the patients was noted during the course of the study until the final evaluation period at 52 weeks. These results suggest a possible steroid-sparing effect of azathioprine in the treatment of giant cell arteritis.

Corticosteroids are considered the treatment of choice for giant cell arteritis, although alternative therapies may need to be considered in selected patients. The initial therapy should be aggressive to prevent the complications related to giant cell arteritis, requiring a minimum of 40 mg/day of prednisone or its equivalent. Once a satisfactory clinical response has been achieved, partially determined by the normalization of the sedimentation rate, a gradual tapering of the dosage of steroid to a low maintenance dosage of about 10 mg/day, may be accomplished in most patients without a flare-up of the disease. In general, the treatment should be continued for at least 6 months in the absence of clinical evidence of the disease. Prolonged therapy, in excess of at least 1 year, may be necessary in these patients. Preventive therapy with calcium carbonate and vitamin D may help decrease the risk of disease complications, such as osteoporosis. Frequent physical examinations and laboratory studies should be performed to monitor the disease progression and complications related to therapy.

SUMMARY

Although headache tends to be a less common occurrence in the elderly, it may continue well into the 70s. Migraine, muscle contraction headache, and cluster diminish in frequency in this aged group. Initial onset of these headache types rarely occurs in the elderly. Organic causes of headache, however, may occur more frequently and are of greater concern in this aged group. Many organic causes of headaches are unlikely to be manifested in patients under the age of 50. Careful evaluations and diagnostic tests are necessary to rule out organic disease. Alterations in drug metabolism and consideration of concomitant medical conditions are important in the treatment of the elderly because drug interactions and side effects are more likely to be critical in this population.

REFERENCES

1. Waters WE. Migraine in general practitioners. Br J Prev Soc Med 1975; 29:48–52.
2. Ziegler DK, Hassanein RS, Couch JR. Characteristics of life headache histories in a nonclinic population. Neurology 1977; 27:265–269.
3. Paulin JM, Waal-Mamming HJ, Simpson FO, Knight RG. The prevalence of headache in a small New Zealand town. Headache 1985; 25:147–151.
4. Lagoe RJ. Hospital stays by diagnosis related group for neurologic patients treated medically. Neurology 1987; 37:139–145.
5. Kaganov JA, Bakal DA, Dunn BE. The differential contribution of muscle contraction and migraine symptoms to problem headache in the general population. Headache 1981; 21:157–163.
6. Goldstein M, Chen TC. The epidemiology of disabling headache. Adv Neurol 1982; 33:377–390.
7. Lance JW. Mechanism and management of headache, 4th ed. Boston: Butterworth 1983:101, 207.
8. Blau NJ. Loss of migraine: when, why and how. J R Coll Physicians Lond 1987; 21:140–142.
9. Bartleson JD. Transient and persistent neurologic manifestations of migraine. Curr Concepts Cerebrovasc Dis Stroke 1984; 15:383–386.
10. Waters WE, Campbell MJ, Elwood PC. Migraine, headache, and survival in women. Br Med J 1983; 287:1442–1443.
11. Hale WE, May FE, Marks RG, Moore MT, Stewart RB. Headache in the elderly: an evaluation of risk factors. Headache 1987; 27:272–276.
12. Serratrice G, Serbanesco F, Sambuc R. Epidemiology of headache in elderly— correlations with life conditions and socio-professional environment. Headache 1985; 25:85–89.
13. Mosnaim AD, Chevesich J, Wolf ME, Freitag FG, Diamond S. Plasma methionine enkephalin, increased levels during a migraine episode. Headache 1986; 26:278–281.
14. Diamond S, Mosnaim AD, Freitag FG, Wolf ME, Lee G, Solomon GD. Plasma methionine-enkephalin levels in patients with cluster headache, longitudinal and

acute studies. In: Rose FC, ed. Advances in headache research. London: Libbey Press, 1987:2209–2215.

15. Genazzani AR, Petraglia F, Facchini V, Facchinetti F. Circulating beta-endorphin levels at various stages of life: possible connections with migraine pathogenesis. Cephalalgia 1983; 3(suppl 1):35–41.

16. Indo T, Naito A, Sobue I. Clinical characteristics of headache in Parkinson's disease. Headache 1983; 23:211–212.

17. Avorn J, Everitt DE, Weiss S. Increased antidepressant use in patients prescribed beta blockers. JAMA 1986; 255:357–360.

18. Scollins MJ, Appel WC, Mann SJ, Graham DJ, Lundin FE, Rosa F, Baum C. Antidepressant use in patients prescribed beta blockers [Letter to the Editor]. JAMA 1986; 255:3248–3250.

19. Chouza C, Caamano JL, Aljanati R, Scaramelli A, DeMedina O, Romero S. Parkinsonism, tardive dyskinesia, akathasia, and depression induced by flunarizine. Lancet 1986; x:1303–1304.

20. Edmeads J. Headache and head pains associated with diseases of the cervical spine. Med Clin North Am 1978; 62:533–544.

21. Wolf RE. Nosteroidal anti-inflammatory drugs. Arch Intern Med 1984; 144:1658–1660.

22. Goldberg M, Murray TG. Analgesic associated nephropathy. N Engl J Med 1978; 299:716–717.

23. Kimberly RP, Plotz PH. Aspirin induced depression of renal function. N Engl J Med 1977; 296:418–424.

24. Emkey RD Mills JA. Aspirin and analgesic nephropathy. JAMA 1982; 247:55–57.

25. Olive DM Stoff JS. Renal syndromes associated with the nonsteroidal anti-inflammatory drugs. N Engl J Med 1984; 310:563–572.

26. Fox DA, Jick H. Nonsteroidal anti-inflammatory drugs and renal disease. JAMA 1984; 251:1299–1300.

27. Ciabattoni G, Cinotti GA, Pierucci A, Simonetti BM, Manzi M, Pugliese F, Barsotti P, Pecci G, Taggi F, Patrono C. Effects of sulindac and ibuprofen in patients with chronic glomerular disease. N Engl J Med 1984; 310:279–284.

28. Levy M. Aspirin use in patients with major upper gastrointestinal bleeding and peptic ulcer disease. N Engl J Med 1974; 290:1158–1162.

29. Traub YM, Korczyn AD. Headache in patients with hypertension. Headache 1978; 17:245–247.

30. Fleetcroft R, Maddocks JL. Headache due to ischemic heart disease. J R Soc Med 1985; 76:676.

31. Das G. Pacemaker headaches. Pace 1984; 7:802–805.

32. Moran JF. Headache following pacemaker implantation. JAMA 1985; 254:1511–1512.

33. Medina J, Diamond S, Rubino F. Headache in patients with transient ischemic attacks. Headache 1975; 15:194–197.

34. Portendy RK, Abissi CJ, Lipton RB, Berger AR, Mebler MF, Baglivo J, Solomon S. Headache in cerebrovascular disease. Stroke 1984; 15:1009–1012.

35. Loeb C, Gandolfo C, Dall'Agata D. Headache in transient ischemic attack (TIA). Cephalagia 1985; 2(suppl):17–19.
36. Edmeads J. The headaches of ischemic cerebrovascular disease. Headache 1979; 19:345–349.
37. Sandock BA, Furlan AJ, Whisnant JP, Sundt TM. Guidelines for the management of transient ischemic attacks. Mayo Clin Proc 1976; 53:665–675.
38. Reding MJ, Orto LA, Winter SW, Fortuna LM, DiPonte P, McDowell FH. Antidepressant therapy after stroke, a double blind trial. Arch Neurol 1986; 43:763–765.
39. Gerber NJ. Giant cell arteritis and its variants. Eur Neurol 1984; 23:410–420.
40. Allen NB, Studenski SA. Polymyalgia rheumatica and temporal arteritis. Med Clin North Am 1986; 70:369–384.
41. Huston KA, Hunder GG, Lie JT, Kennedy RH, Elveback LR. Temporal arteritis, a 25 year epidemiologic clinical and pathologic study. Ann Intern Med 1978; 88:162–167.
42. Koorey DJ. Cranial arteritis, a twenty year review of cases. Aust NZ J Med 1984; 14:143–147.
43. Andersson R, Malmvall B, Bengtsson B. Long-term corticosteroid treatment in giant cell arteritis. Acta Med Scand 1986; 220:465–469.
44. DeSilva M, Hazleman BL. Azathioprine in giant cell arteritis/polymyalgia rheumatica: a double blind study. Ann Rheum Dis 1986; 45:136–138.

15

Treatment of Other Headaches

R. Michael Gallagher

University Headache Center
Moorestown, New Jersey, and
University of Medicine & Dentistry of New Jersey—
School of Osteopathic Medicine
Stratford, New Jersey

INTRODUCTION

Some headaches do not easily fall into one of the typical chronic recurring headache categories. These headaches are often variants and are named for precipitating factors or common characteristics. Francis [1] has categorized over 500 types. Some of the more commonly encountered will be discussed in this chapter.

COMPLICATED MIGRAINE

Migraine headaches, associated with visual or neurological deficits, that are prolonged or continue after the head pain has ceased are referred to as complicated migraine. Some of the more common forms of complicated migraine are hemiplegic, ophthalmoplegic, and basilar. Usually, these associated symptoms resolve entirely. However, on occasion, they may persist or become permanent deficits. Because of this possibility, prophylactic treatment should be considered for all complicated migraine patients.

The management of complicated migraine patients is comprehensive. Non-pharmacologic measures should be taken to reduce triggering or contributing factors (see Chap. 4). Particularly important is the elimination of smoking and the avoidance of estrogen-containing medications. Prophylactic pharmacologic treatment is similar to that of other forms of migraine. Verapamil, various β-blockers (propranolol, nadolol, metaprolol, timolol, atenolol), antidepressants and nonsteroidal anti-inflammatory drugs are often helpful in preventing or lessening the severity of attacks (see Chap. 7).

The abortive pharmacologic treatment of complicated migraine differs somewhat from other forms of migraine. Although the vasoconstrictor medications (ergotamine and isometheptene) probably do not cause significant intracranial constriction [2], they are not recommended. Analgesics, sedatives, and antiemetics can be useful. The addition of a steroid, as in the treatment of status migraine, may be helpful in reducing the severity and length of neurological symptoms (see Chap. 8).

MENSTRUAL MIGRAINE

The majority of migrainous women report increased headaches during menarche, menses, gynecological difficulties, or while taking exogenous hormonal supplements. However, some women experience menstrual migraine, which is characterized by headaches that occur almost exclusively with menses. It is believed that these attacks are related to the natural withdrawal of estrogen in the premenstrual phase of the cycle [3].

The treatment of the menstrual migraine sufferer is often difficult and can be frustrating to the physician and patient. Cyclic pharmacologic therapy has been helpful in reducing the frequency and severity of attacks. Intermittent propranolol [4,5] ergonovine [6], nonsteroidal anti-inflammatory drugs [7] and vasoconstrictors have been reported to be successful in many patients.

I have reported on the improvement of menstrual migraine headaches in studies involving intermittent propranolol [4,5] and intermittent ergonovine [6], respectively. In one study, 22 patients were treated with 60–80 mg of propranolol 1 day before and during menses. Sixty-eight percent of the patients experienced significant improvement after 4 months of therapy. In another study, 40 patients were treated with ergonovine maleate 0.2 mg three to four times daily during menses. Eighty-five percent of the patients experienced significant improvement after 3 months of therapy and 50% after 6 months of therapy.

CYCLIC MIGRAINE

Some patients present with headaches that are in every way characteristic of migraine, with the exception of frequency. The headaches occur frequently for weeks to months and mysteriously disappear for months to years, similar to cluster headache. The intermittent use of migraine prophylactic agents such as β-blockers or nonsteroidal anti-inflammatory drugs, as discussed in Chapter 7, are often helpful.

Medina and Diamond [8] reported on the successful treatment of 27 patients with lithium carbonate. In this study, 19 of the patients experienced significant improvement while taking 900 mg/day. Lithium is often utilized in the treatment of manic–depression and can also be helpful in the treatment of chronic cluster headache. Serum levels should be monitored, and the usual prescribing precautions followed while using this drug.

EXERTIONAL HEADACHE

Headaches can occur as a result of prolonged physical activity such as running, calisthenics, weight lifting, sporting activities, or sexual intercourse ("coital headache"). The headache is vascular and thought to be a variant of migraine. The mechanism is not understood, but may be related to increased cranial venous pressure, sudden release of vasoactive substances, or transient hypertension [2]. It occurs more frequently in males between ages 10 and 70 [9].

The exertional headache is usually throbbing, often unilateral, and can be brief (1–2 hr). Associated symptoms, such as nausea, vomiting, or visual changes, may occur. Some sufferers report a spontaneous resolution of this type of headache after several years of suffering.

Most exertional headaches are benign; however, the physician must be cautious when making this diagnosis. Intracranial lesions, such as tumors, aneurysms, or Arnold-Chiari malformation, must be considered.

Those patients who experience frequent exertional headaches are candidates for prophylactic therapy. Many of the antimigraine drugs can be effective. The nonsteroidal anti-inflammatory drugs and β-blockers are frequently utilized. Diamond reported a dramatic improvement in a study of 15 patients treated with indomethacin (Indocin) 25–150 mg/day [10]. In patients who experience infrequent attacks, headaches may be prevented by preexertion treatment with medication such as indomethacin, β-blockers, small amounts of ergotamine, or isometheptene.

Although many exertional headaches are brief and self-limiting, abortive treatment may be necessary. Mild analgesics or vasoconstrictors are often helpful in prolonged or severe attacks.

ALTITUDE HEADACHE

Headache can be precipitated by exposure to altitude in excess of 8000 ft as part of acute "altitude" or "mountain sickness" (see Chap. 4). The headache resembles migraine and is aggravated by exertion, strain, movement or lying down. It is believed to be caused by a relative hypoxia, with reactive vasodilation or mild cerebral edema [11]. This headache is treated with oxygen inhalation, gradual return to lower altitude, cool fluids, acetazolamide (Diamox) [12], the cautious use of ergotamine or isometheptene and occasionally, corticosteroids.

Some migraine sufferers report the precipitation of attacks when exposed to higher altitudes or air travel. The exact mechanism involved during air travel is not clear, but it is my own opinion that multiple contributing factors, both physiological and psychological, may play a role [13]. These include preflight preparation, delays, excessive flight noise, dryness of the air, dehydration, cramped quarters, and exposure to higher altitude (average airplane cabin pressure is approximately 8000 ft above sea level).

The treatment for altitude-induced migraine can be prophylactic or abortive. Preexposure treatment with various medications has been helpful in preventing or reducing the severity of symptoms in some susceptible patients. These agents include ergotamine, isometheptene [13] acetazolamide (Diamox) [14], diazepam [13], and nonsteroidal anti-inflammatory drugs. Abortively, these headaches are treated as other migraines.

POSTTRAUMATIC HEADACHE

Injuries to the head are a frequent occurrence in our active and mobile society. Whether trauma is trivial or severe, headache can be a significant sequela. It is estimated that 30–50% of head injury patients will develop posttraumatic headache [15]. In most cases, the injury is followed by local soreness and head pain, with resolution in several days or weeks. However, in some patients the headaches become chronic and persist for months to years.

There appears to be little relationship between the severity of the head trauma and length or severity of headache. Many patients with minor injuries go on to experience severe long-lasting headaches, whereas, others with severe injuries experience minimal or no headache. Some physicians have speculated that the less severe injuries result in the more severe headaches. Posttraumatic headache can also result from cervical whiplash in which there is no direct trauma to the head [16]. The onset of headache following injury can be immediate or delayed for months [17].

Following head injury, headache is sometimes one of a more complex set of symptoms known as posttraumatic syndrome. With posttraumatic syndrome, patients commonly report dizziness, cognitive difficulties, anxiety, fatigue, and depression, but a multitude of other symptoms may occur [18] (Table 1). These symptoms can occur to any extent and are not necessarily dependent on the severity of trauma. Usually, posttraumatic syndrome develops within 48 hr of injury, but a more delayed onset is not uncommon. The symptoms may progress with time and persist for months or years.

Various influencing factors must be considered in the evaluation and treatment of posttraumatic headache patients. The individual's occupation, social and

Table 1 Symptoms of Posttraumatic Syndrome

Light-headedness or true vertigo	Easy fatigability
Hyperacusis	Reduced motivation
Tinnitus	Decreased libido
Impaired memory	Alcohol intolerance
Reduced attention span	Increased sensitivity to weather or
Heightened distractibility	temperature change
Inattentiveness	Irritability
Decreased ability to concentrate	Anger outbursts
Forgetfulness	Emotional callousness
Difficulty in turning from one subject to another	Blunting or liability of emotional response
Deterioration of synthetic thinking	Mood swings
Inability to grasp new or abstract concepts	Anxiety, depression, and frustration
Insomnia	Syncope
Lack of spontaneity accompanied by apathy and loss of initiative	

Source: Ref. 18.

economic status, and intelligence may effect his reaction to and ability to cope with the injury. Psychological factors, such as premorbid personality, suppressed hostilities, depressive tendencies, and the possibility of secondary psychological gain, may influence the extent and duration of symptoms. There is no doubt that, in some cases, open legal issues, such as workman's compensation, disability, or pain and suffering claims, will affect the patient's course. However, of interest is that legal issues do not seem to be a substantial determining factor in treatment outcome according to many clinicians [19–21].

Most posttraumatic headaches are of the muscle contraction type and are associated with physical signs of muscle spasm. However, trauma can induce or mimic any of the nontraumatic headache syndromes. Posttraumatic vascular headaches have become increasingly more evident [22–24], although some believe that they occur in patients who are already disposed to the condition.

After excluding serious complications of the head injury, such as subarachnoid hemorrhage, subdural hematoma or bacterial meningitis, the posttraumatic headache patient should be treated in exactly the same fashion as other headache patients. A comprehensive individualized treatment plan should be developed that can include prophylactic or abortive medications, or both, social and personal adjustments, biofeedback, physio- or manipulative therapy, and psychological counseling. The selection of medication and other modalities depends entirely upon the type or types of headaches experienced (e.g., muscle contraction, migraine, mixed, or other). In patients who have daily or near daily headaches, frequent analgesic use is best avoided because of possible habituation and rebound. Treatment of the various types of headaches are discussed elsewhere in this book.

CHRONIC PAROXYSMAL HEMICRANIA

Chronic paroxysmal hemicrania is a cluster variant first described by Sjaastad and Dale [25]. The pain is always unilateral in the periorbital, temporal, or frontal areas and can sometimes be precipitated by flexion of the neck. Patients often describe the pain as severe and piercing. Although many features are shared by cluster headache and chronic paroxysmal hemicrania, the latter is characterized by a greater prevalence in women, shorter but more frequent attacks, and predictable relief with indomethacin.

The dosage of indomethacin (Indocin) will vary with each patient and may require adjustments during the course of treatment. Patients may respond to as little as 25 mg daily or may require as much as 50 mg four times daily. Residual ache or soreness may continue throughout treatment, while the severe attacks are prevented.

PSEUDOTUMOR CEREBRI

The condition, pseudotumor cerebri, is typically characterized by elevated intracranial pressure, papilledema, and deteriorating vision. It is more commonly experienced by obese, young women [26]. The headache is generalized, varies in intensity, and is often unresponsiveness to usual headache medications. When establishing this diagnosis, great care must be taken to exclude intracranial lesions, metabolic disorders, medication causes, and other conditions associated with increased intracranial pressure.

The treatment for pseudotumor cerebri is directed at reducing the intracranial pressure. Osmotic diuretics, lumbar puncture, and salt restriction are sometimes helpful. Some clinicians utilize migraine preparations, with varied results, to treat the associated headaches.

POSTLUMBAR PUNCTURE HEADACHE

Many patients undergoing spinal lumbar puncture will develop headache following the procedure. It is believed to be the result of the leakage of cerebrospinal fluid from the puncture site [27,28]. The headache is usually in the frontal or occipital areas and is worsened in the sitting or standing position. The pain can be incapacitating and is sometimes associated with nausea, vomiting, and stiffness of the neck. Resolution usually occurs within several days, but the headache can persist for prolonged periods. In an occasional patient, the dural puncture site does not spontaneously heal, and the headache continues for months.

The treatment of headache resulting from lumbar puncture poses a difficult problem for clinicians. It has been reported that many of these headaches and associated symptoms can be avoided by the use of smaller caliber needles [29,30], early ambulation [31], precise technique, or possible epidural blood patching [32,33]. For headaches that do occur, various regimens, to include vasoconstrictors, analgesics, sedatives, nonsteroidal anti-inflammatory drugs, and bed rest, have been recommended. However, currently, analgesics and hydration are most frequently utilized.

SINUS HEADACHE

It is extremely common for many headache sufferers to believe that their symptoms are related to sinus disease. Although sinusitis is not infrequent, this condition does not closely resemble other episodic headache disorders and should not be mistaken as such. It is my opinion, as well as others, that the occurrence of sinus headache is greatly overstated.

The symptoms of sinusitis are related to acute infection of the paranasal sinuses. The headache can be severe and located in varying areas of the head, depending on the particular sinus or sinuses involved. The pain is usually pressurelike, constant, more severe on morning awakening, and aggravated by bending over. Associated symptoms include nasal congestion, purulent drainage, elevated temperature, and cough (Table 2).

Sinusitis often follows an acute upper respiratory infection with rhinitis and dental infection. Conditions that can predispose a patient to sinusitis are septal malformation, nasal polys, allergies, trauma, and cystic fibrosis. Treatment consists of appropriate antibiotics, oral decongestants, limited use of vasoconstricting nasal sprays, warm compresses, and increased nasal moisture.

TEMPEROMANDIBULAR JOINT SYNDROME

The temperomandibular joint syndrome (TMJ) is a broad term frequently used in describing pain that is related to the temperomandibular joint and proximal structures. It is often referred to as myofacial pain dysfunction (MPD) and involves

Table 2 Sinusitis Pain

Sinus	Pain	Radiation
Maxillary	Cheek	Ear, teeth
Frontal	Frontal	Eyes, vertex
Ethmoid	Behind eyes	Temporal area
Sphenoid	Eyes, vertex, frontal occipital	Mastoid area

musculoskeletal symptoms resulting from dysfunction of the entire masticatory system [34]. The pain is more often experienced in the area of the ear and may radiate to the temporal or occipital areas. Other associated symptoms include muscle tenderness, clicking of the temperomandibular joint, and limitation of jaw movement.

Temperomandibular joint syndrome has been reported to cause or aggravate various chronic headache conditions, such as cluster, migraine, or tension headache. However, it is the opinion of many headache specialists, as well my own, that TMJ is a distinct entity and is not a major contributing factor in chronic vascular or muscle contraction headache.

Considerable disagreement exists over treatment. Most clinicians agree, however, that destructive or invasive procedures should be avoided, except in the most extreme cases. A comprehensive approach is recommended and may include nonmedicinal measures, such as the altering of eating habits, jaw exercises, intermittent heat packs or ice, and the wearing of a bite plate or night guard. The addition of a nonsteroidal anti-inflammatory agent, such as ibuprofen (Motrin, Rufen) or diflunisal (Dolobid), alone or in combination with muscle relaxants, such as cyclobenzaprine (Flexeril) or carisoprodol (Soma), may be of benefit after several weeks of therapy. These medications are described elsewhere in this book.

REFERENCES

1. Francis JH. Headache classification system: a diagnostic code manual. Irving, Calif: Aardvark, 1989.
2. Kunkel RS. Complicated and rare forms of migraine. In: Diamond S, Dalessio DJ, eds. Practicing physician's approach to headache, 4th ed. Baltimore: Williams & Wilkins, 1986:76–83.
3. Somerville B. The role of estradiol withdrawal in the etiology of menstrual migraine. Neurology 1972; 22:355–365.
4. Gallagher RM. Propranolol HCE in menstrual migraine. Headache 1984; 24:166.
5. Gallagher RM. Menstrual migraine and intermittent propranolol therapy. J Pa Osteo Med Assn 1984; 28:13–14.
6. Gallagher RM. Menstrual migraine and intermittent ergonovine therapy. Headache 1989; 29:366–367.
7. Diamond S, Dalessio DJ. Migraine headache. In: Diamond S, Dalessio DJ, eds. Practicing physician's approach to headache, 4th ed. Baltimore: Williams & Wilkins, 1986:44–65.
8. Medina JL, Diamond S. Cyclical migraine. Arch Neurol 1981; 38:341–344.
9. Rooke ED. Benign exertional headache. Med Clin North Am 1968; 52:801–808.
10. Diamond S. Prolonged benign exertional headache: its clinical characteristics and responses to indomethacin. Headache 1982; 22:96–98.
11. Appenzeller D. Cerebrovascular aspects of headache. Med Clin North Am 1978; 62:478.

12. Larson EB, Roach RC, Schoene RB, Hornbein TF. Acute mountain sickness and acetazolanide. JAMA 1982; 248:328–332.
13. Gallagher RM. Treatment of air travel induced "altitudinal migraine:" a study of diazepam; the combination of isometheptene, dichlorophenazone and acetaminophen; and placebo. Headache 1989; 29:314.
14. Saper JR. Headache disorders. Boston: John Wright & Sons, 1983:176.
15. Appenzeller O. Post-traumatic headache. In: Dalessio DJ, ed. Wolff's headache and other head pain. New York: Oxford University Press, 1987:289–303.
16. Winston KR. Whiplash and its relationship to migraine. Headache 1987; 27:452–457.
17. DeBenedittis G, DeSantis A. Chronic post-traumatic clinical, psychopathological features and outcome determinants. J Neurosurg Sci 1983; 27:176–177.
18. Speed WG. Posttraumatic headache. In: Diamond S, Dalessio DJ, eds. Practicing physician's approach to headache, 4th ed. Baltimore: Williams & Wilkins, 1986:113–119.
19. Elkind AH. Headache and head trauma. Clin J Pain 1989; 5:77–87.
20. Kelly R. Post-traumatic syndrome. Pahlavi Med J 1972; 3:530–547.
21. Lidvall HF, Lindenoff B, Moreen B. Causes of the post-concussional syndrome. Acta Neurol Scand Suppl 1974; 50:56.
22. Kelly R. Headache after cranial trauma. In: Hopkins A, ed. Headache, problems and management. London: WB Saunders, 1988:217–240.
23. Bennett DR, Fuenning SI, Sullivan G, Weber J. Migraine precipitated by head trauma in athletes. Am J Sports Med 1980; 8:202–205.
24. Manzoni GC, Bono G, Lanfranchi M. Cluster headache—clinical findings in 180 patients. Cephalgia 1983; 3:21–30.
25. Sjaastad O, Dale I. A new clinical headache entity "chronic paroxysmal hemicrania." Acta Neurol Scand 1976; 54:140–159.
26. Ryan RE, Ryan RE. Headache and head pain. St Louis: CV Mosby, 1978:341.
27. Vandam LD, Dripps RD. Long-term follow-up of patients who received 10,098 spinal anesthetics, syndrome of decreased intracranial pressure (headache and ocular and auditory difficulties). JAMA 1956; 161:586.
28. Tourtellotte WW, Henderson WG, Tucker RP, Gilland O, Walker JE, Kokman E. Randomized double-blind clinical trial comparing the 22 vs 26 gauge needle in the production of the postlumbar puncture syndrome in normal individuals. Headache 1972; 12:73.
29. Sand T. Which factors affect reported headache incidences after lumbar myelography? Neuroradiol 1989; 31:55–59.
30. Dittmann M, Renkl F. Spinal anesthesia with extremely fine needles [Letter]. Anesthesiology 1989; 70:1035–1036.
31. Vilming ST, Schrader H, Monstad I. Post-lumbar puncture headache: the significance of body posture. Cephalgia 1988; 8:75–78.
32. DiGiovanni AJ, Dunbar BS. Epidural injections of autologous blood for post-lumbar puncture headache. Anesth Analg 1970; 49:268–271.
33. Sengupta P, Bagley G, Lim M. Prevention of postdural puncture headache after spinal anesthesia for extracorporeal shockwave lithotripsy; an essessment of prophylactic epidural blood patching. Anesthesia 1989; 44:54–56.
34. Howell FV. Teeth and jaws as sources of headache and facial pain. In: Dalessio DJ, ed. Wolff's headache and other head pain. New York: Oxford University Press, 1987; 255–265.

16

Analgesics in the Treatment of Headaches

Eugene Mochan
University of Medicine and Dentistry of New Jersey—
School of Osteopathic Medicine
Stratford, New Jersey

INTRODUCTION

Headache is one of the most frequent presenting complaints of patients seen by the primary care physician [1–4]. In most cases, despite the use of the latest diagnostic advances, only a few patients can be identified as having organic causes for their pain symptoms. For most headache patients, the cause and severity of their pain remains difficult to quantify and, consequently, the persistence of their pain is poorly understood by their daily contacts and, in many cases, by their treating physicians.

Through research over the past years, advances have been made in the understanding of the clinical symptomatology associated with headaches, which have led to the identification of various kinds of headaches and helpful therapies [5–8]. Similarly, with recent advances in the understanding of the molecular basis of pain [9–1 1], the physician is now in a position to use drug therapy in the most efficacious manner to selectively modify the pain response by chemical manipulation of the functional activity in these pain pathways.

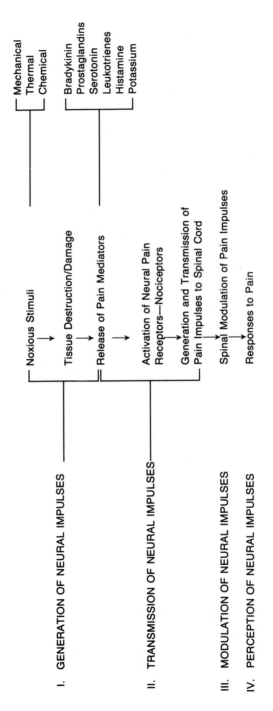

Figure 1 Overview of pain process.

Pharmacotherapy for various kinds of headaches requires expertise in the use of three broad categories of analgesic medications: nonsteroidal anti-inflammatory drugs (NSAIDs), opioid analgesics, and adjuvant analgesics. Although mechanistic details are lacking, these agents appear to act at peripheral or central sites, or both. This chapter reviews the neurophysiological mechanisms at peripheral and central sites involved in pain perception and the current pharmacologic guidelines aimed at providing relief of headache.

PATHOPHYSIOLOGY OF PAIN

Although molecular details of the pain process are still lacking, it appears that most kinds of pain involve at least four basic events (Fig. 1) [9–11]:

1. *Generation of neural impulses*: Noxious stimuli cause tissue damage and release humoral substances that activate neural pain receptors (i.e., nociceptors) to produce neural impulses.
2. *Transmission of neural impulses*: Neural impulses travel up afferent nerves and then through the spinal cord to the brain where the signals are recognized.
3. *Modulation of neural impulses*: Pathways in the central nervous system have been described that selectively inhibit pain transmission cells at the level of the spinal cord.
4. *Perception of neural impulses*: A psychological reaction to these impulses occurs that influences the magnitude and nature of the pain, as well as the emotional response.

Noxious stimuli that are involved in the generation of neural impulses include mechanical, thermal, or chemical events that damage or destroy cells and liberate humoral mediators into the traumatized area. Mediators generated include bradykinin, prostaglandins, serotonin, leukotrienes, histamine, and potassium, and they are believed to be primarily responsible for activating the pain receptors involved in generating neural impulses. Pain receptor activation may be specific for a particular stimulus, or it may be polymodal and able to respond to several types of stimuli. Bradykinin is a particularly potent pain-producing mediator. Although prostaglandins alone cause only mild pain, they can significantly potentiate the discomfort of other pain-inducing substances, particularly the kinins.

Pain impulses initiated at specialized nociceptive pain receptors in the periphery are transmitted to the dorsal horn of the spinal cord via A-delta and C nerve fibers (Fig. 2). An important chemical trigger for the initiation of the pain signal is the polypeptide, substance P. This polypeptide is produced in the cell bodies of the nociceptive nerves and, in addition to being involved in the generation of peripheral nerve impulses, also appears to generate a local inflammatory reaction. As the pain impulses transverse through the dorsal horn,

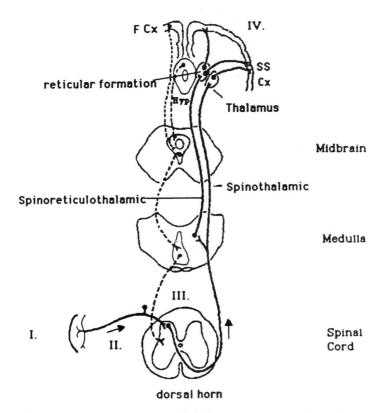

Figure 2 Transmission and modulation networks associated with pain: transmission pathways (———); modulation pathways (--------). I. Generation of neural impulses by noxious stimuli. II. Transmission of neural impulses. III. Modulation of neural impulses. IV. Perception of neural impulses. (Modified from Ref. 10.)

they are modulated by a variety of cells that interact with the incoming pain signal before ascending on the contralateral side of the cord through the spinothalamic and spinoreticulothalamic tracts to the brain. The spinothalamic tract synapses in the thalamus, with third-order neurons ascending to the somatosensory cortex, whereas the spinoreticulothalamic tract synapses in the reticular formation, with neurons going to the thalamus and then to the cerebral cortex. Recent research has demonstrated that pain sensation is also modified by descending central systems that modulate the sensory information that is transmitted from the periphery.

Some evidence suggests that inputs from the frontal cortex and hypothalamus activate cells in the midbrain and medulla that control spinal pain transmission cells through release of enkephalin in the dorsal horn. Evidence also exists that the endogenous opiate peptides, enkephalins and endorphins, liberated by neurons within the dorsal horn may play an important role in reducing the flow of pain along the nerves by inhibiting the amounts of substance P produced.

PHARMACOLOGICAL APPROACH TO MANAGEMENT OF HEADACHE

Despite progress in our understanding of the pain process and the mechanisms of pain relief, too little is currently known about the etiopathogenesis of the various types of headache to develop precise indications for analgesic use. To date, therapies are necessarily empirical and recommended mostly from the study of the modes of action of drugs to which patients have been observed to respond during clinical trials (Table 1) [5–8].

Nevertheless, effective management of most headaches is nearly always possible. Although, the choice of specific pharmacologic intervention may, at many times, be empiric, there are a wide variety of analgesics to choose from. Some guidelines for the effective use of analgesics include the following:

1.   On the basis of the clinical features of the headache, attempt to classify the headache type.

Table 1 Pharmacological Treatment of Headache

Treatment	Nonorganic headache type
Peripheral-acting analgesics	
Nonsteroidal anti-inflammatory drugs (NSAIDS)	Migraine (symptomatic/preventive); cluster (preventive); muscle
Acetaminophen	contraction; mixed
Central-acting analgesics	Severe headache
Opioid analgesics	(short-term management)
Adjuvant analgesics	
Tricyclic antidepressants	Migraine (preventive);
Monoamine oxidase inhibitors	muscle contraction; mixed
Calcium channel blockers	Migraine (preventive); cluster
Corticosteroids	Migraine (supportive); cluster
β-blockers	Migraine (preventive/supportive)
Anxiolytics	
Benzodiazepines	Muscle contraction/cluster
Butalbital	(short-term)
Phenothiazines	Migraine (supportive)
Vasoconstrictors	Migraine (supportive); cluster

2. Choose the appropriate drug class (peripheral-acting, central-acting, other) for the headache.
3. Know the pharmacokinetics of the chosen analgesic drug.
4. Be aware of the side effects and drug interactions of the chosen analgesic agent.
5. Educate the patient and set goals.
6. To maximize the pharmacokinetic factors leading to improved analgesia, administer the analgesic on a fixed time interval.
7. If the chosen drug is unsuccessful, try increasing doses before switching to another agent.
8. Avoid the long-term use of narcotics.
9. Be cautious of developing drug dependency.
10. Be aware of, and utilize when appropriate, nonpharmacologic approaches.

PERIPHERAL-ACTING ANALGESICS

Nonsteroidal Anti-Inflammatory Drugs

The nonsteroidal anti-inflammatory drugs (NSAIDs) and acetaminophen, which is usually classified separately, are the major peripherally acting analgesic agents. These drugs have been shown to be effective in the treatment of several types of headache (see Table 1). The major advantage of these agents is that they provide analgesia without many of the side effects of centrally acting drugs, particularly addiction potential and sedation. However, although lacking these side effects, they have other side effects that the physician should be familiar with [12,13], which are discussed in the following.

The NSAIDs are believed to act primarily by inhibiting the synthesis of prostaglandins by inhibition of the enzyme, cyclooxygenase (Fig. 3). Prostaglandins, as discussed earlier, are important inflammatory mediators that are synthesized from cellular membrane phospholipids following cellular activation or injury, that play a role in facilitation of nociceptor function. The actions, therapeutic advantages, and side effects of a specific NSAID is most likely related to the cellular prostaglandins inhibited. However, recent research indicates that NSAIDs may also inhibit several other metabolic events, which include superoxide production, leukotriene production, and leukocyte migration [14,15].

There is considerable variability among the individual NSAIDs in their pharmacokinetics and toxicity profiles [12,13]. In addition, not all NSAIDs have the same efficacy. In many patients, one NSAID will be effective when others have failed. The NSAIDs differ in structure, potency, duration of action, drug interactions, and side effects. These properties are summarized in Table 2A. Most NSAIDs are rapidly absorbed and peak levels reached within 2 hr. They are

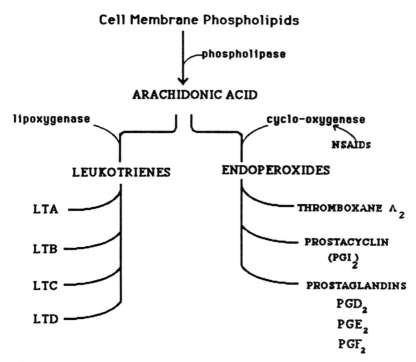

Figure 3   Therapeutic effects of nonsteroidal anti-inflammatory drugs.

metabolized primarily in the liver, are highly protein-bound in the plasma, and are excreted primarily by renal and fecal routes. Most NSAIDs have half-lives of approximately 4–12 hr, the exceptions being piroxicam and phenylbutazone.

Although only a few NSAIDs have approved indications as analgesics, a number of clinical studies suggest that most may be used for this purpose. The analgesia provided by the NSAIDs is characterized by a *ceiling dose*, defined as a dose beyond which additional increments produce no further analgesia. It is important to recognize that the ceiling dose, as well as toxicity, varies among individuals. Another important aspect of the analgesia provided by the NSAIDs is the lack of demonstrable tolerance or physical dependence.

The salicylates include aspirin, choline magnesium trisalicylate, diflunisal, and salsalate. Aspirin has been shown to be effective in the treatment of various types of headaches (see Table 1). However, the high incidence of gastric irritation may limit the use of aspirin. The use of enteric-coated aspirin and nonacetylated salicylates greatly reduces gastrointestinal (GI) distress, as well as many other side effects observed, but these products appear to decrease potency.

Table 2 Pharmacological Properties of NSAIDs

Chemical class	Time to peak (hr)	Onset (hr)	Duration (hr)	Half-life (hr)	Recommended adult dose
A. Analgesic action					
Acetylated salicylates					
Acetylsalicylic acid (aspirin)	0.75			2–30	650 mg q6h
Nonacetylated salicylates					
Choline magnesium trisalicylate (Trilisate)	1–2			9–17	1500 mg q12h
Diflunisal (Dolobid)	2–3			12	500 mg q12h
Magnesium salicylate (Magan)	1.5			2	1000 mg q8h
Salsalate (Disalcid)	4			4–16	1000 mg q8h
Pyrole acetic acids					
Indomethacin (Indocin)	1–2	1.0	4	4.5	25–50 mg q6h
Sulindac (Clinoril)	1–2			8–16	200 mg q12h
Tolmetin (Tolectin)	0.5–1			1–6	400 mg q6–8h
Propionic acids					
Fenoprofen (Nalfon)	1–2				300 mg q6h
Flurbiprofen (Ansaid)	0.5–2	0.5	4–6	2–4	200 mg q4–6h
Ibuprofen (Motrin, Rufen, Advil, Nuprin, Medipren)	1–2	0.5	4–6	2	400–600 mg q6h
Ketoprofen (Orudis)	0.5–2	0.5	6	3–5	75 mg q8h
Naproxen (Naprosyn)	3–4	1.0	6–8	13	375 mg q12h
Naproxen sodium (Anaprox)	1–2	1.0	6–8		375 mg q8–12h
Anthranilic acids (fenamates)					
Meclofenamate (Meclomen)	0.5–2			2–4	100 mg q6h
Mefenamic acid (Ponstel)	2–4			2–4	250 mg q6h

Oxicams					
Piroxicam (Feldene)	3–5	1.0	> 12	50	10–20 mg q24h
Pyrazoles					
Phenylbutazone (Butazolidin)	2			50–60	100 mg q6h
Quinazolinone					
Proquazone (Biarsan)	1.5–2	0.5	4–6	13	75–150 mg q8h

B. Side effects

Gastrointestinal
Dyspepsia
GI or intestinal ulceration
GI hemorrhage
Diarrhea
Constipation
Stomatitis
Nausea

Dermatological
Rashes
Urticaria
Pruritus

Renal
Azotemia
Hyperkalemia
Acute renal failure
Fluid retention

Central nervous system
Headache
Tinnitus
Dizziness
Cognitive dysfunction

Hematological
Leukopenia
Thrombocytopenia
Anemia

Hepatic
Elevated transaminases
Hepatitis

Source: Physicians Desk Reference. Oradell, NJ: Medical Economics, 1989.

The pyrole acetic acids include indomethacin, sulindac, and tolmentin. These drugs are potent inhibitors of cyclooxygenase and have a relatively rapid onset. It should be noted, however, that psychotomimetic effects and headache ocur with the use of indomethacin.

The propionic acids are also useful NSAIDs with rapid onset of action. The approval of over-the-counter use of low-dose ibuprofen attests to the minimum of side effects observed with this NSAID.

The pyrazoles include phenylbutazone and oxyphenylbutazones. These NSAIDs are potent cyclooxygenase inhibitors and have several serious effects (e.g., bone marrow depression), which have essentially replaced their use by other drugs.

The oxicam, piroxicam, is unique among NSAIDs because of its extremely long half-life. Consequently, the time required for peak analgesic effects is longer than the other NSAIDs.

Acetaminophen

Acetaminophen has long been used as a treatment for mild to moderate headache. There are approximately 200 over-the-counter preparations that contain this drug. In contrast with NSAIDs, acetaminophen is a poor inhibitor of peripheral cyclo-oxygenase and, consequently, it has weaker anti-inflammatory effects and fewer side effects. The mode of action of acetaminophen is uncertain and, most likely, also involves prostaglindin inhibition in the central nervous system. Acetaminophen is rapidly absorbed from the GI tract, reaches peak levels in 30–60 min, lasts up to 6 hr and has a plasma half-life of 2–4 hr. Side effects are rarely associated with therapeutic doses. However, extended use (e.g., 650 mg four times daily for 1–2 weeks) may slightly potentiate action of oral anticoagulants. The major toxicity occurs with overdose (> 150 mg/kg), which can lead to fatal hepatic necrosis. The maximum dosage should not exceed 1000 mg every 4 hr.

Side Effects of Nonsteroidal Anti-Inflammatory Drugs

The NSAIDs may have adverse effects on gastrointestinal (GI) function, renal function, the central nervous system, the skin, the hematological system, and the hepatic system (see Table 2B). The major adverse effect associated with NSAIDs is on the GI tract. Less frequent side effects include alterations in renal function, hepatic toxicity, pancreatitis, blood dyscrasias, cutaneous reactions, fluid retention, and hypersensitivity reactions.

Adverse effects to the GI tract include dyspepsia, nausea, GI bleeding, and peptic ulcers. There is evidence that the adverse GI effects are related to the degree of inhibition of gastric prostaglandin production. Although all NSAIDs inhibit gastric prostaglandin production, they do so to varying degrees. For example, a higher incidence of GI effects occurs with patients treated with aspirin than nonacetylated derivatives and acetaminophen. Food, antacids, histamine antagonists (e.g., cimetidine, ranitidine, famatidine), or synthetic prostaglandins (e.g., misoprostol) have been used to improve GI tolerance. There is also evidence that sucralfate is effective, and that its mode of action may be by enhancing gastric prostaglandin E_2 production.

Renal side effects with the use of NSAIDs can also occur. The NSAIDs have been reported to impair renal function, cause acute renal failure, or exacerbate chronic renal failure. This is believed to occur because renal prostaglandins are important in regulating renal blood flow, glomerular filtration rate, renin release, electrolytes and water transport, and vessel tone. Risk factors for developing NSAID-induced renal impairment include patients with renal disease, decreased cardiac output, hepatic disease, and extracellular volume depletion. The renal impairment associated with NSAID use is generally reversible following discontinuation of the drug, but permanent renal failure can occur. Some studies have reported indomethacin, fenoprofen, and phenylbutazone as the most likely NSAIDs associated with acute renal impairment, with aspirin and sulindac as the least likely. Therefore, these latter NSAIDs should be considered in those high-risk patients requiring analgesic agents. A list of side effects of the various NSAIDs are summarized in Table 2B.

Drug Interactions of Nonsteroidal Anti-Inflammatory Drugs

Few drug interactions of major importance occur with NSAIDs. Those that do most likely reflect the high affinity of NSAIDs for plasma proteins. Consequently, NSAIDs may displace oral anticoagulants and oral hypoglycemics from protein-binding sites. Some evidence suggests that ibuprofen, flurbiprofen, naproxen, tolmentin, and acetaminophen do not displace other protein-bound medications and, therefore, should be used in patients taking warfarin or oral hypoglycemic agents. Other drug interactions of NSAIDs are summarized in Table 3.

Guidelines for Nonsteroidal Anti-Inflammatory Drug Use

Most NSAIDs can be used to effectively treat headaches, but differences in efficacy and toxicity have been reported. There is now no superior NSAID available, and many factors should be considered in prescribing these drugs. These include age of the patient, concurrent diseases, the use of other drugs, the drug pharmacokinetic profile, compliance issues, and psychosocial issues.

In general, relatively low doses should be started initially for mild to moderate pain, although loading doses have been well-tolerated and effective for severe pain. Dosing should proceed as each drug's pharmacokinetic profile predicts. Particular attention should be paid to the drug's half-life. It has been estimated that four to five half-lives are required for steady-state plasma levels to be approached and, similarly, the same time is needed after stopping the drug to almost remove

Table 3 NSAIDs–Drug Interactions

Drug	Interaction
Antacids	Decreases NSAID absorption
Anticoagulants	NSAIDs can cause anticoagulant toxicity
Antirheumatic agents	NSAIDs may enhance bone marrow toxicity caused by these agents
Antihypertensive agents	NSAIDs may decrease antihypertensive effects of β-blockers, ACE inhibitors, or diuretics
Lithium	NSAIDs may elevate serum levels
Oral hypoglycemic agents	NSAIDs may displace from plasma-binding sites
Phenytoin (Dilantin)	NSAIDs may displace from plasma-binding sites
Probenecid	May decrease the excretion of NSAIDs; NSAIDS may antagonize uricosuric action of probenecid

it from the body. In elderly patients, the NSAID half-life may be prolonged and, thereby, reach toxic levels under average dosing.

Most NSAID side effects occur relatively soon after initiating therapy and are most common in the elderly. To assure safety, a complete blood count, serum creatinine levels, and liver enzyme levels should be periodically obtained.

CENTRAL-ACTING ANALGESICS

Overview

The opioid analgesics are the major central-acting analgesic agents. These agents, with morphine as the prototype, are believed not to alter noxious stimuli in the periphery but, instead, to bind receptors in the brain that interfere with the processing of the pain impulse as it moves to the brain.

Opioid receptors are located throughout the central nervous system, with high concentrations in the limbic system, thalamus, and hypothalamus. There is a strong correlation between high affinity of opioid analgesics for opiate receptors and their analgesic properties. These opioid receptors also appear to be the normal sites for the endogenous opioid substances—met-enkephalin, leu-enkephalin, and β-endorphin. There are at least five known opioid receptors: μ, σ, $\varkappa$, δ, and ϵ. The μ- and κ-receptors appear to be responsible for analgesia, whereas the others may be responsible for the adverse effects.

Opioid Analgesics and Headaches

Opioid analgesics that are commonly used alone, or in combination with peripheral-acting agents, for the treatment of headache are summarized in Table 4. Generally, these drugs should be avoided except for severe headache and be used only for brief courses (1–2 days). All opioid analgesics produce analgesia by the mechanism just described, but differ in their potency and are usually classified as agonists or agonist–antagonists. Agonists bind opiate receptors and produce morphinelike actions. On the other hand, agonist–antagonists have agonist action at some opiate receptors and antagonist action at other receptors. This group appears to possess fewer side effects than pure agonists. It is important to realize that all of these drugs have similar efficacy. That is, at appropriate doses, all of these drugs produce the same degree of pain relief. Therefore, if an adequate dose of one of these drugs is ineffective, then it is unlikely that an equivalent dose of any of the others will be effective. The pharmacokinetics of the various opioid analgesics are listed in Table 4.

There is evidence that the adverse effects of opioid drugs are related to activation of specific receptors. Hence, all of these drugs have similar patterns of side effects, which include nausea and vomiting, respiratory depression, sedation, and constipation. In addition, for reasons not well understood, these drugs have the potential to induce tolerance and dependence and have significant cross-tolerance between them.

Opioid agonists include morphine, codeine, meperidine, oxycodone, and propoxyphene. Parenteral morphine or meperidine, alone or with hydroxyzine (Vistaril), will abolish most acute severe nonorganic headaches commonly seen in the emergency room. Here, the physician should be sure that the patient does not regularly require or seek medical attention for their headaches. If drug-seeking behavior is suspected, parenteral butorphanol (Stadol), or nalbuphine (Nubain) can be used. Because these drugs are potent antagonists, as well as agonists, narcotic withdrawal symptoms will appear in the drug-dependent patient.

Oral opioid agonists are also indicated for brief treatment (i.e., 1–2 days) of severe nonorganic headaches. Codeine in combination with acetaminophen or aspirin is commonly used. Because codeine is a weak opiate, the addiction

Table 4 General Properties of Opioid Analgesics

Drug	Time to peak (hr)	Duration (hr)	Half-life (hr)	Recommended daily dose
Morphine agonists				
Codeine	1.5–2	4	3	32–65 mg
Oxycodone	1.5–2	3	3	5–10 mg
Meperidine (Demerol)	1.5–2	2–3	3	50–100 mg
Propoxyphene (Darvon)	2–2.5	3	12	65–130 mg
Mixed agonist–antagonist				
Pentazocine (Talwin)	1.5–2	2–3	2–3	50–100 mg

Source: Physicians Desk Reference. Oradell, NJ: Medical Economics, 1989.

Table 5 Combination Products Use in the Treatment of Headache

Produce name	Aspirin	Acetaminophen	Narcotic	Other
Ascription w/codeine	+		Codeine	Magnesium–aluminum hydroxide
Axotal	+			Butalbital
Bancap HC		+	Hydrocodone	
Capital w/Codeine		+	Codeine	
Co-Gesic		+	Hydrocodone	
Darvocet N-100		+	Propoxphene	Caffeine
Darvon	+		Propoxphene	Caffeine
Empirin w/Codeine	+		Codeine	
Empracet		+		
Empracet w/Codeine		+	Codeine	
Equagesic	+			Meprobamate
Esgic		+		Butalbital, Caffeine
Esgic w/Codeine		+	Codeine	Butalbital, Caffeine
Fioricet		+		Butalbital, Caffeine
Fiorinal	+			Butalbital, Caffeine
Fiorinal w/Codeine	+		Codeine	Butalbital, Caffeine
Hydrocet		+	Hydrocodone	
Hy-Phen		+	Hydrocodone	
Percocet		+	Oxycodone	
Percodan	+		Oxycodone	
Percogesic		+		Phenyltolaxamine
Phenaphen w/Codeine		+	Codeine	
Phrenlin		+		Butalbital
Phrenlin w/Codeine		+	Codeine	Butalbital
Synalgos-DC	+		Dihydrocodeine	Caffeine
Talacen		+	Pentazocine	
Talwin Compound	+		Pentazocine	
Tylenol w/Codeine		+	Codeine	
Tylox		+	Oxycodone	
Vicodin		+	Hydrocodone	
Wygesic		+	Propoxyphene	

Source: Physicians Desk Reference. Oradell, NJ: Medical Economics, 1989.

potential is considered low. Similarly, propoxphene is often effective and also has low addiction potential. Oxycodone is available only in combination with either aspirin (Percodan) or acetaminophen (Percocet). Because oxycodone is completely absorbed orally, it is as potent as injected morphine and, therefore, has a high addiction potential.

The mixed agonist–antagonist include pentazocine (Talwin), nalbuphine (Nubain), and butorphanol (Stadol). Only pentazocine, in combination with the antagonist naloxone (Talwin Nx), is present in oral form. Generally, mixed agonist–antagonists opiates cause less respiratory depression and have a lower abuse potential than agonist opiates. However, their tendency to cause dysphoria has reduced their usefulness as analgesics.

Guidelines for the Use of Opioid Analgesics

Because of their abuse potential, opioid analgesics are generally recommended for use only for severe nonorganic headache on a short-term basis. In selected cases for whom narcotics may represent the most appropriate and safest treatment, the tendency for dependency must be considered. The physician should be cautious of somatic expression of psychosocial problems and drug-seeking behavior presenting through the complaint of headache. These agents should not be used unless standard drugs have failed or are contraindicated. Additionally, the headaches should be infrequent. On the other hand, although controversial, some studies have suggested that opioid maintenance therapy can be successfully employed to manage chronic pain, provided that the administration of these drugs is carefully supervised.

ADJUVANT ANALGESICS

Adjuvant analgesics are drugs that have primary indications other than pain and have been shown to be effective in the treatment of headaches. These include antidepressants, anxiolytics, corticosteroids, β-blockers, calcium channel blockers, vasoconstrictors, and antihistamines. These agents do not produce analgesia by an effect on the opioid-receptor system, but some may achieve analgesia by altering peripheral nociception. In addition, some appear to have independent direct or indirect analgesic properties, but all are particularly effective because of their synergistic interaction with other analgesics.

Current evidence suggests that depression can lower pain tolerance and increase analgesic requirements. The most likely mechanism of action of antidepressant drugs is through alteration of the monoamine-dependent endogenous pain-modulating systems found in the brain. It is currently believed that these drugs increase central monoamine levels, which leads to activation of descending pathways (e.g., endorphin- and serotonin-mediated) involved in modulation of incoming nociceptive information in the dorsal horn of the spinal cord.

The efficacy of tricyclic antidepressants (e.g., amitryptiline, imipramine, dox-epin) in the treatment of tension headache, migraine, and psychogenic headache has been documented in well-controlled trials. Monoamine oxidase inhibitors have been reported to be effective in the treatment of migraine. However, these drugs are to be used cautiously because of their risk of hypertensive crisis.

Although the choice of tricyclic antidepressant is largely empiric, some guidelines for their use have been developed. Generally, much lower doses of antidepressants are required for the treatment of headaches than for the treatment of depression. Patients should be alerted to developing dry mouth and transient sedation on starting therapy with these drugs. To decrease early toxicity, the initial doses should be low and the dose increased slowly. If there is an absence of clinical benefit or the side effects become intolerable, it may be worthwhile to try an alternative antidepressant.

Several clinical trials point to the possible benefit of anxiolytics, corticosteroids, calcium channel blockers, β-blockers, and vasoconstrictors in the treatment of headache. Although the use of these drugs may be useful for management of a specific headache type, there is evidence that some of them are coanalgesics when combined with other drugs.

DRUG COMBINATIONS

In view of the complex nature of the pain processes discussed in the foregoing, various combinations of peripheral-acting, central-acting, and adjuvant analgesics have been successfully employed as treatments for headache. A list of some of the more common combinations is presented in Table 5. There is good evidence that the individual drugs provide an additive analgesic effect. Thus, relatively low doses of the analgesics in the combination drugs can provide a superior level of analgesia, with fewer side effects than using one drug alone at a relatively high dose. Therefore, when used appropriately, these combinations allow the physician to utilize less of the narcotic analgesics, without affecting efficacy of treatment.

MEDICATION OVERUSE AND DEPENDENCY

Medication overuse and drug dependency occur frequently in chronic headache sufferers [16]. Commonly abused substances include (a) aspirin and other NSAIDs, (b) acetaminophen, (c) barbiturates, (d) tranquilizers, (e) narcotics, and (f) ergotamine derivatives. This abuse can lead to serious medical complications as discussed in the listed side effects.

In addition to these toxic side effects, several reports of a "rebound" phenomenon have recently appeared, in which excessive use of these agents has been shown to enhance headache frequency [17,18]. In a clinical study of chronic muscle contraction headache, Kudrow [18] presented evidence that analgesic overuse can increase the frequency of these headaches in many patients, and that restricting analgesics in these patients diminished headache frequency. Similar findings were reported by Rowsell and colleagues [17] with the use of ergotamine in the treatment of migraine patients. These types of clinical observations may, therefore, account for treatment refractoriness often seen in long-standing headache patients. It is also noteworthy that some studies have linked both prophylactic use [19] and overuse [17] of ergotamine in migraine patients with increased frequency of headaches (i.e., rebound headache) upon withdrawal of this drug.

The treatment of the headache patient who overuses medication presents a difficult management problem. A comprehensive intervention program as an outpatient, or inpatient if indicated, is necessary. Restriction of current drugs, prophylactic use of new drugs, psychotherapy, dietary counseling, occupational therapy, and behavioral modification are helpful aids in treatment.

SUMMARY AND CONCLUSIONS

At present, because of the poor understanding of its etiopathogenesis, headache, like other pain syndromes, is difficult to treat. In a few patients with demonstrable pathology (e.g., temporal arteritis), specific pharmacologic treatment can be successfully employed. For the vast majority of patients with headache, however, essentially empirical pharmacologic approaches, based on numerous on-going clinical trials, have been commonplace. In these patients, the use of analgesics should be considered as one arm of a multimodal approach.

Most patients with occasional attacks of headache respond well to over-the-counter analgesics intended to suppress each attack as it occurs. Although analgesic control of chronic recurrent headaches is more difficult to achieve, much success has been noted. This success is partly based on the indirect influence on the mechanism of headache by the pharmacologic agents described in this chapter.

Despite the foregoing limitations, analgesic drug therapy is a major approach for managing chronic headaches. This approach involves the use of peripheral-acting (nonnarcotic), central-acting (narcotic), and adjuvant analgesics, alone or in combinations, titrated to the needs of the individual patient. The choice of specific analgesic follows a full physical and psychological assessment, with an attempt to clarify the headache type as summarized in Table 1 [also, see Ref. 5]. When this is not feasible, another approach is to select the appropriate analgesic based on the intensity of the pain. On this basis, analgesics can be separated into (a) nonnarcotic, (b) "weak" narcotic (e.g., codeine, oxycodone, propoxyphene), (c) combinations of nonnarcotics and narcotics, and (d) "strong" narcotic (e.g., morphine, meperidine, pentazocine).

For patients who require mild analgesia, acetaminophen, aspirin, or other NSAIDs are the usual drugs of choice. These drugs have the advantages that tolerance and physical dependence do not occur with repeated administration, and their side-effects are well known. They should be prescribed in low doses, on a regular basis, with the dosing interval determined by the pharmacokinetic properties of the analgesic selected. A major objective of this approach is to attempt to prevent the recurrence of disabling pain as the prerequisite for receiving further medication. This latter behavioral pattern is felt by many to encourage drug abuse. Despite having essentially the same mechanism of action, an individual NSAID appears to have different effectiveness in various patients. Therefore, an adequate trial period of one NSAID on a regular basis should be made before switching to another. In view of the fact that two different peripheral-acting agents compete with each other for plasma protein-binding sites and, thereby, clinically diminish the analgesic effectiveness of each other, their concurrent use is to be discouraged.

If a peripheral-acting, nonnarcotic drug is ineffective or poorly tolerated, adjuvant drugs, "weak" narcotics, or combination drugs are alternative approaches. Adjuvant analgesic drugs may be used alone (e.g., antidepressants for muscle contraction headaches) or as a second drug added to a peripheral-acting drug. Because of their low addiction potential, codeine, oxycodone, and propoxyphene are generally considered to be "weak" narcotics. However, they are morphinelike agonist drugs and, thereby, exhibit the desirable and undesirable effects of morphine. These weak narcotics are used most commonly in combination with nonnarcotic analgesics. The advantages of the combinations include (a) enhanced analgesia, (b) decreased tolerance and physical dependence, and (c) decreased narcotic side effects (e.g., sedation, constipation). Despite these advantages, the use of narcotic analgesics should be generally avoided, except for brief therapeutic courses when the headache is severe. Similarly, other combinations that contain anxiolytics (e.g., barbiturates, benzodiazepines) can also be helpful, but should be used only for short-term management of headaches. The use of strong narcotics should be limited to acute nonorganic headaches with severe intractable pain.

Medication overuse and development of drug dependency are common and serious problems associated with pharmacologic management of headaches. These problems frequently require referral to a headache center for inpatient management. The primary care physician needs to be cognizant of preventive measures aimed at minimizing these problems.

Although the standard therapies specifically designated for a particular kind of headache (see Table 1) are usually successful, headaches refractory to these therapies occur and should be referred to a headache center for further management. As our knowledge into the pathophysiology of headache continues to grow, newer therapies are currently under investigation. Current research includes drugs aimed at altering (a) production of noxious stimuli, (b) activation of nociceptors, (c) transmission of neural impulses, (d) modulation of neural impulses, and (e) perception of pain. As research progresses and knowledge in the neurophysiology of pain increases, it is anticipated that new drugs will be developed that produce effective specific analgesia, with avoidance of side effects, tolerance to its analgesic effects, and without physical dependence.

REFERENCES

1. Diamond S, Dallessio DJ. The practicing physicians approach to headache, 4th ed. Baltimore: Williams & Wilkins, 1986.
2. Dalessio DJ. Wolff's headache and other head pain. New York: Oxford University Press, 1980.
3. Saper JR. Headache disorders: current concepts and treatment strategies. Littleton, Mass: John Wright & Sons, 1983.
4. Peatfield R. Headache. New York: Springer-Verlag, 1986.
5. Diamond S, Freitag FG. Diagnosing common headache disorders. Fam Pract Recertif 1989; 11:67-72.
6. Diamond S, Freitag FG. Current treatments for headache. Fam Pract Recertif 1989; 11:25-51.
7. Diamond S, Medina JL. Headaches. Ciba Clin Symp 1989; 41:2-32.
8. Saper JR. Drug treatment of headache: changing concepts and treatment strategies. Semin Neurol 1987; 7:178-191.
9. Condouris GA. Drug therapy in the treatment of chronic pain. In: Wu WH, Smith LG, eds. Pain management. Human Sciences Press, 1987:127-136.
10. Fields HL. Pain New York: McGraw-Hill, 1987.
11. Paris PM, Uram M, Ginsburg MJ. Physiological mechanisms of pain. In: Paris PM, Steward RD, eds. Pain management in emergency medicine. Norwalk, Conn: Appleton & Lange, 1988:3-15.
12. Arnold W, Beaver WT, Kantor TG, Wilkens RF. When NSAIDs are the right choice. Patient Care 1988; 26:190-207.
13. Amadio P, Cummings DM. Nonsteroidal anti-inflammatory agents: an update. Am Fam Pract 1986; 34:147-154.
14. Gall EP. NSAIDS—Guidelines for use in arthritic patients. Drug Ther 1987; 17:30-47.
15. Hochberg MC. NSAIDs: mechanism and pathways of action. Hosp Pract 1989; 24:139-156.
16. Elkind AH. Drug abuse in headache patients. Clin J Pain 1989; 5:111-120.
17. Rowsell AR, Neylan C, Wilkinson M. Ergotamine induced headaches in migrainous patients. Headache 1973; 13:65-67.
18. Kudrow L. Paradoxical effects of frequent analgesic use. Adv Neurol 1982; 33:335-341.
19. Gallagher RM. Ergotamine withdrawal causing "rebound headache." J Am Osteopath Assoc 1983; 677:109.

17

Headache Drug Interactions

Frank J. DiSerio
Sandoz Research Institute
East Hanover, New Jersey

In headache therapy as in the rest of medicine, each time a patient takes a drug it is like a controlled scientific experiment, with the drug as the independent variable. On the basis of years of personal and collective experience, we can be confident that such an "experiment" should yield a particular response or set of responses. We hope this response will be positive, but we try to be prepared for the known negative side effects as well. As any scientist will tell you, experiments with just one independent variable are usually relatively easy to control. But when you add one or more other variables to the mix, all bets are off. The reason can be summed up in one word: interaction.

Every time a physician treating a headache patient adds a new drug to those a patient is already taking for headache or some other illness, he is creating a novel combination and opening the door to a drug interaction. A *drug interaction* can be defined as a change in the pharmacologic effects of a therapeutically administered drug caused by the presence of another drug. In more clinical terms, a drug interaction is a response to pharmacologic treatment that is not due to the action of a single drug, but is the result of two or more drugs acting together.

It is not inconceivable for a patient to be taking 10 or even 20 drugs at a time; the average hospitalized patient takes six to eight drugs concurrently [1]. Just as important, and even less controllable, is patient self-medication with over-the-counter (OTC) drugs, other people's prescriptions, or even seemingly innocuous substances such as antacids or vitamins. All can result in alteration of the intended therapeutic effect, either by intensifying one or more expected drug effects, even to the point of toxicity, by neutralizing one or more of these effects, or by producing an altogether new effect.

If you know which other drugs a patient is taking, it is often possible to draw on the known pharmacology of the individual agents to predict the risks of the combination. For example, drugs that inhibit or facilitate a particular enzyme system can produce broad and fairly predictable interactions. A common culprit is cimetidine, the H_2-blocker that inhibits the cytochrome P_{450} microsomal hydroxylating system in the liver. The fact that numerous different drugs are catalyzed by this enzyme system gives cimetidine an important role in drug interactions. Among medications used for the treatment of headache, concomitant administration of cimetidine alters the activity of propranolol, amitriptyline, meperidine, phenytoin, carbamazepine, and metoclopramide. Similarly, monoamine oxidase inhibitors (MAOIs), which block the enzyme that degrades catecholamines and other key substances, interact with a wide range of other drugs, including propranolol, amitriptyline, meperidine, opioids, cyproheptadine, metoclopramide, and isometheptane. In some cases (e.g., propranolol, amitriptyline, or meperidine), the interaction with an MAOI can be life-threatening.

Often though, it is impossible to predict a drug interaction. There is no way to remember, let alone systematically study, all the possible combinations and their consequences. To complicate matters, as noted in the foregoing, patients may well be taking more than two drugs. In addition to those you have prescribed, they may be taking drugs prescribed by another physician for the same or other illnesses, and they may also be taking OTC remedies they "prescribe" for themselves.

The best way to minimize the impact of a drug interaction is to prevent it in the first place. Toward this end, there are a number of routine steps the physician should take when beginning treatment of a patient with headaches.

DRUG HISTORY AND PHYSICAL EXAMINATION

A thorough physical examination and history, including a drug history is essential. When a patient presents with some form of headache, the physician should ascertain whether he or she is also being treated for the same or other medical problems by another physician and whether he or she is taking any medication(s) for those other conditions. If the answer is yes, you should check to see if any interactions are possible between those drugs and the drug(s) you may prescribe (see Table 1).

Just as important is finding out which OTC medications a patient may be taking. At one time or another almost everyone takes OTC analgesics, antacids, vitamins, antihistamines, and others. Many of these drugs can have a profound effect on the disposition of other drugs; and do not forget about three of the most common drugs in use, alcohol, nicotine, and caffeine. Alcohol, in particular, can interact with some drugs with devastating consequences.

Predisposing Physical Conditions

Certain types of patients are particularly prone to drug interactions, either because of their physical condition *per se* or because that condition causes them to take certain drugs with a propensity for interaction with common headache medications. The most important of these conditions is the patient's age.

More than any other aged group, the elderly are likely to have other illnesses that require medication, often chronically. And even if they are relatively healthy, elderly patients are likely to have reduced functioning in the organs that absorb, distribute, metabolize, and eliminate drugs. Otherwise normal patients over aged 65 may have a 30% reduction in renal tubular function and glomerular filtration rate. At aged 90, renal function may be down by 50% [2]. Their altered physiology, in turn, alters the pharmacokinetics of the drugs they take. This makes many elderly patients more sensitive to the intended effects of some drugs and to the unwanted effects of others. Consequently, the doses of general anesthetics, analgesics, benzodiazepines, β-blockers, and sedative–hypnotics, among others, often must be reduced. Increased sensitivity also means that an interaction that might not be noticeable in a younger person would be manifest in an elderly patient.

The physician who is treating elderly patients for headaches should be aware of these issues. He or she should also be on the lookout for poor compliance with prescribed regimens and for patients taking OTC medications along with their prescriptions.

These factors all conspire to increase the likelihood of drug interactions in the elderly. With this in mind, Kofoed has recommended that clinicians have an "index of suspicion" with elderly patients because of the likelihood that they may be taking multiple medications, especially OTC drugs. He even suggests that, in some cases, physicians should seek multiple sources of information, interview family members, obtain urine toxicologies, and critically analyze routine laboratory data, to ascertain which nonprescribed drugs an elderly person might be taking [3].

Another factor that should alert physicians to the possibility of drug interactions, in all aged groups, is the presence of chronic illness. In the first place, alterations in drug distribution, metabolism, or excretion may be inherent to these conditions. In the second place, chronic disorders, such as diabetes, arthritis, heart disease, gastrointestinal disease, kidney disease, or mental illness or retardation, usually mean long-term medication. The nature of this medication may well dictate which headache drugs a patient can and cannot safely take.

BASIC MECHANISMS OF DRUG INTERACTIONS

Drugs are complex chemical substances, and their interactions reflect this complexity. Interactions can be based on the similar chemical structures of two drugs, on their physiological effect, on their physical site of action, on their effect on the metabolism, absorption, protein-binding, or excretion of another drug. The following is a brief summary of some of the more common mechanisms of drug interaction, particularly as they relate to common headache medications.

Gastrointestinal Absorption

It is relatively common for drugs to interact in the gastrointestinal tract. The absorption of some drugs, for example, is dependent on the pH of this tract. Salicylates (aspirinlike drugs) are absorbed more rapidly at low pH because more of the drug is present in a readily diffusible, lipid-soluble state. When a patient takes an antacid along with aspirin, thus raising the pH of the gut, he effectively slows the absorption of the drug. The same is true for H_2-blockers, which also raise gastric pH. In the face of such an interaction, timing of the administration of aspirin and antacids or aspirin and H_2-blockers becomes important [1,2].

Protein Binding

Interactions involving protein binding are most important for those drugs that are extensively bound at therapeutic concentrations to plasma proteins such as albumin. Competition for these albumin-binding sites by another drug effectively raises the free concentration of both competing agents over what you would expect if each drug were given alone. A prime example here is the interaction between aspirin (or other nonsteroidal anti-inflammatory drugs) and an anticoagulant, such as warfarin. The excessive free anticoagulant that results from the coadministration of these two receptor-site competitors can cause occult gastrointestinal bleeding, reduce plasma prothrombin, and decrease platelet adhesiveness, in addition to a range of other hemorrhagic consequences [1,2].

Receptor-Site Displacement Interactions

Drugs may also antagonize each other directly by competing for the same effector site. For example, isoproterenol stimulates β-adrenergic receptors and propranolol blocks them. Drugs can also interact indirectly by affecting separate but physiologically related sites. For example, propranolol keeps muscles from releasing lactate, leaving less lactate to be converted into glucose. This increases the efficacy of a given dose of an antidiabetic drug. It also suggests that once a stable balance between the two interacting drugs has been achieved, the alert physician should not overlook the danger of antidiabetic drug overdose if the propranolol is withdrawn. Such rebound reactions occur in other interactions as well [1,2].

Metabolic Interactions

Many drugs interact by enhancing or inhibiting the metabolism of other drugs. One example is cimetidine, which was noted previously. Another is the common OTC antihistamine chlorpheniramine, which inhibits the metabolism of phenytoin, leading to ataxias, diplopia, drowsiness, headache, and other symptoms of phenytoin toxicity. On the other hand, cyclosporine *enhances* the metabolism of phenytoin, decreasing the level of free drug and *reducing* its effectiveness [1,2].

Renal Excretory Interactions

Because most drugs are excreted through the kidneys, interferences with this mechanism can lead to higher-than-normal serum levels of a drug. One mechanism of interaction involves urinary pH. Amitriptyline, for example, is a weak base that is excreted more rapidly in acidic urine. The pH of urine can be lowered by many compounds, from the salicylates to vitamin C, effectively raising the dose and perhaps prolonging the action of the antidepressant drug [1,2].

TABLE OF HEADACHE DRUG INTERACTIONS

The following compendium of drug interactions includes the drugs most commonly used in the treatment of headache, along with most of their important interactions. In all cases, the interactions shown have been documented in human patients or clinical study subjects. Interactions known only *in vitro* or *in vivo* in laboratory animals have not been included. Although it is theoretically possible they could occur in people, because of cross-species differences in drug metabolism and other variables, they must remain theoretical until they actually do occur. Also not here are interactions that might occur, but are highly unlikely, given common guidelines on drug use. The most important examples are the anticonvulsants phenytoin and carbamazapine. In addition to their widespread use in epilepsy, these drugs are sometimes used to treat headache in children. Thus, the present summary of interactions includes only those drugs a child might also be taking.

It should also be borne in mind that although many drug interactions are extremely well documented, others are based on only one or two published cases. This does not necessarily invalidate them, but speaks primarily to the likelihood or to the special conditions under which they might occur.

Table 1 is arranged in alphabetical order according to the generic names of the drugs most commonly used to treat headache. Also shown under each heading are the brand names by which these drugs are usually known. In going through this table, keep in mind that many of the drugs used to treat headache are combination products (e.g., Fiorinal and Darvocet). Thus, to determine the possibilities of interactions involving these drugs, it is necessary to check each of the compounds that make up the combination.

Table 1 Drug Interactions

Primary headache drug	Interacting drug	Results of interaction
Acetaminophen	Alcohol	Enhanced hepatotoxicity [4]
Anacin-3, Darvocet-N, Datril, Esgic, Excedrin, Fioricet, Hydrocet, Medigesic, Midrin, Migralam, Panadol, Percocet, Percogesic, Phenaphen with Codeine, Phrenilin, Repan, Roxicet, Sedapap, Sine-Aid, Sinubid, Sinulin, Talacen, Tylenol, Tylox, Unisom Dual Relief, Vanquish, Vicodin, Wygesic, Zydone	Antidiuretic hormone	Enhanced action of ADH caused by sensitization of the kidney to reabsorb water at a lower concentration [2]
	Anticoagulants	May potentiate anticoagulant effects [2,5] (controversial)
	Azidothymidine (AZT)	Higher frequency of hematological toxicity in AIDS patients [6]
	Caffeine	Enhanced analgesia [7]
	Chloramphenicol	Decreased chloramphenicol clearance owing to acetaminophen competition; enhanced chloramphenicol-induced agranulocytosis [8]
	Doxylamine	Enhanced postoperative sleep and analgesia [9]
	Ethyl alcohol	Hepatic necrosis [14]
	Metoclopramide	Accelerated absorption of acetaminophen [11]
	Pentazocine	Delayed gastric emptying and absorption of acetaminophen [12]
	Propoxyphene	Enhanced analgesia [13]
Amitriptyline *(and other tricyclic antidepressants)*	Alcohol	Additive sedative or CNS depressive effects [1,14,15]
	Antihistamines	Enhanced anticholinergic side effects of amitriptyline, especially in the elderly [2]
Elavil, Endep, Etrafon, Limbitrol, Triavil	*Antihypertensives*	Inhibition of antihypertensive action [2]
	Antipsychotics	Increased plasma levels of tricyclic drug, possible CNS side effects [2]
	Barbiturates	Reduced effectiveness of amitriptyline; withdrawal of barbiturates from an effective combination may lead to amitriptyline overdose [1,2,14]
	Benzodiazepines	Enhanced sedation; enhanced anticholinergic effects [2]
	Cimetidine	Elevated amitriptyline plasma levels owing to interference with hepatic metabolism; increased side effects, especially anticholinergic effects [14]
	Clonidine	Reduced hypotensive efficacy [2]

CNS depressants

Enflurane — Enhanced CNS depression [1]; Seizures caused by enhancement of enflurane-induced motor activity [2]

Sympathomimetic amines (epinephrine, norepinephrine) — Enhanced, possibly hazardous cardiovascular effects caused by inhibition of norepinephrine uptake [2,14]

Lithium — Enhanced urinary retention [1]; memory impairment [16]; epileptiform seizures [17]

MAOIs

Meperidine — Hyperpyretic crises, severe convulsions, death [1,2,14,18]

Meprobamate — Enhanced meperidine-induced respiratory depression [2]

Orphenadrine — Enhanced CNS depressant effects [1]

Phenytoin *(and other anticonvulsants)* — Enhanced anticholinergic side effects; possible urinary retention, acute glaucoma, adynamic ileus in elderly patients [2]; Epileptiform seizures in susceptible patients [1,2]

Physostigmine — Bradycardia, asystole [2]

Thioridazine — Life-threatening ventricular arrhythmias [19]

Acetaminophen — Increased plasma levels of both drugs [20]

Acetazolamide — Reduced renal clearance of acetazolamide owing to competition for plasma protein-binding sites [21]

Alcohol — Potentiation of aspirin-induced prolonged bleeding time [22]

Anticoagulants — Potentiation of anticoagulant action; reduced plasma prothrombin (high doses of aspirin); decreased platelet adhesiveness; occult bleeding from superficial gastric erosions [2]

Antidiabetic agents — Reduced insulin requirements; some reports of profound hypoglycemia associated with sulfonylurea drugs [2]

Corticosteroids — Increased glomerular filtration rate resulting in decreased blood levels of salicylate [23]; possibility of salicylism (nausea, vomiting, tinnitus) if dosage of corticosteroid is reduced; additive ulcerogenic effects [2]

Aspirin *(and other salicylates)*

Alka-Seltzer, Anacin, Ascriptin, Axotal, B-A-C Tablets, Bufferin, Carisoprodol, Darvon, Easprin, Empirin, Equagesic, Excedrin, Fiogesic, Fiorinal, Norgesic, Percodan, Persistin, Robaxisal, Soma Compound, Synalgos-DC, Talwin, Van-quish, Zorprin

(continued)

Table 1 Continued

Primary headache drug	Interacting drug	Results of interaction
	Dichlorphenamide	Severe salicylate intoxication, possibly due to synergistic effect of both drugs on cerebrovascular regulation [24]
	Fenoprofen	Impaired intestinal absorption, reduced plasma concentrations and efficacy of fenoprofen following concomitant administration [2]
	Meclofenamate	Increased GI blood loss [25]
	Methotrexate	Increased methotrexate toxicity resulting from inhibited renal tubular excretion of methotrexate [2,26]
	Pentazocine	(See pentazocine)
	Phenylbutazone	Increased serum urate levels [2]
	Probenecid	Antagonism of uricosuric action of probenecid [2,26]
	Spironolactone	Reversal of spironolactone-induced natriuresis [2]
	Sulfinpyrazone	Inhibited uricosuric action of sulfinpyrazone [2]
	Sulfonamides	Enhanced effects of sulfonamides owing to displacement from plasma protein binding by aspirin [2]
	Valproic acid	Possibly toxic levels of valproic acid, tremors, ataxia; caused by competition for active transport sites in renal tubules or liver [2,27]
Benzodiazepines	Alcohol	Enhanced CNS depression, death [2]
Ativan, Centrax, Dalmane, Halcion, Librium, Limbitrol, Serax, Tranxene, Valium, Xanax	Aminophylline	Antagonism of sedation [2]
	Tricyclic antidepressants	Enhanced sedation, atropinelike effects [2]
	Cimetidine	Enhanced effects of chlordiazepoxide, diazepam, and triazolam, owing to reduced hepatic metabolism [2]
	Dextropropoxyphene	Potentiation of alprazolam owing to reduction of metabolic clearance and synergistic CNS effects [2]
	Levodopa	Reduction in antiparkinsonian response with chlordiazepoxide [2]
	Oral contraceptives	Potentiation of diazepam effects [2]
	Penicillamine	Phlebitis [2]
	Phenytoin	(See phenytoin)

Carbamazepine **Tegretol**	*Skeletal muscle relaxants*	Increased duration of neuromuscular block produced by gallamine; decreased duration of block produced by suxamethonium [2]
	Thyroid hormone	Temporary elevation of free thyroxine levels [2]
	Valproate	Inhibited metabolism and competitive protein binding of diazepam [2]
	Diphenhydramine	Possible stillbirth with temazepam/diphenhydramine [2]
	Anticoagulants	Potentiation of anticoagulant effect [2]
	Cimetidine	Increased plasma concentrations of carbamazepine, neurologic toxicity [2]
	Danazol	Increased serum levels, acute toxicity of carbamazepine [28]
	Dextropropoxyphene	Sharp increase in carbamazepine plasma concentrations, severe side effects [2]
	Diltiazem, verapamil	Carbamazepine toxicity [2]
	Doxycycline	Increased rate of clearance, decreased efficacy of doxycycline [14]
	Erythromycin	Increased plasma concentrations of carbamazepine, neurological toxicity [2,29,30]
	Isoniazid	Increased plasma concentrations of carbamazepine, neurological toxicity [2,31]
	Lithium	(See lithium)
	Phenytoin	(See phenytoin)
	Theophylline	Very rapid metabolism, reduced efficacy of theophylline [32]
	Troleandomycin	Increased plasma concentrations of carbamazepine, neurological toxicity [2]
Clonidine **Catapres-TTS**	Alcohol	Enhanced CNS depression [2]
	Barbiturates	Enhanced CNS depression [2]
	Sedatives	Enhanced CNS depression [2]
	Tricyclic antidepressants	Reduced clonidine efficacy [2]

(continued)

Table 1 Continued

Primary headache drug	Interacting drug	Results of interaction
Cyproheptadine	*Antianxiety drugs*	Additive CNS depressant effects [14]
Periactin	Alcohol	Additive CNS depressant effects [14]
	Hypnotics	Additive CNS depressant effects [14]
	MAOIs	Prolonged anticholinergic effects of cyproheptadine [14]
	Sedatives	Additive CNS depressant effects [14]
	Tranquilizers	Additive CNS depressant effects [14]
	Antianxiety drugs	Additive CNS depressant effects [14]
Dihydroergotamine	Erythromycin	Severe peripheral vasoconstriction (ergotism) [33]
D.H.E.		
Ergot alkaloids	Caffeine	Increased GI absorption of ergotamine; increased vasoconstriction; enhanced therapeutic effects [1]
Ergotamine	Propranolol	Severe peripheral vasoconstriction with pain and cyanosis, increased migraine headache pain [26,34–37]
Bellergal, Cafergot, Ergomar, Ergostat, Medihaler Ergotamine, Wygraine	Troleandomycin	Severe peripheral vasospasm [38]
Ibuprofen *(and other nonsteroidal anti-inflammatory drugs)*	*Anticoagulants*	May potentiate ibuprofen-induced GI bleeding [14]
	Baclofen	Increased baclofen toxicity [39]
	Diuretics	Attenuation of hypotensive effects, probably by inhibiting renal prostaglindin synthesis; can induce cardiac failure [2,14]
Advil, Medipren, Midol-200, Motrin, Nuprin, Rufen	Lithium	Elevation of plasma lithium levels, reduction of renal lithium clearance; may induce lithium toxicity [14,40]
	Methotrexate	May reduce tubular secretion of methotrexate [14]
	Verapamil + propranolol	Life-threatening hypotension from sinus arrest [41]
Isometheptane		
Isocom, Midrin, Migralam	MAOIs	Enhanced toxicity [14]

Lithium		
Cibalith, Eskalith, Lithane, Lithobid		
	Antipsychotics	
	Aminophylline	Decreased lithium effects from increased renal excretion of lithium ions [2]
		Possible increase in blood sugar levels [2]
	Acetazolamide	Decreased lithium effects from increased renal excretion of lithium ions [2]
	Carbamazepine	Ataxia, dizziness, blackout, agitation, restlessness, confusion, feelings of unreality [2,42]
	Chlorpromazine	Reduced effectiveness of chlorpromazine; sudden chlorpromazine toxicity when lithium is withdrawn [2]
	Cisplatin	Reduction in serum lithium levels [2]
	Diclofenac	Increase in plasma lithium concentration [43]
	Diuretics (thiazides, loops)	Elevated, possibly toxic plasma lithium levels [2,44–46]
	Fluphenazine decanoate	Acute, irreversible neurotoxic reaction [47]
	Haloperidol	Extrapyramidal side effects [48]; severe encephalopathic symptoms [49]
	Mazindol	Enhanced lithium toxicity [2]
	Methyldopa	Enhanced lithium intoxication owing to reduced renal clearance of lithium [2]
	Metronidazole	Long-term renal damage [50]
	NSAIDs (indomethacin, piroxicam, sulindac)	Sharply increased plasma lithium concentration owing to reduction in renal clearance with indomethacin or piroxicam [2,51]; drop in lithium levels with sulindac [52]
	Phenytoin	Enhanced lithium toxicity [2]
	Sodium bicarbonate	Increased renal excretion of lithium [2]
	Tetracycline	Sharp rise in serum lithium levels owing to tetracycline-induced nephrotoxicity [2]
Meperidine		
Demerol, Mepergan	Acyclovir	Additive toxicities [53]
	Alcohol	Enhanced sedation [14]
	Barbiturates and other sedative hypnotics	Enhanced sedation [2,54]
	Phenothiazines	Marked, debilitating lethargy; depressed blood pressure [2,14,55]

(continued)

Table 1 Continued

Primary headache drug	Interacting drug	Results of interaction
	Cimetidine	Enhanced sedation, depression [2,56]
	General anesthetics	Enhanced sedation [2]
	Isoniazid	Hypotension [57]
	MAOIs	Excitation, rigidity, coma, hyper- or hypotension, death [2,14]
	Oral contraceptives	Possible increased analgesia, CNS depression owing to inhibition of meperidine metabolism [2]
	Phenytoin	Decreased analgesia owing to increased metabolism of meperidine [2,58]
	Tricyclic antidepressants	Possible enhanced respiratory depression [2]
Methysergide Sansert	*Narcotic analgesics*	Reversal of analgesic effect [26]
Metoclopramide Reglan	Acetaminophen	Enhanced intestinal absorption of acetaminophen [14]
	Alcohol	Additive CNS depressant effects [14]
	Anticholinergic drugs	Inhibition of metoclopramide-induced increased GI motility [14]
	Cimetidine	Reduced availability of cimetidine [2]
	Hypnotics	Additive CNS depressant effects [14]
	Insulin	Mistiming of insulin administration owing to enhanced stomach clearance of food [14]
	Levodopa	Enhanced intestinal absorption [14]
	MAOIs	Enhanced toxicity [14]
	Narcotics	Additive CNS depressant effects [14]
	Sedatives	Additive CNS depressant effects [14]
	Tetracycline	Enhanced intestinal absorption [14]
	Tranquilizers	Additive CNS depressant effects [14]

Opioids (e.g., codeine, butorphanol, nalbuphine)	Alcohol and other CNS depressants	Enhanced depressant effects [1]
Empirin with Codeine, Fiorinal with Codeine, Nubain, Percodan, Stadol, Tylenol with Codeine	MAOIs	Enhanced depressant effects [1]
	Phenothiazines	Enhanced depressant effects [1]
	Tricyclic antidepressants	Enhanced depressant effects [1]
Pentazocine	Acetaminophen	(See acetaminophen)
Talwin	Aspirin	Renal papillary necrosis [59]
	Hydroxyzine	Enhanced respiratory depression [60]
Phenobarbital	Anticoagulants	Reduced anticoagulant effect [2,61]
	CNS depressants	Enhanced CNS depressant activity [2,61]
	Corticosteroids	Increased metabolism, decreased efficacy of corticosteroids [61]
	Cyclosporine	Enhanced cyclosporine metabolism, reduced efficacy [2]
	Dextropropoxyphene	Possibly enhanced barbiturate activity [2]
	Digitoxin	Enhanced metabolism, decreased efficacy of digitoxin [61]
	Disulfiram	Inhibition of phenobarbital metabolism, increased toxic effects [61]
	Doxycycline	Enhanced metabolism, reduced efficacy of doxycycline [2,61]
	Griseofulvin	Impaired griseofulvin absorption, possibly decreased efficacy [61]
	MAOIs	Inhibition of barbiturate metabolism, increased efficacy [61]
	Meperidine	Enhanced sedation [2]
	Metronidazole	Enhanced metabolism, reduced efficacy of metronidazole [2]
	Oral contraceptives	Enhanced metabolism, decreased efficacy of contraceptive [61]
	Phenytoin	(See phenytoin)
	Valproate	Reduced metabolism, increased toxicity of phenobarbital [2]
	Vitamin D_3	Higher risk of bone fractures, osteomalacia owing to enhanced metabolism of vitamin D_3 [2]

(continued)

Table 1 Continued

Primary headache drug	Interacting drug	Results of interaction
Phenytoin	*Anticoagulants*	Potentiation of anticoagulant effect [2,62]
Dilantin	*Benzodiazepines*	Inhibition of phenytoin metabolism [2]
	Cancer chemotherapeutic agents	Reduction of serum concentrations of phenytoin [63]
	Carbamazepine	Increased metabolism, lower serum levels of carbamazepine [2,64]; increased levels of phenytoin [65]
	Chloramphenicol	CNS toxicity of phenytoin [2,66]
	Chlorpheniramine	Inhibition of phenytoin metabolism leading to phenytoin toxicity: ataxia, diplopia, drowsiness, headache, tinnitus, vomiting [2]
	Cimetidine	Increased serum phenytoin concentrations; phenytoin toxicity [2,67]
	Cyclosporine	Enhanced metabolism, reduced efficacy of cyclosporine [68]
	Co-trimoxazole	Increased rate of metabolism, decreased efficacy of co-trimoxazole [2]
	Dexamethasone	Increased blood concentrations of dexamethasone [2]
	Diazoxide	Decreased efficacy of phenytoin [69]
	Folic acid	Reduced plasma levels of phenytoin [70]
	Halothane	Phenytoin toxicity [2]
	Imipramine	Increased serum phenytoin concentrations; phenytoin toxicity [2,71]
	Influenza vaccine	Increased serum concentration of phenytoin [2,72,73]
	Isoniazid	Increased serum phenytoin concentrations; phenytoin toxicity [2]
	Mexilitine	Reduced plasma concentrations of mexilitine [2]
	Meperidine	(See meperidine)
	Phenobarbital	Increased metabolism, decreased efficacy of phenytoin [2]
	Phenothiazines	Phenytoin intoxication [74]

Rifampin	Increased clearance, reduced efficacy of phenytoin [2,75]
Sucralfate	Reduced absorption, decreased efficacy of phenytoin [76]
Sulfadiazine	Potentiation of phenytoin effects, increased risk of toxicity [2]
Sulfamethiazole	Inhibition of hepatic metabolism, potentiation of phenytoin effects [2]
Tetracyclines	Accelerated metabolism, reduced efficacy of tetracyclines [2,77]
Theophylline	Increased rate of clearance, decreased efficacy of theophylline [2,78]
Thioridazine	Reduced metabolism, increased toxicity of phenytoin [2]
Valproate	Drowsiness, stupor or coma [2]; inhibition of phenytoin binding to plasma protein, increased plasma levels [79]
Prednisone	
Deltasone, Liquid Pred Syrup, Sterapred	
Phenytoin	Increased rate of metabolism, decreased efficacy of predisone [2]
Cyclosporine	Increased levels of cyclosporine leading to nephrotoxicity [2]
Magnesium-containing antacids	Decreased bioavailability, decreased efficacy of prednisone [1]
Prochlorperazine	
Compazine	
Phenytoin	Enhanced effects of phenytoin [2]
Propoxyphene	
Darvon, Darvocet-N, Dolene, Wygesic	
Acetaminophen	(See acetaminophen)
Alcohol	Enhanced, dangerous CNS depressant effects [2,80,81]
Alprazolam	Potentiation of alprazolam owing to reduction in drug clearance [2,82]
Antidepressants	Enhanced antidepressant effects owing to reduced drug metabolism [14]
Barbiturates	Enhanced sedation [2,14]
Carbamazepine	Enhanced carbamazepine toxicity owing to sharp increase in drug levels [2,83]
Smoking	Loss of analgesic efficacy [84]
Warfarin	Increased anticoagulant response [85]

(continued)

Table 1 Continued

Primary headache drug	Interacting drug	Results of interaction
Propranolol *(and other β-adrenergic blockers)* Inderal	Aluminum hydroxide gel	Greatly reduced intestinal absorption of propranolol [14]
	Antidiabetic drugs	Potentiation of hypoglycemic action; may prolong insulin hypoglycemia (reduction in dosage of antidiabetic drug may be necessary) [26]
	Antihypertensive drugs	Potentiation of antihypertensive effect [26]
	Antipyrine	Reduced antipyrine clearane [14]
	Calcium-channel blockers (especially verapamil IV)	Synergistic depression of myocardial contractility or atrioventricular conduction [1]
	Chlorpromazine	Decreased plasma levels of both drugs [14]
	Cimetidine	Delayed elimination and increasing blood levels of propranolol [2]
	Digitalis glycosides (digoxin, digitoxin)	Potentiation of digitalis-induced bradycardia [2]
	Epinephrine	Potentiation of pressor effect of epinephrine; profound reflex bradycardia, atrioventricular block; sharply increased blood pressure [26]
	Ergotamine	(See ergotamine)
	Ethanol	Slowed propranolol absorption [14]
	General anesthetics and CNS depressants	Exaggerated hypotension; cardiac depression; possibly death [2,26]
	Indomethacin	Reduced or abolished antihypertensive effects of propranolol [26]
	Lidocaine	Reduced lidocaine clearance; increased toxicity [14]
	MAOIs	Severe hypertensive crisis [2]
	Morphine	Synergistic CNS depressant action [26]
	Nicotine	Increased blood pressure, heart rate, contractility, conduction velocity; decreased cardiac output [26]

Phenobarbital	Accelerated propranolol clearance [1,14]
Phenytoin	Accelerated propranolol clearance; potentiation of cardiac depression [14]
Quinidine	Synergistic antiarrhythmic activity; enhanced bradycardia [2]
Reserpine (or other catecholamine-depleting drugs)	Hypotension, marked bradycardia, vertigo, syncope, orthostatic hypotension, excessive sedation [26]
Rifampin	Accelerated propranolol clearance [1,14]
Sympathomimetics (phenylephrine isoproterenol, etc.)	Reversal of bronchial-relaxing effect of sympathomimetics; exacerbation of asthma; increased hypertension [26]
Theophylline	Decreased theophylline clearance [14]
Thyroxine	Lower than expected T_3 concentrations [14]
Tubocurarine	Potentiation of paralysis [26]
Trimethobenzamide Stemetic, Tigan	
Alcohol	Additive CNS depressant effects [14]
Verapamil (and other calcium-channel blockers) Calan, Isoptin	
Calcium-containing drugs (e.g., calcium adipinate, calciferol)	Atrial fibrillation [2]
Digoxin	Possible inhibition of digoxin clearance; increases in digoxin serum concentration [2]
Rifampin	Reduced efficacy of verapamil [2]
Terfenadine	Acute anginal attack due to possible potentiation of calcium-channel blockade [2]

CONCLUSIONS

If a physician fears that a drug he is administering, or is about to administer, might interact with another drug the patient is taking, he has a number of resources: a search through the medical literature describing the feared interaction, a phone call to the manufacturer(s) of the drugs involved, or a consultation with a pharmacist with either a good knowledge of drug interactions or a computer program that shows them.

A consideration in all drug administration is the balance between benefit and risk. Before administering a drug, it is important that the physician have certain expectations of its effects, potential interactions, and the limits of toxicity beyond which he will discontinue its use. If an unexpected, apparently drug-related incident does occur, he or she should be able to judge if it is an interaction and, if so, how serious its consequences might be. Such an alertness to the symptoms of common drug interactions could help save precious time and possibly avoid serious consequences in the event of an interaction.

We are taught to think of medicine as a science, and indeed, the information on drug interaction presented here is a result of careful scientific observation. But anyone who has practiced medicine knows that in treating patients, art also plays a major role. No amount of literature can tell you how a particular pair of drugs will react in a particular patient. An experienced physician will use all the information at hand to make a therapeutic decision that is best for this patient, at this time. Although you might not want to avoid a particular drug because only one or two cases of interaction have been reported, you might want to use this evidence as an alarm to be extra alert to potential adverse effects. Usually, if an interaction is possible or has occurred, one or the other of the drugs can be replaced, the doses can be adjusted and balanced, or the timing of the dose(s) can be altered to head off the interaction. That is the art.

REFERENCES

1. Gilman AG, Goodman LS, Rall TW, Murad F. Goodman and Gilman's the pharmacological basis of therapeutics, 7th ed. New York: Macmillan, 1985.
2. Griffin JP, D'Arcy PF, Speirs CJ. A manual of adverse drug interactions, 4th ed. London: John Wright & Sons, 1988.
3. Kofoed LL. OTC drug overuse in the elderly: what to watch for. Geriatrics 1985; 40:55-60.
4. McClain CJ, Kromhout JP, Peterson FJ, Holtzman JL. Potentiation of acetaminophen hepatotoxicity by alcohol. JAMA 1980; 244:252-253.
5. Boeijinga JK, Boestra EE, Ris P, Breimer DD, Jeletich Bastiaanse A. Influence of paracetamol on anticoagulant therapy with coumarin derivatives. Pharm Weekbl 1983; 118:209-212.
6. Richman DD, Fischl MA, Grieco MH, et al. Toxicity of azidothymidine (AZT) in the treatment of patients with AIDS and AIDS-related complex: double-blind controlled trial. N Engl J Med 1987; 317:192-197.

7. Laska EM, Sunshine A, Zighelboim I, et al. Effect of caffeine on acetaminophen analgesia. Clin Pharmacol Ther 1983; 33:498–509.

8. Buchanan N, Moodley GP, Interaction between chloramphenicol and paracetamol. Br Med J 1979; 2:307–308.

9. Smith GM, Smith PH. Effect of doxylamine and acetaminophen on postoperative sleep. Clin Pharmacol 1985; 37:549–557.

10. Kartsonis A, Reddy KR, Schiff ER. Alcohol, acetaminophen, and hepatic necrosis. Ann Intern Med 1986; 105:138–139.

11. Nimmo J, Heading RC, Tothill P, Prescott LF. Pharmacological modification of gastric emptying: effects of propantheline and metaclopramide on paracetamol absorption. Br Med J 1973; 1:587–589.

12. Nimmo WS, Heading RC, Wilson J, Prescott LF. Reversal of narcotic-induced delay in gastric emptying and paracetamol absorption by naloxone. Br Med J 1979; 2:1189.

13. Messick RT. Evaluation of acetaminophen, propoxyphene, and their combination in office practice. J Clin Pharmacol 1979; 19:227–230.

14. Physicians' Desk Reference, 43nd ed. Oradell, NJ: Medical Economics, 1989.

15. Seppala T, Linnoila H, Elonen E, Mattila MJ, Maki M. Effect of tricyclic antidepressants and alcohol on psychomotor skills related to driving. Clin Pharm Ther 1975; 17:515–522.

16. Worral EP, Gillham RA. Lithium-induced constructional dyspraxia. Br Med J 1983; 286:189.

17. Solomon JG. Case report: seizure during lithium–amitriptyline therapy. Postgrad Med 1979; 66:145–146.

18. Schuckit M, Robins E, Feighner J. Tricyclic antidepressants and monoamine oxidase inhibitors. Arch Gen Psychiatry 1971; 24:509–514.

19. Heiman E. Cardiac toxicity with thioradizine–tricyclic antidepressant combination. J Nerv Ment Dis 1977; 165:139–143.

20. Gennaro AR, Packman EW, Delong AF. Plasma levels of aspirin and acetaminophen produced by single combined dose of aspirin and acetaminophen in man. Am J Pharmacol 1981; 153:12–18.

21. Sweeney KR, Chapron DJ, Brandt JL, Gomolin IH, Kramer PA, et al. Toxic interaction between acetazolamide and salicylate: case reports and a pharmacokinetic explanation. Clin Pharm Ther 1986; 40:518–524.

22. Deykin D, Janson P, McMahon L. Ethanol potentiation of aspirin-induced prolongation of the bleeding time. N Engl J Med 1982; 306:852–854.

23. Koren G, Roifman C, Gelfand E, et al. Corticosteroids–salicylate interaction in a case of juvenile rheumatoid arthritis. Ther Drug Monit 1987; 9:177–179.

24. Hurwitz GA, Wingfield W, Cowart TD, Jollow DJ. Toxic interaction between salicylates and a carbonic anhydrase inhibitor. Vet Hum Pharmacol 1980; 22(suppl 2):42–44.

25. Baragar FD, Smith TC. Drug interactions with sodium meclofenamate (Meclomen). Curr Ther Res Clin Exp 1978; 23:S51–S59.

26. Martin EW. Hazards of medication, 2nd ed. Philadelphia: JB Lippincott, 1978.

27. Anonymous. Anticonvulsant may be dangerous with aspirin. Am Pharm 1987; NS27:26.

28. Zielinski JJ, Lichten EM, Haidukewych D. Clinically significant danazol–carbamazepine interaction. Ther Drug Monit 1987; 9:24–27.

29. Goulden KJ, Camfield P, Dooley JM, et al. Severe carbamazepine intoxication after coadministration of erythromycin. J Pediatr 1986; 109:135–138.

30. Wroblewski BA, Singer WD, Whyte J. Carbamazepine–erythromycin interaction: case studies and clinical significance. JAMA 1986; 255:1165–1167.

31. Valsalan VC, Cooper GL. Carbamzepine toxication caused by interaction with isoniazid. Br Med J 1982; 285:261–262.

32. Reed RC, Schwartz HJ. Phenytoin–theophylline–quinidine interaction. N Engl Med 1983; 308:724–725.

33. Leroy F, Asseman P, Pruvost P, et al. Dihydroergotamine–erythromycin induced ergotism. Ann Intern Med 1988; 109:249.

34. Baumrucker JF. Drug interaction—propranolol and Cafergot. N Engl J Med 1973; 288:916–917.

35. Diamond S. Propranolol and ergotamine tartrate. N Engl J Med 1973; 289:159.

36. Blank NK, Reider MJ. Paradoxical response to propranolol in migraine. Lancet 1973; 2:1336.

37. Venter CP, Joubert PH, Buys AC. Severe peripheral ischaemia during concomitant use of beta blockers and ergot alkaloids. Br Med J 1984; 289:288.

38. Matthew NT, Havill JH. Ergotism with therapeutic doses of ergotamine tartrate. NZ Med J 1979; 89:476–477.

39. Dahlin PA, George J, George J. Baclofen toxicity associated with declining renal clearance after ibuprofen. Drug Intell Clin Pharm 1984; 18:805–808.

40. Kristoff CA, Hayes PE, Barr WH, et al. Effect of ibuprofen on lithium plasma and red blood cell concentrations. Clin Pharm 1986; 5:51–55.

41. Lee TH, Salomon DR, Rayment CM, Antman EM. Hypotension and sinus arrest with exercise-induced hyperkalemia and combined verapamil/propranolol therapy. Am J Med 1986; 80:1203–1204.

42. Ghose K. Interaction between lithium and carbamazepine. Br Med J 1980; 280:1122.

43. Reiman IW, Frolich JC. Effect of diclofenac on lithium kinetics. Clin Pharmacol Ther 1982; 30:348–352.

44. Ramsay LE. Interactions that matter, part 2. Diuretics and antihypertensive drugs. Prescr J 1984; 24:60–65.

45. Michaeli J, Ben-Ishay D, Kidron R, Dasberg H. Severe hypertension and lithium intoxication. JAMA 1984; 251:1680.

46. Kerry RJ, Ludlow JM, Owen G. Diuretics are dangerous with lithium. Br Med J 1980; 281:371.

47. Singh SV. Lithium carbonate/fluphenazine decanoate producing irreversible brain damage. Lancet 1982; 2:278.

48. Loudon JB, Waring H. Toxic reactions to lithium and haloperidol. Lancet 1976; 2:1088.

49. Cohen WJ, Cohen NH. Lithium carbonate, haloperidol, and irreversible brain damage. JAMA 1974; 230:1283–1287.

50. Teicher MH, Altesman RI, Cole JO, Schatzberg AF. Possible nephrotoxic interaction of lithium and metronidazole. JAMA 1987; 257:3365–3366.

51. Frolich JC, Leftwich R, Ragheb H, et al. Indomethacin increases plasma lithium. Br Med J 1979; 1:1115–1116.

52. Furnell MM, Davies J. Effect of sulindac on lithium therapy. Drug Intell Clin Pharm 1985; 19:374–376.

53. Johnson R, Douglas J, Corey L, Krasney H. Adverse effects of acyclovir and meperidine. Ann Intern Med 1985; 103:962–963.

54. Stambaugh JE, Hemphill DM, Wainer IW, Schwartz I. Potentially toxic drug interaction between pethidine (meperidine) and phenobarbitone. Lancet 1977; 1:398–399.

55. Stambaugh JE, Wainer IW. Drug interaction: meperidine and chlorpromazine, a toxic combination. J Clin Pharmacol 1981; 21:140–146.

56. Guay DRP, Meatherall RC, Chalmers JL, Grahame GR. Cimetidine alters pethidine disposition in man. Br J Clin Pharmacol 1984; 18:907–914.

57. Gannon R, Pearsall W, Rowley R. Isoniazid, meperidine, and hypotension. Ann Intern Med 1983; 99:415.

58. Pond SM, Kretschzmar KM. Effect of phenytoin on meperidine clearance and normeperidine formation. Clin Pharmacol Ther 1981; 30:680–686.

59. Muhalwas KK, Shah GM, Winer RL. Renal papillary necrosis caused by long-term ingestion of pentazocine and aspirin. JAMA 1981; 246:867–868.

60. Gasser JC, Bellville JW. Interaction of the effects of hydroxyzine and pentazocine on human respiration. Anesthesiology 1975; 43:599–601.

61. American Hospital Formulary Service. AHFS No: 12.16, 1989.

62. Nappi JM. Warfarin and phenytoin interaction. Ann Intern Med 1979; 90:852.

63. Jarosinski PF, Moscow JA, Alexander MS, et al. Altered phenytoin clearance during intensive chemotherapy for acute lymphoblastic leukemia. J Pediatr 1988; 112:996–999.

64. Wang RB, Yiu CH, Liu CY, Chang TY. Evaluations of carbamazepine and phenytoin blood levels in epileptic patients in Taiwan. ASHP Midyear Clinical Meeting 1988, 23:P-168.

65. Zielinski JJ, Haidukewych D. Dual effects of carbamazepine–phenytoin interaction. Ther Drug Monit 1987; 9:21–23.

66. Harper JM, Yost RL, Stewart RB, Ciezkowski J. Phenytoin–chloramphenicol interaction: retrospective study. Drug Intell Clin Pharm 1979; 13:425–429.

67. Hetzel DJ, Bochner F, Hallpike JF, Shearman DJC, Hann CS. Cimetidine interaction with phenytoin. Br Med J 1981; 282:1512.

68. Freeman DJ, Laupacis A, Keown PA, Stiller CR, Carruthers SG. Evaluation of cyclosporine–phenytoin interaction with observations of cyclosporine metabolism. Br J Clin Pharmacol 1984; 18:887–893.

69. Roe TF, Podosin RL, Blaskovics ME. Drug interaction: diazoxide and diphenylhydantoin. J Pediatr 1975; 87:480–484.

70. Baylis EM, Crowley JM, Preece JM, Sylvester PE, Marks V. Influence of folic acid on phenytoin blood levels. Lancet 1971; 1:62–64.

71. Perucca E, Richens A. Interaction between phenytoin and imipramine. Br J Clin Pharmacol 1977; 4:485–486.

72. Smith CD, Bledsoe MA, Curran R, Green L, Lewis J. Effect of influenza vaccine on serum concentrations of total and free phenytoin. Clin Pharm 1988; 7:828–832.

73. Jann MW, Fidone GS. Effect of influenza vaccine on serum anticonvulsant concentrations. Clin Pharm 1986; 5:817–820.

74. Vincent FM. Phenothiazine-induced phenytoin intoxication. Ann Intern Med 1980; 93:56-57.
75. Kay L. Kampmann JP, Svendsen TL, et al. Influence of rifampicin and isoniazid on the kinetics of phenytoin. Br J Clin Pharmacol 1985; 20:323-326.
76. Smart HL, Somerville KW, Williams J, Richens A, Langman MJS. Effects of sucralfate upon phenytoin absorption in man. Br J Clin Pharmacol 1985; 20:238-240.
77. Pentilla O, Neuvonen PJ, Aho K, Lehtovaara R. Interaction between doxycycline and some antiepileptic drugs. Br Med J 1974; 2:470-472.
78. Miller M, Cosgriff J, Kwong T, Morken DA. Influence of phenytoin on theophylline clearance. Clin Pharmacol Ther 1984; 35:666-669.
79. Isanclis LM, Allen J, Perucca E, Routledge PA, Richens A. Effects of valproate sodium on free plasma phenytoin concentrations. Br J Clin Pharmacol 1985; 18:17-20.
80. D'Arcy PF. Alcohol and dextropropoxyphene. Pharm Int 1985; 6:244.
81. Whittington RM, Barclay AD. Epidemiology of dextropropoxyphene (Distalgesic) overdose fatalities in Birmingham and West Midlands. J Clin Hosp Pharm 1981; 6:251-257.
82. Abernethy DR, Greenblatt DJ, Morse DS, Shader RI. Interaction of propoxyphene with diazepam, alprazolam and lorazepam. Br J Clin Pharmacol 1985; 19:51-57.
83. Dam M, Christiansen J. Interaction of propoxyphene with carbamazepine. Lancet 1977; 2:509.
84. Miller RR. Effects of smoking on drug action. Clin Pharmacol Therap 1977; 22:749-756.
85. Smith R, Prudden D, Hawkes C. Propoxyphene and warfarin interaction. Drug Intell Clin Pharm 1984; 18:822.

18

Treatment of Facial and Scalp Neuralgias

James R. Couch
Southern Illinois University
School of Medicine
Springfield, Illinois

LANCINTING NEURALGIAS

Trigeminal Neuralgia

Neuralgic pain is one of the most intense pains known [1–4]. Typically the pain is illustrated by that occurring in trigeminal neuralgia or "tic douloureux," the most common form of the facial neuralgias. The pain is lighteninglike or paroxysmal, occurring for less than 1 sec and is of very high intensity. Patients usually live in fear of the next paroxysm of pain, which is both agonizing and intolerable. The pain is always unilateral and is triggerable by light touch, with trigger zones usually located around the mouth or the nares. Firm pressure will not trigger the spasms. The pain usually occurs in the distribution of the maxillary or mandibular branches of the trigeminal nerve; however, in approximately 10% of patients it is located within the distribution of the ophthalmic branch. Most patients will usually manifest one trigger zone, although occasionally more than one zone may be seen.

The paroxysms of pain typically occur in bursts over a short period and may be followed by a refractory period after each paroxysm of pain consisting of a period of a few seconds or more during which the pain is not triggerable. This may correspond to the absolute refractory period of the nerve itself. Patients typically will report having a burst of pain paroxysms, often followed by periods of up to 1 hr during which they are pain-free. The physical examination of the patient is entirely within normal limits for the typical trigeminal neuralgia patient who has had no prior surgical therapy for this condition. There is no sensory loss or motor loss on the face. A trigger zone for the pain can usually be demonstrated, as can the refractory period.

The effect of this pain upon the patient's behavior is absolutely remarkable. The patient's entire life centers around pain avoidance. Patients will go to great lengths to avoid any kind of stimulation of the face or mouth. For those patients with a trigger zone on the lips or inside the mouth, weight loss of significant proportions may occur, as they will markedly diminish oral intake of food to avoid.

It is not uncommon for the paroxysms of pain to occur in a cyclic fashion. Patients may have periods during which the pain occurs very frequently, followed by periods during which there is no occurrence of the pain.

The pain of trigeminal neuralgia may be associated with organic processes involving the fifth cranial nerve in a small percentage of patients. Tumors and vascular malformations affecting the nerve itself have been reported. Approximately 2% of the patients with trigeminal neuralgia will have multiple sclerosis or may develop multiple sclerosis later. It has been postulated that this may relate to a plaque lesion at the trigeminal root entry zone. In a series reported by Sweet [1,2], atypical features of the trigeminal neuralgia were reported in 36% of patients with multiple sclerosis, as opposed to 25% of the other patients. Sweet also noted that in those with multiple sclerosis, bilateral tic pains were seen in 30%.

Patients with trigeminal neuralgia will frequently have periods of exacerbation of the pain, followed by periods in which they are pain-free. These cycles may last for months or years. As the condition persists, however, the tendency is for the cycles to become more frequent, and the patient may need a more interventive approach for pain relief.

Trigeminal neuralgia is usually a condition of middle or late life, but can occur at any age. Females are affected more often than males. The incidence is about 4:100,000 per year with a prevalence of 155:1 million. These figures would suggest that there are approximately 40,000 patients with trigeminal neuralgia in the United States at any given time.

Glossopharyngeal (Vagoglossopharyngeal) Neuralgia

This syndrome refers to a lancinating, paroxysmal pain occurring in the throat and ear on one side [1-3]. The pain may be triggered by yawning, swallowing, or contact of food with the tonsillar area. In addition to lancinating pain, the patient may suffer bradycardia or even asystole caused by discharge in the carotid sinus nerve which joins the glossopharyngeal nerve en route to the brain stem. Convulsions have been reported as part of this syndrome, probably relating to the bradycardia and subsequent cerebral hypoxia.

The occipital, geniculate, and postherpetic neuralgias reviewed later constitute a somewhat different syndrome (Table 1). These are conditions in which a lancinating type of pain may occur, but the intensity of the pain is significantly less than that for trigeminal neuralgia and not as specifically triggerable. In addition, the patient will usually manifest some sensory changes in the distribution of the involved nerve in between the paroxysms of pain.

MECHANISM OF NEURALGIA

Despite that this terribly painful condition has received a great deal of attention from both neurologists and neurosurgeons, little is known about the actual mechanism of the neuralgia pain. It is known that approximately 2% of patients with trigeminal neuralgia have or will develop multiple sclerosis. As noted in the foregoing, Sweet [2] reported that atypical features of trigeminal neuralgia were more common in patients with trigeminal neuralgia who also had multiple sclerosis. Others have suggested that the syndrome may be related to infection of the neurons of the trigeminal ganglion with herpes simplex virus [5,6], but confirmatory data has yet to be presented.

Fromm has published extensively on physiological studies of the trigeminal system and has suggested that the physiological mechanism of trigeminal neuralgia is a deficit in polysnynaptic inhibition at the trigeminal nucleus [7]. Fromm has carried this hypothesis one step further and found that drugs that inhibit the firing of interneurons in the trigeminal sensory nuclei will be effective in therapy of trigeminal neuralgia. Fromm found that both carbamazepine and phenytoin were effective in reducing interneuron firing. He then went one step further to postulate that baclofen would be of therapeutic use in trigeminal neuralgia because it affected the experimental preparation in the same way as carbamazepine. Clinical trials have shown that baclofen is, indeed, effective, although generally not as effective as carbamazepine [8,9].

In the other syndromes of glossopharyngeal neuralgia and geniculate neuralgia, it can be assumed that the same mechanism that produces the lancinating pains in trigeminal neuralgia probably produces these latter two syndromes.

In the postherpetic neuralgias and occipital neuralgias, the mechanism is probably different. In these neuralgias, there is usually recognizable damage to the nerve from some source, and there is recognizable alteration of nerve function manifested by diminished sensation in the distribution of that nerve. Stimulation of the skin with light touch in the distribution of that nerve will usually produce

Table 1 Classification of Neuralgias

Type	Location of pain	Characteristics of pain	Neurological findings
Trigeminal neuralgia (tic douloureaux)	Mandibular maxillary distribution of fifth nerve, rarely ophthalmic division, virtually always unilateral	Lightninglike lancinating; very severe, triggerable	Facial sensation normal
Glossopharyngeal neuralgia	Posterior pharynx and external auditory canal on same side, unilateral	Lancinating, very severe, triggerable	No weakness in pharynx; sensation normal
Geniculate neuralgia	External auditory canal	Lancinating, triggerable	No weakness or sensory loss
Postherpetic neuralgia	In distribution of branch of trigeminal nerve involved	Burning dysesthesia/paresthesia; exacerbation by light touch	Numbness and sensory loss in distribution of involved nerve with herpetic lesions or postherpetic scarring in distribution of involved nerve
Geniculate neuralgia (Ramsay Hunt)	In external auditory canal	Burning dysesthesia and exacerbation by light touch	Vesicular eruption in the external auditory canal with a small area of sensory loss; seventh nerve palsy may occur
Carotidynia	Neck, jaw, or one side; possibly hemicranial pain	Throbbing, aching, pressure	Tenderness over carotid artery
Occipital neuralgia	Occipital and parietal scalp, jaw, retroorbital area	Aching, boring, at times triggerable by turning head or tapping occipital nerve	Tenderness or dyesthesia over ipsilateral parietal and occipital scalp and over occipital nerve; tapping on occipital nerve may elicit Tinel's sign

additional discomfort and dysesthesia, consisting of a burning or "raw skin" sensation. Patients with these syndromes, however, do not usually experience the intense lancinating pains typical for trigeminal neuralgia.

The syndrome of anesthesia dolorosa is one which develops in patients who have had multiple lesioning procedures of the trigeminal nerve as an attempt for therapy for trigeminal neuralgia. In this syndrome, patients have alterations of sensory function with demonstrable loss of sensation. They experience a chronic aching, boring discomfort of variable intensity. Again, this particular syndrome is not associated with lancinating pains, although the patient may have lancinating pains that appear to be residual from the underlying trigeminal neuralgia. The anesthesia dolorosa, however, appears to be a direct result of the trigeminal nerve lesion.

THERAPY OF NEURALGIAS ASSOCIATED WITH LANCINATING PAINS

The syndromes of trigeminal neuralgia, glossopharyngeal neuralgia (vagoglossopharyngeal neuralgia), and certain forms of geniculate neuralgia or vidian neuralgia are associated with a triggerable, lancinating type of pain without any neurological findings or sensory loss in the area affected by the lancinating pain. Therapy for these conditions is basically the same and is reviewed in Table 2.

The medications that are useful in treating trigeminal neuralgia are those that have an effect of inhibiting polysynaptic firing within the nervous system. Theoretically, these drugs may act to diminish a positive-feedback type of augmentation within the sensory nucleus that results in transient activation of neurons involved in the pain system.

Carbamazepine (Tegretol) is the drug of choice for first-line therapy of trigeminal neuralgia [1–4]. Use of this drug for trigeminal neuralgia was first reported by Blom [10] in 1962. A very large percentage of patients will respond to this drug with a high degree of relief. It has been stated by some authorities that absence of response to carbamazepine puts the diagnosis of trigeminal neuralgia in doubt.

Investigation of the mechanism of action of carbamazepine reveals that it can inhibit maximal electroshock seizures and can abolish focal discharges elicited by penicillin or alumina cream in the brain. It is effective in reducing interneuron firing in the trigeminal nucleus, but has little effect on postsynaptic potentiation in the spinal cord [11]. The biochemical mechanism of action for carbamazepine is unknown. The mechanism by which carbamazepine affects trigeminal neuralgia is unknown. Fromm [7] has shown that carbamazepine can increase interneuron inhibitory activity and diminish excitatory transmission in the trigeminal nucleus in cats. He has postulated this to be the mechanism of action in carbamazepine and also for phenytoin and baclofen in treating trigeminal neuralgia.

Carbamazepine is absorbed rapidly after an oral dose. The half-life in the naive patient may be as long as 65 hr. With long-term administration, however,

Table 2 Drugs for Therapy of Trigeminal Neuralgia

Drug	Dosage (mg/day)	Blood levels (μg/ml)	Serum half-life (hr) (long-term use)	Toxic and side effects
Carbamazepine	400–2000	4–12	12–17	Major: agranulocytosis, aplastic anemia, thrombocytopenia, leukopenia, hepatic dysfunction Minor: ataxia, sedation, nausea, vomiting, confusion, headache, personality change
Phenytoin	200–600	10–20	18–24	Major: agranulocytosis, aplastic anemia, thrombocytopenia, leukopenia, hepatic dysfunction, lymphadenopathy, fetal malformations, neuropathy, cerebellar degeneration Minor: ataxia, sedation, nausea, vomiting, confusion, headache, personality change
Baclofen	10–80	Not known	3–4	Major: abrupt withdrawal may produce hallucinations, hepatic dysfunction Minor: headache, insomnia, euphoria, sedation, confusion, weakness, fatigue, nausea, urinary frequency, altered hepatic function, constipation, urinary frequency
Chlorphenesin	800–2400	Not known	Not known	Major: rare leukopenia, thrombocytopenia, agranulocytosis, anaphylactoid reactions Minor: sedation, dizziness, confusion, nausea

a half-life of 12–17 hr is seen. The drug demonstrates first-order kinetics. Patients being treated for trigeminal neuralgia will often require dosing three to four times a day and will usually find that they know right away when the medication is beginning to "wear off," and it is time for the next dose.

The dose of carbamazepine that is effective in trigeminal neuralgia is frequently lower than the dose required for seizure therapy. It is not uncommon for patients to respond well to dosages of 400–600 mg/day. These patients may, however, become refractory to these low dosages over time and require escalation of the dosage. The dosage range for carbamazepine varies from 400 to 2000 mg/day. Serum blood levels should be monitored and are approximately the same as those employed for control of seizures, with a range of 4–12 μg/ml. In my experience, most patients who are going to respond to carbamazepine will respond to dosages of under 1000 mg/day. Patients who do not respond to dosages of this level usually show little response to increasing the dosage further. On the other hand, it is categorically necessary to push the dose level to the point at which the patient has a trough blood level of close to 12 μg/ml before declaring carbamazepine a failed therapy.

The major side effects of carbamazepine are those associated with blood dyscrasias and hepatic dysfunction [11] (see Table 2). Anemia, leukopenia, and thrombocytopenia, all have been reported with carbamazepine. Severe blood dyscrasias, such as aplastic anemia and agranulocytosis, occur rarely, but are a major concern. There is a debate over whether the blood dyscrasias are dose-related or idiosyncratic and similar to the severe bone marrow arrest that rarely occurs with the antibiotic, chloramphenicol.

A significant number of patients will experience a mild leukopenia in association with carbamazepine therapy. If the leukopenia develops, it will usually be seen within 4 weeks. The white blood cell count may drop into the range of 3500–4000/mm^3 and then stabilize. In other patients, the white blood count may continue to fall, necessitating cessation of the drug. The drug should always be discontinued if the white cell count falls below 3000–3500 cells/mm^3. Patients whose white blood cell count remains above 3500 will be able to continue taking carbamazepine, but should continue to have monthly determinations of blood cell count for the first 6 months and then every 3 months, thereafter.

Carbamazepine may cause drug-induced hepatitis; consequently, the patients should have periodic determinations of hepatic function. This is a reversible process if the medication is discontinued, but potentially serious hepatic dysfunction may occur if the carbamazepine is continued.

Rashes of an allergic type may occur with carbamazepine, and the Stevens-Johnson syndrome has been reported as a rare complication. The patient should be watched for these types of allergic reactions.

Minor side effects of carbamazepine include ataxia, sedation, nausea, vomiting, confusion, headache, and personality change. These are generally dose-related, not idiosyncratic, and remit if the dose is lowered.

Phenytoin (Dilantin) has been effective in trigeminal neuralgia [1-4] and remains the drug of second choice. Phenytoin is effective in therapy of seizures and acts to prevent the spread of seizure activity within the nervous system [11]. Experimentally, phenytoin can modify maximal electroshock therapy, but has little effect on seizures induced by pentylenetetrazol. Phenytoin also enhances postsynaptic potentiation within the spinal cord and can enhance the activity of inhibitory efferents from the cerebellum which, in turn, help to diminish the risk of seizure. At the cellular and membrane level, phenytoin decreases sodium flux and delays activation of potassium current following the action potential, thus preventing the rapid repetitive depolarization that may be necessary for seizure genesis. As noted, phenytoin can diminish excitatory transmission in the trigeminal nucleus [7].

Phenytoin is absorbed slowly and somewhat variably. Peak concentration after an oral dose is achieved in 2-6 hr. The half-life for phenytoin in the extended administration state is between 18 and 24 hr. Patients may need at least two doses per day to maintain an adequate effect.

The dosage of phenytoin is quite variable from one individual to another. It may vary between 200 and 600 mg/day, usually in divided doses, and it is usually necessary to give the medication on a twice-to three-times-a-day schedule. Serum blood levels should be monitored and kept between 10 and 20 μg/ml. It is important to note that phenytoin has second-order kinetics because of its protein binding. As a result, patients may have little change in blood level until serum protein binding is saturated, and then a rapid escalation of blood level may occur with a minimal increase in dosage. Toxicity may occur rapidly and unpredictably in some patients.

The side effects of phenytoin are similar to those outlined for carbamazepine [11]. Blood dyscrasias are less of a problem, and the idiosyncratic aplastic anemia mentioned as a possibility for carbamazepine is not associated with phenytoin. Other major side effects include lymphadenopathy syndrome that may resemble lymphoma or leukemia, often requiring lymph node biopsy. In this situation, phenytoin should be discontinued and not restarted.

A fetal hydantoin syndrome has been reported in up to 5% of infants born to women taking phenytoin during pregnancy. This syndrome generally is manifested by minor morphological changes, such as wide-set eyes, low-set ears, and a fingerlike thumb. This syndrome may also be associated with an apparent significant decrease in mental capabilities. Usage of phenytoin in pregnant females should be undertaken only with great caution.

Minor side effects, again, are those of ataxia, sedation, confusion, headache, and personality change. Nausea and vomiting may occur at higher doses. Gum hypertrophy frequently occurs in children and adolescents, but is much less common in adults. Acneiform skin eruptions may occur in adolescents and produce very significant dermatological problems for the patient.

Finally, the neurodegenerative features of phenytoin appear to be relatively unique to this drug. Long-term use of phenytoin is associated with a fairly high frequency of neuropathy. This appears to be a cumulative problem, and it is one that a large percentage of patients taking phenytoin will manifest if they take the drug long enough. This neuropathy is potentially reversible if the patient discontinues the phenytoin, depending on the severity of the neuropathy at the time of discontinuance of the drug.

Cerebellar degeneration is an even more serious condition that may be seen in long-term use of phenytoin. This is a very uncommon problem, and there is relatively little information on the mechanism of pathogenesis. If the patient develops substantial truncal ataxia, the medication should be discontinued.

Baclofen (Lioresal) has been investigated by Fromm as a therapy for trigeminal neuralgia [8,9]. The background and basic pharmacology were reviewed in the foregoing. Baclofen is a γ-aminobutyric acid (GABA) analogue. GABA is a major inhibitory neurotransmitter within the central nervous system and baclofen may exert some of its effect by acting as a GABA agonist. The exact mechanism by which this medication affects trigeminal neuralgia is unknown, but may relate to diminishing excitatory transmission in the trigeminal nucleus [7]. The main use for baclofen currently is in therapy of spasticity associated with central nervous system lesions. The medication is absorbed rapidly from the gastrointestinal tract and is excreted unchanged by the kidneys. The ability to determine blood levels is not now available for guiding therapy.

The initial dosage for baclofen is 5–10 mg twice a day. The dosage may be increased every 3–7 days to a maximum of 80 mg/day in a divided dose of three to four times per day. It is difficult to ascertain a half-life, as the absorption of baclofen is dependent upon the dose, and absorption may be reduced with increasing doses.

The major side effects of baclofen include hallucinations and seizures associated with abrupt withdrawal [11]. Baclofen should be used with caution in patients with impaired renal function because the drug is excreted by the kidney. The less severe side effects include drowsiness, dizziness, confusion, headache, insomnia, nausea, abdominal pain, vomiting, diarrhea, and urinary urgency and frequency. Overdosage produces vomiting, drowsiness, difficulty with accommodation, and hypotonia. More severe intoxication can produce respiratory depression and seizures.

In his work with baclofen, Fromm reported that up to 75% of patients with trigeminal neuralgia received significant relief from use of baclofen [8,9]. On longer-term follow-up, however, the efficacy of the medication as a single therapeutic agent dropped rather dramatically. After 1–18 months, 50% of patients became refractory to the medication.

Baclofen can be used in combination with either carbamazepine or phenytoin. Its usefulness may be greater as a combined-therapy agent than as a monotherapy agent.

Chlorphenesin (Maolate) is a congener of mefenesin, which was one of the earliest muscle relaxants. It appears to act by inhibiting polysynaptic reflexes. Neuronal conduction, neuromuscular transmission, and muscle excitability are not affected by this drug at therapeutic doses.

Chlorphenesin is useful primarily as an adjunctive agent for trigeminal neuralgia, in combination with carbamazepine or phenytoin, and has relatively limited usefulness as a primary agent [4]. The dosage of chlorphenesin ranges between 800 and 2400 mg/day. Major side effects are those of drowsiness and sedation. The usual allergic reactions can occur.

The foregoing medications may also be used for glossopharyngeal or geniculate neuralgias, which are manifested by lancinating type of pains [1–4,12]. In patients with anesthesia dolorosa, use of these medications in various combinations may be helpful to diminish the primary dysesthetic pain or to diminish the lancinating neuralgic pain that may also occur in this syndrome.

Other anticonvulsants, such as phenobarbital, have been tried in trigeminal neuralgia and have been unsuccessful. Valproic acid (Depakene) has received an anecdotal trial. Results, so far, are not particularly promising, but further work needs to be done. Certainly, new medications are needed to treat these syndromes that produce such excruciating pain.

SURGICAL THERAPY FOR NEURALGIAS

Surgical therapy for neuralgia has evolved over many years [1,2,13–17]. Cushing and Dandy worked on this problem, reporting on various procedures dealing with trigeminal nerve. Sjöqvist [15] described bulbar trigeminal tractotomy as an approach to this problem in 1938. In more recent years, two surgical procedures have been developed, which constitute almost all of the surgical therapy for neuralgias. These include neurolysis, at the level of the trigeminal ganglion, and vascular decompression, in the posterior fossa. Other procedures are still employed occasionally; however, these two procedures are the major ones now being used.

Neurotomy

Neurotomy at the level of the geniculate ganglion was developed by Sweet and his colleagues [1,2]. The usual method for neurotomy is to undertake radiofrequency lesioning through a needle introduced into the trigeminal ganglion through the foramen ovale from a percutaneous puncture. A thermal lesion is induced through the needle by radiofrequency heating. The lesion can be tailored to produce hypoalgesia, but not analgesia, and can be directed at the particular branch of the trigeminal nerve in which the trigger zone lies, sparing the other branches. The patient can be allowed to awaken after the needle is once placed to cooperate with the surgeon in making the lesion. The goal of the surgeon is to produce loss of pinprick sensation with preservation of light touch.

Theoretically, the operation is possible because the smaller C fibers that carry pain are more sensitive to the thermal lesion than are the heavily myelinated fibers that carry light touch. During the operation, the patient can be tested for light touch and pinprick sensation after each burst of radiofrequency energy, to limit the extent of the lesion.

Sweet has reviewed the results of this operation in 7333 patients collected from 11 centers in recent years [2]. In his review, Sweet chose those centers with active services carrying out significant numbers of these operations. He included results from 11 centers with 550–1100 patients per center. He found that more than 96% of the patients received early relief from the operation, and the degree of relief was usually very good. On the other hand, recurrence of pain requiring reoperation was also fairly high. Pain recurrence was reported in 8–31% of the patients, with an average of about 20%. In Sweet's own series of 702 patients, 31% of the patients required reoperation. For those patients who had at least a 5-year follow-up, the rate of reoperation ranged from 21 to 28%. In my experience, recurrence of pain after 2–5 years has not been an uncommon occurrence, and this often requires a repeat neurological procedure.

Operative complications for this procedure are relatively few and decline significantly with experience of the surgeon. The early complications include possibility of bacterial meningitis or subarachnoid hemorrhage. Masseter dysfunction and other cranial nerve lesions, including that of the 3rd, 4th, or 6th cranial nerves have been reported [1,2]. Death occurred in 1 of 726 patients in Sweet's series [2]. A major complication that can be serious, if not controlled, is that of increased blood pressure occurring at the time of the radiofrequency lesion. This can be controlled with the use of nitroprusside.

Complications relating to the nerve lesion include corneal anesthesia, dysesthesias, anesthesia (analgesia) dolorosa. Sweet found corneal anesthesia in 2–8% of outpatients in his multicenter review. This, of course, is a very serious complication that can lead to corneal ulceration and possibly to loss of sight.

Dysesthesias in the area of the trigeminal nerve occurred in 18% of patients. In 5%, the dysethesia produced major discomfort for the patient, whereas in 13%, discomfort was only minor. Anesthesia dolorosa is a condition in which the patient develops a persistent burning, aching pain in the distribution of the lesioned nerve. The intensity of this problem may range from minor to very serious, with severe disruption of the patient's life. In Sweet's series, the incidence varied from 0.2 to 25% with most centers reporting 0.5–3% occurrence of this problem. Sweet points out that production of complete anesthesia is more likely to be associated with anesthesia dolorosa, whereas hypoesthesia only has a lower incidence of this problem.

Microvascular Decompression

The idea for microvascular decompression was initiated by Dandy, who developed the procedure of transecting the sensory root of the fifth nerve for trigeminal neuralgia [16]. Dandy observed that many patients had a blood vessel in close proximity to this structure in 45% of his 215 cases. Between 1955 and 1970, Gardner, Rand, Jannetta, and Taarnhöj began to utilize this concept by separating the proximate blood vessel from the fifth nerve root with materials, such as a gelatin sponge [13,14,17]. Jannetta has been the major proponent of this procedure during the past 20 years.

For this procedure the cerebropontine angle is approached through a retromastoid incision and craniectomy. With present day microscopic surgery, the craniectomy can be relatively small. The junction of the sensory root of the fifth nerve with the pons is then explored for vascular contact. If such contact is identified, a soft material such as Ivalon or Teflon is inserted between the offending blood vessel and the nerve to maintain separation. It is felt that the movement of the blood vessel with the pulses of blood flow from the cardiac cycle provides ballottement of the vessel against the nerve and damage to the nerve. Insertion of the buffer prevents this ballottement and prevents further nerve damage, allowing the nerve to recover.

Wilkin, in his series of 105 operations, identified arterial contact with distortion of the fifth nerve in 70% of these patients [13]. In addition, 5% had venous contact with the nerve and 2% had a venous angioma impinging on the nerve, whereas in 23%, there was no vascular contact noted. Relative to the arterial contact, Wilkin found that 23% of patients had wedging of the superior cerebellar artery between the fifth nerve root and the pons, 14% showed anatomical distortion of the nerve, and 33% had some other type of arterial contact. Wilkin reported that of his 68 patients with arterial contact, 72% had excellent results, 6% had good results, and 22% were either not relieved or were early failures. In an additional 13 patients, arterial contact was not clearly identified or the patient had apparent venous contact with division of the vein at surgery. Only 54% of these patients had good or excellent results.

In the remaining patients, Wilkin carried out a partial sectioning of the posterior half of the main sensory root of the trigeminal nerve and reported that 86% of these patients had good or excellent results in a 21-month follow-up.

Complications of this procedure are those of crainectomy and manipulation of the brain stem itself. Hemorrhagic infarct of the brain stem, epidural hematoma, subdural hematoma, and cerebral spinal fluid leak have been reported. Facial weakness and auditory nerve damage likewise have been reported. The frequency of auditory nerve damage has been diminished by the use of intraoperative auditory-evoked potentials.

Various workers have reported on use of this procedure in atypical facial pain. Jannetta reported that 50% of patients with this diagnosis had relief by microvascular decompression [17]. This procedure has also been used in geniculate neuralgia and glossopharyngeal neuralgia; the experience does not allow a judgment about whether or not this should be adopted as standard therapy. This material has been reviewed recently by Wilkin [13].

The microvascular decompression procedure has found several proponents in the major neurosurgical centers. The procedure has the advantage that it does not produce a neural lesion, and there is the possibility that the patient will have relief without the feared complications of corneal anesthesia or anesthesia dolorosa. On the other hand, the operation is technically demanding, and there is a risk of life-threatening complications. Currently, many centers will proceed with microvascular decompression as a first surgical procedure. If the patient has recurrence of pain, they will use neurotomy as a follow-up operation. The field remains in a state of flux because it is still too early for a compilation of a truly long-term follow-up on numerous patients. Further experience is necessary to determine if microvascular decompression can offer long-term relief to the patient with trigeminal or other neuralgia.

NONLANCINATING NEURALGIC CONDITIONS

Inflammatory Neuralgias

In addition to the lancinating neuralgias, there is another group of syndromes that produce head and facial pain with features of more persistent, but less intense, neuralgic pain. This is a somewhat diverse group that includes syndromes in which there is definite nerve damage, periodic nerve irritation, and vascular syndromes associated with pain. These syndromes are outlined in Table 1.

Postherpetic Neuralgia

A small, but significant, number of patients experiencing herpes zoster in the trigeminal distribution will develop a postherpetic neuralgic syndrome [3]. This syndrome consists of a burning, aching dysesthesia in the distribution of the trigeminal branch in which the herpes zoster eruption occurred. The course of this problem is variable. Many patients experience significant relief over time; however, occasional patients will have continuing pain over many years. Physical examination generally reveals evidence of some decreased sensation to pinprick and light touch in the distribution of the involved nerve. At the same time, the patient will report that banal stimuli such as light touch will produce a burning, aching sensation or will intensify an underlying, already present, burning sensation.

Treatment for this condition is generally relatively unsatisfactory. The use of carbamazepine and phenytoin in the usual doses has produced relief for some patients. In other patients, use of amitriptyline (Elavil, Endep) in dosages ranging from 75 to 250 mg/day has produced some relief. Amitriptyline may be combined with fluphenazine (Prolixin) which, at times, may enhance the analgesic effect. Amitriptyline may also be combined with phenytoin or carbamazepine. Limited success has been reported with transcutaneous nerve stimulation (TNS), but generally I have not found this to produce long-term beneficial results.

Sweet has reported use of either thermal or glycerol lesioning of the trigeminal ganglion, in an attempt to help these unfortunate patients [2]. He notes, however, that patients not infrequently have initial success, with recurrence of the pain over time. He feels that the success rate for this procedure is marginal, at best.

Finally, the use of steroids in this syndrome has been reported. Steroid therapy must be started early while patients still have the herpetic eruption. This therapy has been called into question, and the data on its usefulness are conflicting at this point. With early use of steroids, there is the possibility that the herpes infection might spread to produce corneal involvement or a herpes encephalitis. Currently, the use of steroids in conjunction with herpes zoster should be approached with some caution.

Ramsay Hunt Syndrome

A second herpes zoster infection, which is rare but well-described, is the Ramsay Hunt syndrome. In this syndrome, a herpetic eruption is seen in the ear, with origin in the geniculate ganglion. Examination of the ear reveals a herpetic lesion along the external auditory canal. The syndrome may be associated with facial palsy and also with alteration in hearing from loss of the stapedius muscle. At onset of the acute phase, there is a deep, aching pain in the ear that may spread to the jaw and retroauricular area. This pain may precede the herpetic eruption. The patient may go on to develop a postherpetic neuralgia. Treatment is symptomatic as outlined in the foregoing.

Tic Convulsif

Tic convulsif refers to a syndrome of otalgic and ipsilateral hemifacial spasm [3,17]. In this syndrome, a deep aching continuous pain is noted in the ear. The pain may radiate to the cheek or jaw. The hemifacial spasm may develop concomitantly or apparently independently. Yeh and Tew reported a patient in whom vascular decompression of the geniculate nerve relieved both conditions [18].

Tolosa-Hunt Syndrome

The Tolosa-Hunt syndrome [19] is an inflammatory syndrome of unknown origin. In this syndrome, there is a painful unilateral headache, which is deep and boring or aching. The syndrome may come on rapidly and is associated with variable degrees of paresis of cranial nerves III, IV, and VI. It has been postulated that the origin of the syndrome is related to a periostitis of the superior orbital fissure. Alternatively, an inflammatory reaction in the cavernous sinus has also been proposed. However, these patients do not progress to developing a cavernous sinus thrombosis or other cavernous sinus pathology. The diagnosis of Tolosa-Hunt syndrome is one of exclusion. The possibilities of an orbital or parasellar tumor or granuloma or aneurysm of the carotid artery in the area of the cavernous sinus must be ruled out [20]. The treatment is with corticosteroids in moderate to high doses initially, with tapering over several weeks to a low dose. Tapering is based on a continued absence of pain and cranial nerve palsy as the dose is lowered. There is rapid recovery from the pain and total remission of the cranial palsies.

Gradenigo's Syndrome

Gradenigo's syndrome results from an epidural abscess at the tip of the petrous pyramid. Part of the syndrome may involve the fifth and sixth cranial nerves, producing sixth nerve palsy and impairment of facial sensation. The patient may have severe pain in the ipsilateral ear, as well as over the side of the face and temporal region. Therapy is directed at the infectious process at the epidural abscess itself.

Upper Cervical Neuralgias with Facial Pain

Occipital Neuralgia

Occipital neuralgia was described by Hunter and Mayfield [21], who reported a group of patients with recurrent attacks of hemicranial pain. In these patients, the pain began in the suboccipital region and radiated to the vertex. Frequently, a deep aching pain occurred in the temporal region, periorbital area and, at times, a superficial pain was described in the lower jaw. These authors also noted that the pains could be associated with lacrimation, facial flushing, and even nasal stuffiness. During the attacks, patients were acutely ill, and there was tenderness over the course of the greater occipital nerve. Rotary movements of the neck or hyperextension at the neck intensified the symptoms, and traction of the head provided relief. Local block of the greater occipital nerve or the second and third cervical nerve roots provided relief. The authors reported that section of the greater occipital nerve or the second and third sensory roots produced relief in those patients with trauma underlying the origin of the pain, but not in other patients.

Other descriptions of this condition have included a much less dramatic [3,22,23] syndrome, with pain localized primarily to the distribution of the greater occipital nerve. The pain has been described as a constant, aching pain or a positionally related paroxysmal pain that occurs with neck movement. In those patients with the lower-grade constant, aching pain, there is often a component of triggerable exacerbation elicited by movement of the head or neck or by tapping of the greater occipital nerve at the occipital ridge [3,22-24].

This syndrome, as an isolated cause of headache, is a relatively unusual one. The diagnosis is made by confirming sensitivity of the greater occipital nerve to pressure or tapping or precipitation of the pain syndrome by specific neck movement. Blockade of the greater occipital nerve with local anesthetic should produce complete relief. This procedure can be employed to confirm the diagnosis.

Greater occipital neuralgia occasionally can be treated with nonsteroidal anti-inflammatory agents [24]. In those patients with a demonstrable neuralgic component, use of carbamazepine or phenytoin may be helpful; in those in whom the pain does not appear to be truly neuralgic, the possibility of a posterior facet syndrome involving the first, second, or third cervical vertebrae should be considered [23]. Nonsteroidal anti-inflammatory agents may be very useful in these patients. Amitriptyline in modest doses may also be useful in the true neuralgic syndrome or in the posterior facet syndrome.

Surgical therapy has been attempted, with section of the greater occipital nerve, but the failure rate is high [22,23]. In my own limited experience (one case), a severe denervation neuralgic type of persistent pain resulted that responded to carbamazepine.

Superior Laryngeal Neuralgia and Neck–Tongue Syndrome

O'Neil et al. [25] reported a case of a man with right anterior neck pain that would extend into the right shoulder, cheek, face, retroauricular, and retroorbital region. The pain was intermittent and was initiated by mouth opening, yawning, or turning the head. The patient also noted that singing or prolonged talking would exacerbate the pain. The patient was found to have a palsy of the superior laryngeal nerve. Block of this nerve produced complete relief of the pain and superior laryngeal neurectomy produced a permanent relief. The patient's pain was refractory to antimigraine and antineuralgic medication.

The neck–tongue syndrome [26,27] is another rare syndrome in which movement of the neck produces pain in the side of the neck, which can spread to the ipsilateral ear or occiput. The pain is also associated with a hemiglossal and ipsilateral hemiglossal paresthesia and may have a component of suboccipital paresthesia and even numbness in the hand. The headache is precipitated by turning the head. Relief is obtained by stabilizing the neck with a cervical collar. In this syndrome, mobility of the tongue and taste sensation are both normal. The source of neuralgic pains is still unclear; however, it is felt that this involves the upper cervical roots, as well as the pharyngeal plexus. In some patients, immobilization of the neck with a cervical collar may be helpful. If so, pathology of the upper cervical spine, such as disk protrusion or minor atlantoaxial dislocation, should be considered. In this small minority of cases, cervical disectomy and fusion may be appropriate therapy, but a clear relation between the anatomical picture and the pain needs to be established before such a procedure is undertaken [26,27].

Vascular Conditions Associated with Facial Pain

Carotodynia

Carotodynia is a syndrome of swelling and tenderness in the cervical triangle, with pain referred to the eye and retroorbital area, retroauricular region, and deep in the malar region [28–30]. The swelling noted may be due to a tender carotid artery at the bifurcation, but angiography is normal. There is a constant pain in the neck over the carotid artery in most cases, and jaw pain on that side is frequent. The patients often have periodic exacerbations of head pain in the periorbital, retroauricular, or maxillary area similar to migraine. The pain exacerbation in other patients may be more focal in the neck and jaw. The pain may be associated with nausea and vasomotor phenomena, similar to migraine. The carotid arteries are tender to palpation in these patients, which is one of the key diagnostic features.

In Lovshin's report of 100 cases [28], he noted a greater female preponderance and noted that the problem was most common in the fourth and fifth decades, but could occur at any age.

The syndrome may respond to simple analgesics or nonsteroidal anti-inflammatory agents. In other cases, the use of antimigraine agents, such as ergotamine preparations, ergonovine, or methysergide, produced a beneficial response [3,29].

Oculosympathetic Palsy and Pericarotid Syndrome

Oculosympathetic palsy was originally described by Raeder, and the eponym Raeder's syndrome has persisted. This syndrome has evolved to include those patients who have oculosympathetic palsy along with varying degrees of facial pain [3]. Because of confusion with other syndromes, this has been a difficult entity to define. The term should be used in those situations for which no other etiology for the oculosympathetic palsy is identified.

In the pericarotid syndrome described by Vijayan and Watson [31], an oculosympathetic palsy, ipsilateral headache, and anhidrosis of the forehead were noted. Facial sweating was otherwise intact. This was felt to be due to lesioning of the upper sympathetic fibers of the paracarotid plexus, although this was only proved in one of the cases reported by Vijayan and Watson. It is unclear whether this represents a variant of the oculosympathetic palsy.

ATYPICAL FACIAL PAIN

The syndrome of atypical facial pain is one that has caused a deal of consternation to physicians, as well as patients, and is one that defies definition. This syndrome refers to those patients who have facial pain that is of obscure origin and for whom no clear etiology of the pain can be defined. Solomon and Lipton [32] and Raskin [33] have reviewed this problem recently.

In this syndrome the patient usually complains of a pain involving the face, which may be of variable location in the 1st, 2nd, or 3rd branches of the trigeminal nerve or may involve the entire face. The pain is usually described as a deep, aching type of pain that is present most or all of the time. It is not a lancinating type of pain but may be enhanced or exacerbated by physical maneuvers such as chewing or by contact of cold or warm air with the face. The pain is usually of moderate intensity, but occasionally may be quite severe. The constant pain, although moderate in intensity, usually leads the patient to seek medical attention and may lead to habituation problems with narcotic–analgesic medications if the patient's medication usage is not monitored carefully by the physician.

In these patients, a thorough investigation should be undertaken to look for underlying etiologic problems, which may range from inflammatory conditions to tumors, to bony cysts in the jaw lying below the root of a tooth. Raskin feels that extensive investigation will elucidate an etiology in most cases. In those cases where extensive investigation reveals no etiology, Jannetta has postulated that the syndrome is a specific syndrome of the trigeminal nerve, relating to the same mechanisms that produce typical trigeminal neuralgia [17].

Therapy of this syndrome is difficult. Intensive efforts should be directed toward identifying a specific cause for the pain. If no cause can be found, treatment with the same medications employed for trigeminal neuralgia is sometimes beneficial. In general, surgical procedures should be undertaken only as a last resort and after other attempts at specific diagnosis or medical therapy have failed, because surgical treament in this syndrome has been associated with a fairly high rate of failure.

REFERENCES

1. Sweet WH. The treatment of trigeminal neuralgia (tic douloureux). N Engl J Med 1986; 315:174–177.
2. Sweet WH. Percutaneous methods for the treatment of trigeminal neuralgia and other faciocephalic pain: comparison with microvascular. Semin Neurol 1988; 8:272–279.
3. Dalessio DJ. The major neuralgias, postinfectious neuritis, intractable pain, and atypical facial pain. In: Dalessio DJ ed. Wolff's headache and other head pain. New York: Oxford University Press, 1972:233–255.
4. Dalessio DJ. Medical treatment of the major neuralgias. Semin Neurol 1988; 8:286–290.
5. Baringer JR, Swoveland P. Recovery of herpes-simplex virus from human trigeminal ganglion. N Engl J Med 1973; 288:648–50.
6. Wepsic JG. Tic douloureux: etiology, refined treatment. N Engl J Med 1973; 288:680–681.
7. Fromm G, Chattha AS, Terrence CF, Glass JD. Role of inhibitory mechanisms in trigeminal neuralgia. Neurology 1981; 31:683–687.
8. Fromm GH, Terrence CF, Chattha AS. Baclofen in the treatment of trigeminal neuralgia: double-blind study and long-term follow-up. Ann Neurol 1984; 15:240–244.
9. Fromm GH, Terrence CF. Comparison of L-baclofen and racemic baclofen in trigeminal neuralgia. Neurology 1987; 37:1725–1728.
10. Blom S. Trigeminal neuralgia: its treatment with a new anticonvulsant drug (G-32883). Lancet 1962; 1:839–840.

11. Gilman A, Goodman LS, Gilman A, eds. Goodman and Gilman's the pharmacological basis of therapeutics, 6th ed. New York: MacMillan, 1980:452-455, 459-460, 488-490.
12. Ringel RA, Roy EP. Glossopharyngeal neuralgia: successful treatment with baclofen. Ann Neurol 1987; 21:514-515.
13. Wilkins RH. Surgical therapy of neuralgia: vascular decompression procedures. Semin Neuro 1988; 8:280-285.
14. Jannetta PJ. Neurovascular compression in cranial nerve and systemic disease. Ann Surg 1980; 192:518-525.
15. Sjöqvist O. Studies on pain conduction in the trigeminal nerve, a contribtion to the surgical treatment of facial pain. Acta Psychiatry Neurol 1938; 17:1-139.
16. Dandy WE. Section of the sensory root of the trigeminal nerve at the pons: preliminary report of the operative procedure. Bull Johns Hopkins Hosp 1925; 36:105-106.
17. Jannetta PJ. Observations on the etiology of trigeminal neuralgia, hemifacial spasm, acoustic nerve dysfunction and glossopharyngeal neuralgia. Definitive microsurgical treatment and results in 117 patients. Neurochirurgia 1977; 20:145-154.
18. Yeh H, Tew JM. Tic convulsif, the combination of geniculate neuralgia and hemifacial spasm relieved by vascular decompression. Neurology 1984; 34:682-684.
19. Hunt WE, Meagher JN, LeFever HE, Zeman W. Painful ophthalmoplegia: its relation to indolent inflammation of the cavernous sinus. Neurology 1961; 11:56-62.
20. Spector RH, Fiandaca MS. The "sinister" Tolosa-Hunt syndrome. Neurology 1986; 36:198-203.
21. Hunter CR, Mayfield FH. Role of the upper cervical roots in the production of pain in the head. Am J Surg 1949; 78:5, 743-751.
22. Kerr FWL. Mechanisms, diagnosis, and management of some cranial and facial pain syndromes. Surg Clin North Am 1963; 43:951-961.
23. Pawl RP. Headache, cervical spondylosis, and anterior cervical fusion. In: Nyhus LM, ed. Surg Ann 1977; 9:391-408.
24. Dalessio DJ. Occipital neuralgia. Headache 1980; 20:107.
25. O'Neill BP, Aronson AE, Pearson BW, Nauss LA. Superior laryngeal neuralgia: carotidynia or just another pain in the neck? Headache 1982; 22:6-9.
26. Lance JW, Anthony M. Neck-tongue syndrome on sudden turning of the head. J Neurol Neurosurg Psychiatry 1980; 43:97-101.
27. Fortin CJ, Biller J. Neck tongue syndrome. Headache 1985; 25:255-258.
28. Lovshin LL. Vascular neck pain—a common syndrome seldom recognized. Cleve Clin Q 1960; 27:5-13.
29. Roseman DM. Carotidynia. Arch Otolaryngol 1967; 85:103-106.
30. Raskin NH, Prusiner S. Carotidynia. Neurology 1977; 27:43-46.
31. Vijayan N, Watson C. Pericarotid syndrome. Headache 1978; 18:244-254.
32. Solomon S, Lipton RB. Atypical facial pain: a review. Semin Neurol 1988; 8:332-338.
33. Raskin N. Facial pain. In: Headache, 2nd ed. New York: Churchill Livingston, 1988:333-373.

Index

275

About the Editor

R. Michael Gallagher is Director of the University Headache Center, Moorestown, New Jersey, Assistant Dean for Clinical Affairs and Professor of Clinical Medicine at the University of Medicine and Dentistry of New Jersey—School of Osteopathic Medicine, Stratford, New Jersey, and formerly a Clinical Associate Professor at the Philadelphia College of Osteopathic Medicine, Philadelphia, Pennsylvania. The author or coauthor of numerous medical journal articles on headache management and the treatment of pain, he is a Fellow of the Alliance of Air National Guard Flight Surgeons, and a member of the American Association for the Study of Headache, International Headache Society, American Osteopathic Association, American College of General Practitioners, and American Academy of Pain Management. Certified in family medicine and pain management, Dr. Gallagher serves on the editorial board of *Headache Quarterly* and on the board of directors for the National Headache Foundation. He received the D.O. degree (1976) from the Philadelphia College of Osteopathic Medicine, Philadelphia, Pennsylvania.